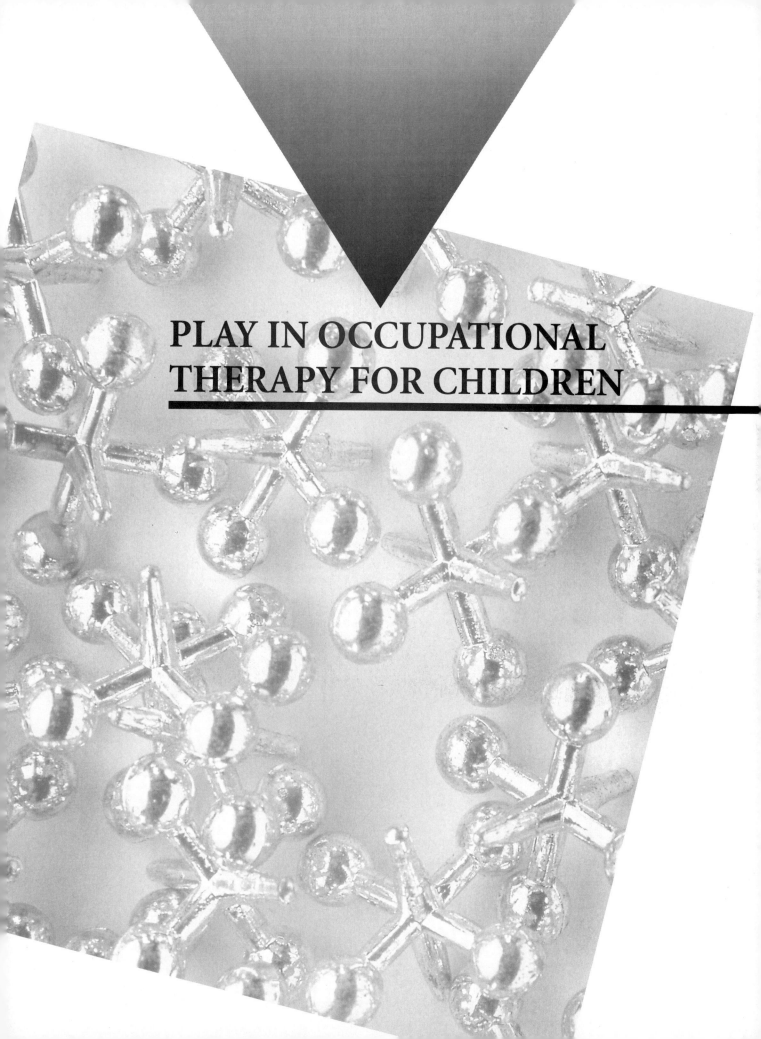

PLAY IN OCCUPATIONAL THERAPY FOR CHILDREN

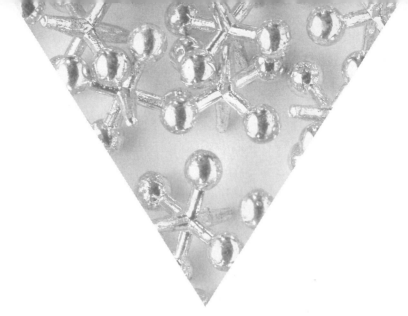

PLAY IN OCCUPATIONAL THERAPY FOR CHILDREN

Edited by

L. DIANE PARHAM, PhD, OTR, FAOTA
Associate Professor
Department of Occupational Therapy
University of Southern California
Los Angeles, California

LINDA S. FAZIO, PhD, OTR, FAOTA
Professor of Clinical Occupational Therapy and Assistant Chairperson
Department of Occupational Therapy
University of Southern California
Los Angeles, California

with **20** *contributors*
with **126** *illustrations*

Primary photographer: Shay McAtee

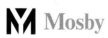 Mosby

St. Louis Baltimore Boston Carlsbad Chicago Naples New York Philadelphia Portland
London Madrid Mexico City Singapore Sydney Tokyo Toronto Wiesbaden

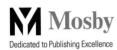

Mosby
Dedicated to Publishing Excellence

**A Times Mirror
Company**

Publisher: Don Ladig
Executive Editor: Martha Sasser
Associate Developmental Editor: Amy Dubin
Project Manager: Carol Sullivan Weis
Project Specialist: Pat Joiner
Designer: Sheilah Barrett
Manufacturing Supervisor: Andrew Christensen
Cover Photos: Shay McAtee

Printed in the United States of America
Composition by Graphic World, Inc.
Editing and Production by Graphic World Publishing Services
Printing and Binding by R.R. Donnelley & Sons Company

Mosby–Year Book, Inc.
11830 Westline Industrial Drive
St. Louis, MO 63146

Library of Congress Cataloging in Publication Data

Play in occupational therapy for children / edited by L. Diane Parham,
   Linda S. Fazio; primary photographer, Shay McAtee
        p.   cm.
   Includes bibliographical references and index.
   ISBN 0-8016-7838-2
      1. Occupational therapy for children.   2. Play therapy.
   I. Parham, L. Diane.   II. Fazio, Linda S.
   RJ53.025P53   1996
   615.8′5153′083—dc20   96-15085
                                                          CIP

    97 98 99 00 / 9 8 7 6 5 4 3 2

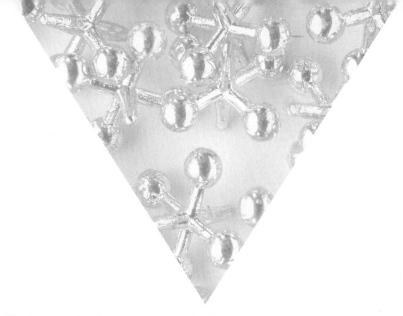

CONTRIBUTORS

ERNA I. BLANCHE, MA, OTR
Therapy West
Culver City, California

KIMBERLY C. BRYZE, MS, OTR/L
Assistant Professor
Occupational Therapy Program
Midwestern University
Downers Grove, Illinois

ANITA BUNDY, ScD, OTR, FAOTA
Associate Professor
Colorado State University
Department of Occupational Therapy
Fort Collins, Colorado

JANICE POSATERY BURKE, MA, OTR, FAOTA
Assistant Professor
Department of Occupational Therapy
Thomas Jefferson University
Philadelphia, Pennsylvania

JEAN CROSETTO DEITZ, PhD, OTR/L, FAOTA
Associate Professor and Graduate Program Coordinator
Department of Rehabilitation Medicine
University of Washington
Seattle, Washington

JULIE ANDERSEN EWALD, MA, OTR/L
Private Practice
Portland, Maine

LINDA S. FAZIO, PhD, OTR, FAOTA
Professor of Clinical Occupational Therapy and Assistant
   Chairperson
Department of Occupational Therapy
University of Southern California
Los Angeles, California

LINDA L. FLOREY, MA, OTR, FAOTA
Chief, Rehabilitation Services
UCLA Neuropsychiatric Institute and Hospital
Los Angeles, California

SANDRA GREENE, MA, OTR
Senior Occupational Therapist
Rehabilitation Services
UCLA Neuropsychiatric Institute and Hospital
Los Angeles, California;
Private Practice
Santa Monica, California

JIM HINOJOSA, PhD, OTR, FAOTA
Associate Professor
Occupational Therapy Department
New York University
New York, New York

ELISE HOLLOWAY, MPH, OTR
Occupational Therapy Clinical Specialist, Neonatology
Huntington Memorial Hospital
Pasadena, California;
Associate Faculty
Brazelton Center for Infants and Parents
Boston, Massachusetts

BONNIE KENNEDY, PhD (Cand.), OTR
Assistant Professor
Occupational Therapy Program
University of Wisconsin-Milwaukee
Milwaukee, Wisconsin

SUSAN KNOX, PhD (Cand.), OTR, FAOTA
Private Practice
Los Angeles, California

PAULA KRAMER, PhD, OTR, FAOTA
Professor and Chair
Department of Occupational Therapy
Kean College of New Jersey
Union, New Jersey

ZOE MAILLOUX, MA, OTR, FAOTA
Director of Administration and Practice
The Ayres Clinic
Torrence, California;
Adjunct Instructor
Department of Occupational Therapy
University of Southern California
Los Angeles, California

ANN NEVILLE-JAN, PhD, OTR, FAOTA
Associate Professor
Department of Occupational Therapy
University of Southern California
Los Angeles, California

L. DIANE PARHAM, PhD, OTR, FAOTA
Associate Professor
Department of Occupational Therapy
University of Southern California
Los Angeles, California

DORIS PIERCE, PhD, OTR
Private Practice
LaVerne, California

LOREE A. PRIMEAU, PhD, OT(C), OTR
Assistant Professor
School of Occupational Therapy
Dalhousie University
Halifax, Nova Scotia
Canada

ROSEANN C. SCHAAF, MeD, OTR/L
Instructor
Department of Occupational Therapy
Thomas Jefferson University
Philadelphia, Pennsylvania

CAROLYN SNYDER, MHS, MA, OTR
Assistant Professor of Clinical Occupational Therapy
Department of Occupational Therapy
University of Southern California
Los Angeles, California

YVONNE SWINTH, MS, OTR/L
Occupational Therapy Department
University Place School District
University of Puget Sound
Tacoma, Washington

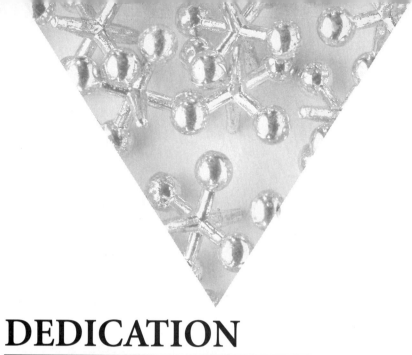

DEDICATION

To the spirit of play in our daughters
April, Holly, and Dorothy Helen

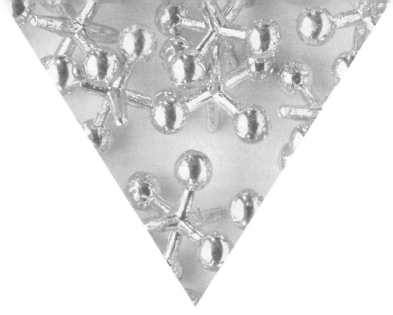

FOREWORD

A revolution is occurring that promises to transform occupational therapy in the twenty-first century. Its impetus has come from scholars, researchers, and practitioners who do not wish to see the profession's commitment to occupation irretrievably lost in the current climate of health care reform. These courageous individuals are generating scholarly papers, developing intervention models, and producing research that powerfully address the linkages of occupation to health. They are giving us hope in the midst of the more depressing aspects of health care reform that occupational therapy will be able to continue safeguarding the public good, not by abrogating its traditional focus, but instead by expanding its knowledge base on occupation. The seemingly overwhelming pressures of health care today coupled with the fear that occupation may vanish from health care seem to be stimulating the production of scholarly works that are sufficiently compelling to secure a vital place for occupational therapy in the future.

Diane Parham, Linda Fazio, and their contributors are to be commended for creating a book that is in this league. The focus of the book is on play, the primary occupation in which children engage. Although this focus, in and of itself, is not new to our profession, how it is presented in *Play in Occupational Therapy for Children* is revolutionary. In occupational therapy, we have traditionally thought of play within the framework of role theory, we have understood play through the theoretical lenses of psychologists and play theorists from other disciplines, and our application of play in the treatment context have tended to be prescriptive and deficit-oriented.

In sharp contrast, the content of this book successfully challenges these conventional notions and approaches. Role theory is critiqued primarily for its tendency to homogenize engagement in occupation and for its inadequacy in addressing diversity. Play theories and assessments imported from other disciplines are carefully presented; alongside of them, however, we are introduced to the unique theories and assessments that have resulted from research conducted by occupational therapists and occupational scientists that lead to a reconsideration of practice. Finally, a detailed picture unfolds, revealed in the numerous case studies contained in the book on how pediatric occupational therapy (1) is shaped when it is guided by state-of-the-art occupational therapy theory on play, (2) is context sensitive, and (3) is non-prescriptive.

A book on play and play-centered occupational therapy runs the risk of being accused of oversimplification or not presenting anything new. There is a tendency to assume that new scientific and intellectual advances of relevance to pediatric occupational therapy are typically made in the neurosciences, whereas the ordinariness of play renders new discoveries unlikely. The content of *Play in Occupational Therapy for Children,* fortunately, belies such an assumption. For example, Bundy's chapter on play and playfulness not only contains a highly innovative model that addresses the primary elements of play in an entirely fresh way, but also includes the first published presentation of a standardized instrument for assessing playfulness. In the chapters by Knox and Bryze, convincing rationales are provided for modifying our standard operating procedures for administering the Preschool Play Scale and The Play History. As a result, we come to see the necessity for change, even in the use of instruments we have routinely employed. Other chapters, such as Pierce's spellbinding presentation on the power of object play, expose us to highly elaborated and original theory with elegant examples of how it can be applied in treatment. In many of the chapters, the voices of master clinicians make explicit the tacit knowledge they have acquired through their years of practice. Florey and Greene, for example, provide insights on how to read, interpret, and adjust therapeutic play strategies with children with emotional and behavior disorders; Blanche describes how children with cerebral palsy can be encouraged to engage in genuine play rather than a motor performance with an educational toy; and Deitz and Swinth exercise their imaginations while grounded on the solid turf of research and clinical experience to give us a vision of the potential of technology to encourage play. Subtle insights of this kind are not typically included in textbooks; it is fortunate that so many have been assembled in this work.

It is fascinating that so many of the chapters in this book ultimately deal with the situatedness of play. They are thematically unified by their emphasis on context, though this concern takes on a variety of appearances. In the chapter by Holloway, we are provoked to think about whether play should be addressed with medically fragile infants in neonatal intensive care units. Holloway not only justifies the need to do so, but provides illustrations in case examples of how this is done, despite the constraints of the highly technological and threatening hospital context. Pierce, on the other hand, forces us to acknowledge the limitations of clinic-based occupational therapy through the elaboration of a practice theory that can guide therapists in harnessing sources of therapeutic power that are indigenous to home settings. Finally, in the chapter by Hinojosa and Kramer, a compelling argument is made that it is insufficient to address a child's play in isolation of his family's play patterns. They describe the therapeutic benefits of including the child with a disability in family play, and, vice versa, family members in the play of the child with disabilities. Just as Marjorie Devault (1991), in her acclaimed ethnography, demonstrated that feeding the family was essential to the social construction of a family "as family," so too do Hinojosa and Kramer convince us of the absolute necessity of including family play in intervention that claims to meet the needs of the family.

Although the focus of this book is clearly on play and context, it is not surprising that most of the chapters also address the therapeutic relationship between the parent, the child with disability, and the therapist. It seems that the contributors believe that a prescriptive, deficit-focused, directive approach will inevitably undermine play-focused interventions. Holloway, for example, advocates embracing a non-prescriptive stance in which parents are sensitized to the infant's adaptive capacities rather than informed about deficits or dysfunction. Burke and Schaaf suggest storytelling as an approach for building connective knowing in which the therapist's assessment can be tied to the parent's concern. Similarly, Bryze discusses how parents and therapists can work together to find shared meaning in the child's play. Finally, Fazio recommends storytelling as a playful occupation through which the therapist can develop a keener understanding of the life world of the child. All of these methods, it would seem, cast parent, therapist, and child as co-collaborators in a fluid, spontaneous, and improvisational relationship, the kind of relationship that seems particularly well suited for interventions centered on play.

It is hard for me to a imagine a better example of the kinds of books occupational therapy needs to enrich and secure its place in serving the public good. We are much in debt to the editors and contributors for demonstrating how the time-honored occupational therapy focus on play, newly illuminated through state-of-the-art theory, can be reforged to meet the health care challenges of these times.

REFERENCE

DeVault, M. L. (1991). *Feeding the family.* Chicago, Ill: The University of Chicago Press.

FLORENCE CLARK, PhD, OTR, FAOTA
Professor and Chair
Department of Occupational Therapy
University of Southern California
Los Angeles, California

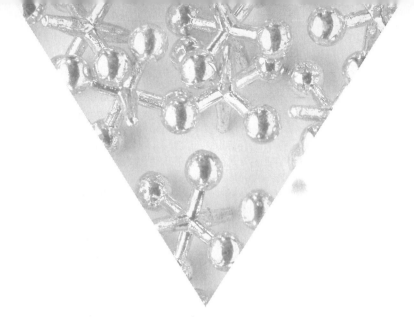

PREFACE

We dance around in a ring and suppose but the secret sits in the middle and knows.

Robert Frost

P lay is a secret that occupational therapists have danced around for many years. Since the early twentieth century, the profession has declared that play is essential to a healthy lifestyle (Meyer, 1922) and has identified play as a primary domain of concern in official documents (e.g., American Occupational Therapy Association, 1994). It has long been part of the profession's folk knowledge that play has a magical power to open up human potentials locked away by disability, disadvantage, or illness. Yet play has been kept a secret by occupational therapists, in part because of its low status within the scientific and medical establishments, and in part because, until relatively recently, so little was understood by any discipline regarding the nature of play.

The secret of play's power remained enshrouded in mystery as long as therapists were embarrassed by it. Afraid of being dismissed as frivolous or trivial through association with play, mid–twentieth century occupational therapists turned their efforts in professional development toward more clearly scientific endeavors, and the problems of play—what it is, why it works, and how to assess and apply it systematically in clinical practice—remained unexamined.

It was not until Mary Reilly published *Play as Exploratory Learning* in 1974 that the problem of play became a focus of serious study and theory-based clinical application in the profession. That work became a stimulus for a new generation of clinicians and scholars who are intrigued by the mystery of play's power and who, benefiting from the foundation laid by Reilly and her students, are no longer embarrassed to claim play as both a therapeutic agent and a critical outcome of intervention. Poised on the threshold of the twenty-first century, contemporary occupational therapists have a variety of theoretical interpretations, assessment approaches, and treatment models on which to draw that are uniquely suited for play applications in occupational therapy.

This book brings together these diverse contemporary approaches to play in occupational therapy for children. Until now, these resources have been scattered across different sources, and, in many cases, they are not available in any other publication. In this book, traditional ideas on play in occupational therapy are represented, as well as work on the cutting edge of theory and practice concerning play.

The book is divided into four main parts. Part I, Introduction to Play and Occupational Therapy, provides a historical and conceptual backdrop for the rest of the book. It consists of one chapter that provides an extensive review of multidisciplinary play theories, a historical overview of play in occupational therapy practice, and a discussion of current streams of theory and practice concerning play in occupational therapy. The remaining sections of the book focus on ideas and guidelines for clinical assessment and treatment that are grounded in theory and research, as well as in clinical experience. Part II, Assessment of Play, presents specific assessment instruments and discussions of how to incorporate a family-centered, narrative approach into the assessment process. Part III, Play As a Means for Enhancing Development and Skill Acquisition, addresses play as a means to an end. Chapters in this section focus on play as a tool to promote perceptual, motor, cognitive, self-care, and social skills; environmental negotiation; sensory integrative development; and adaptation to transitions within the school setting. Finally, Part IV, Play As a Goal of Intervention, focuses on play as an end in itself. Chapters in this section describe ways to expand the child's play life by making it more accessible, satisfying, and meaningful. Authors discuss strategies for facilitating play within the context of the family, and within the context of specialized areas of practice, such as early intervention, therapy for children with neuromotor disabilities or emotional disorders, and assistive technology.

The four parts of the book are organizational devices that call the reader's attention to different angles on the topic of play, but the parts are not entirely discrete and their boundaries are not rigid. For example, some ideas regarding assessment are presented in chapters outside of Part II (assessment); many of the chapters that are placed in Part III (play as a means) include some discussion of play as an end, and vice versa for chapters in Part IV.

This book is intended to meet the needs of several audiences. First, it is intended to be used in the professional entry-level occupational therapy curriculum. Chapter 1 provides important theoretical background on play for entry-level students, and additional chapters provide extensive assessment and treatment guidelines to demonstrate clearly how theory may be put into practice. The inclusion of ample case illustrations is intended to be particularly useful in helping the student or novice clinician to visualize what assessment or treatment may look like in a clinical situation. Although most occupational therapy curricula do not include a specific course on play, this book gives faculty a tool with which to infuse play concepts throughout the curriculum. Because the chapters can stand alone as individual readings, separate chapters may be assigned in courses on human development, pediatric practice, assessment, psychosocial dysfunction, physical dysfunction, and practice skills. For example, the chapter on assistive technology would be an excellent way to relate this topic to occupation in a course on treatment of physical dysfunction.

This book is also intended to be used by graduate students. The extensive literature reviewed, the original ideas presented, and the innovations in assessment and treatment described in many of the chapters are hoped to serve as a springboard for seminar discussions, research, and scholarship.

Experienced occupational therapists who work with children may find this valuable as a reference volume. Because most occupational therapists did not receive adequate theoretical preparation or practical skill development regarding play in their formal professional education, this book can become the backbone of a postgraduate study process that fills the void in their knowledge base. Even clinicians who already are formally educated or self-taught experts on play will find much that is stimulating and novel within the covers of this book.

Scholars and clinicians from other fields who are interested in play may find that the notion of play as occupation puts a new twist on an old topic and thus opens up new avenues for thinking about play. The instruments and intervention programming ideas, although originally conceived for use in occupational therapy, may very well lend themselves to interdisciplinary applications.

An important final note is that the focus of this book is on applications to children simply because most of the work on play in our profession (and in other disciplines) has focused on this portion of the lifespan. We do endorse play in occupational therapy for adults, and we hope to see the occupational therapy play literature expand in the coming years to include life after adolescence.

REFERENCES

American Occupational Therapy Association (1994). Uniform terminology for occupational therapy—third edition. *American Journal of Occupational Therapy, 48,* 1047-1054

Meyer, A. (1922). The philosophy of occupation therapy. *Archives of Occupational Therapy, 1,* 1-10.

Reilly, M. (Ed.) (1974). *Play as exploratory learning.* Beverly Hills, CA: Sage Publications.

L. DIANE PARHAM
LINDA S. FAZIO

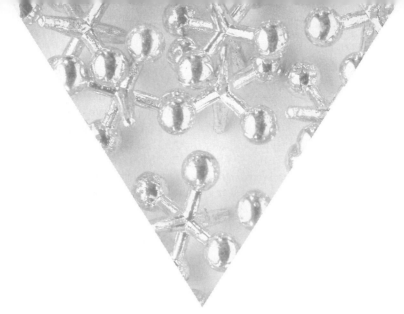

ACKNOWLEDGEMENTS

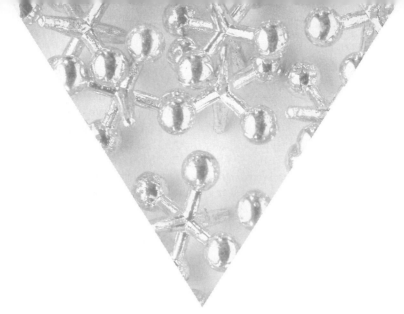e are grateful for the willingness of the contributors to write what, in most cases, was a very new synthesis of abstract material and further, to make theory come to life with case illustrations and a "how to" orientation. They are applauded for their contributions to the profession's literature on play.

The talent of photographer Shay McAtee, and her commitment to the book, is deeply appreciated. She tirelessly shot roll after roll of film when we needed to illustrate an idea or concept, and she always seemed to know just what we wanted to show. (Being an occupational therapist as well as a photographer helped!) Shay truly has a gift for capturing the essence of play in photography. The assistance of the other photographers, many of whom were graduate students, and the illustrator is also acknowledged. The willingness of the pictured children and families to allow Shay and the other photographers to intrude on their schedules and turf, and to give permission for their photographs to be published, is appreciated.

We are well aware that we are standing on the shoulders of Mary Reilly and her colleagues, whose work paved the way for us to create a textbook on play in occupational therapy in the 1990s. Her courage and foresight in bringing play out of hiding and into the light as a serious topic of scholarship are honored. The inspiration of occupational therapists who are expert players is also acknowledged. In particular, the memory of A. Jean Ayres, who was a genius at using play to engage a child in therapy, is treasured.

Discussions with many colleagues have been an important influence in this work. Diane especially acknowledges the comments and discussions of doctoral students in her play course in the Occupational Science PhD program at USC. Stimulating conversations on play and playfulness with Erna Blanche, Susan Knox, Doris Pierce, Loree Primeau, and Wendy Wood, who all were esteemed colleagues before they were graduate students, are especially appreciated. The comments and observations of Canadian visiting scholars Francine Ferland and Barbara O'Shea are also acknowledged as an influence.

Although other faculty at USC did not directly contribute to our ideas on play, they had an impact on our ideas about play as occupation. Florence Clark, Jeanne Jackson, and Ruth Zemke are particularly appreciated in this regard. The inspiration and leadership of Elizabeth Yerxa, whose vision shaped the doctoral program in occupational science at USC, continues to be tremendously influential.

We appreciate the hard work of the editors at Mosby, especially Amy Dubin and Martha Sasser, who gave us just the right amount of pressure along with support to keep us going. It has been a pleasure to work with them.

We thank our families and our colleagues at the University of Southern California and the Ayres Clinic for their tolerance while we were occupied with this book, which sometimes required that we postpone or give up other activities.

We have become experts at enfolding play into work occupations, but nevertheless look forward now to the possibility of having blocks of time devoted entirely to play.

Work on this book was partially supported through the U.S. Department of Health and Human Services, Public Health Service, Health Resources and Services Administration, Maternal and Child Health Bureau, Grant No. MCJ 009048-11, and through an author's grant from the publisher, Mosby–Year Book.

L. DIANE PARHAM
LINDA S. FAZIO

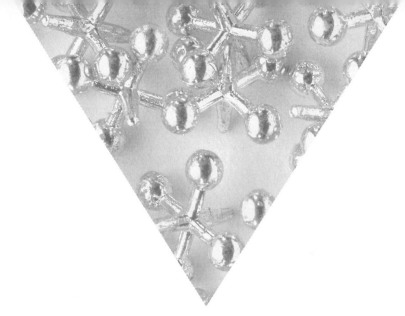

CONTENTS

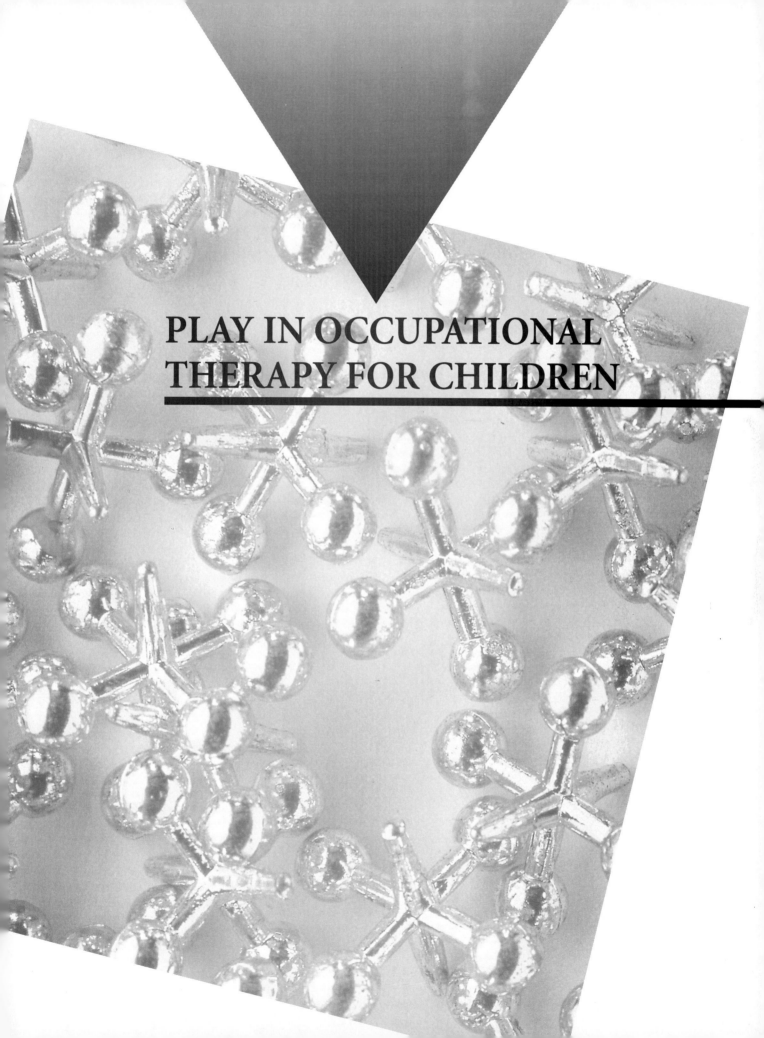

PLAY IN OCCUPATIONAL THERAPY FOR CHILDREN

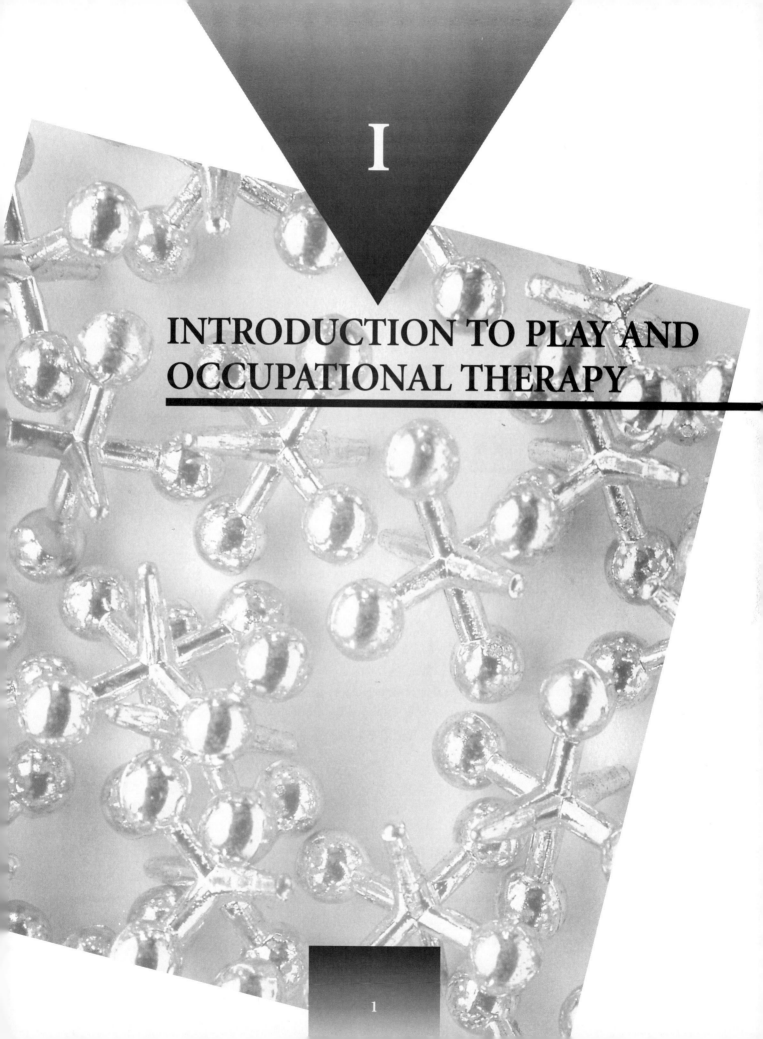

I

INTRODUCTION TO PLAY AND OCCUPATIONAL THERAPY

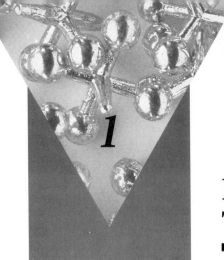

PLAY AND OCCUPATIONAL THERAPY

L. Diane Parham and Loree A. Primeau

> Play is a child's way of learning and an outlet for his innate need of activity. It is his business or his career. In it he engages himself with the same attitude and energy that we engage ourselves in our regular work. For each child it is a serious undertaking not to be confused with diversion or idle use of time. Play is not folly. It is purposeful activity. (Alessandrini, 1949, p. 9).

These are the opening lines from an article written nearly 50 years ago by an occupational therapist, Norma Alessandrini. At the time that she wrote this, she was Director of Children's Recreation Service at Bellevue Hospital in New York City. Interestingly, the philosophy of play that Alessandrini outlined in this paper resounds with a core idea that is being explored by contemporary occupational therapy leaders: that play is a significant and primary occupation of children.

The purpose of this chapter is to provide the reader with a broad overview of how play is approached in the profession of occupational therapy, particularly in relation to children. It begins with questions regarding the nature of play: how it is defined, and how it has been explained from the diverse perspectives of many disciplines. It then moves on to examine how play historically has been viewed and used within the field of occupational therapy. The chapter concludes with a review of contemporary streams of ideas on play in occupational therapy.

A caveat is in order before this discussion of play is continued. The focus of this chapter, and of this entire book, is on children's play solely because the topic of play has been addressed in the literature predominantly in relation to childhood. Concepts of play are indeed relevant throughout the lifespan and offer a potentially rich field of knowledge that, for the most part, has not yet been explored or applied by occupational therapists in a systematic manner. Many of the ideas that have sprung from research and clinical work with children may be applicable to adults as well.

WHAT IS PLAY?

"It's child's play." This colloquial expression is used to denote a task that is so simple it does not require effort. To scholars, however, the study of child's play is not a simple task. Play is an elusive concept and is difficult (some would say impossible) to define. Before reading further, the reader should try the exercise shown in Box 1-1.

▼
| Box |
| 1-1 |
EXERCISE 1: DEFINING PLAY

Write down two activities that were favorite play occupations for you when you were a child. Next, write down two activities that you consider to be play.

Now, consider what the critical ingredients may be that make you think of these four occupations as play. Write a definition of play that captures these critical ingredients, beginning it with the phrase "Play is...." You may consider additional examples of play occupations if this helps you to formulate your ideas about what constitutes play.

Save your definition and refer to it as you read further on the nature of play. How do your ideas compare with those of the distinguished scholars who have struggled with this problem of defining play?

In everyday use, the meaning of "play" seems clear enough, but its boundaries are fuzzy (Garvey, 1990). Even when people easily agree that what they are observing is play, they may struggle with how to articulate what play is. Scholars over the years have attempted to define it, explain it, suggest criteria for it, and relate it to other types of behaviors, but the fuzzy boundaries of play remain (Saracho, 1991). One reason for this, no doubt, is the wide range of meanings that the word "play" takes on in the English language. *Merriam-Webster's Collegiate Dictionary* (1994) lists 84 definitions of play, including a recreational activity, the spontaneous activity of children, the absence of serious or harmful intent, to take part in a game, and to toy or fiddle around with something.

The philosopher Ludwig Wittgenstein dealt with the problem of defining elusive concepts in his discussion of games. His view was that the multifarious activities that people call games have no one thing in common that makes them all games, yet they are related to each other in a variety of ways. The same idea can apply to the diverse occupations that are called play.

> Consider for example the proceedings that we call "games." I mean board games, card-games, ball-games, Olympic games, and so on. What is common to them all?... Look for example at board games.... Now pass to card-games; here you find many correspondences with the first group, but many features drop out, and others appear. When we pass next to ball-games, much that is common is retained, but much is lost.—Are they all "amusing"? Compare chess with noughts and crosses. Or is there always winning and losing, or competition between players?... In ball games there is winning and losing; but when a child throws his ball at the wall and catches it again, this feature has disappeared.... Think now of games like ring-a-ring-a-roses; here is the element of amusement, but how many other characteristic features have disappeared!... The result of this examination is: we see a complicated network of similarities overlapping and criss-crossing: sometimes overall similarities, sometimes similarities of detail.... I can think of no better expression to characterize these similarities than "family resemblances"... And I shall say: "games" form a family. (Wittgenstein, 1958, pp. 31-32)

Drawing from Wittgenstein's ideas, many of the efforts to define play can be seen as involving an identification of the types of "family resemblances," or groups of related characteristics, that encompass the broad domain of play. For example, Rubin, Fein, and Vandenberg (1983), three psychologists who are experts on play, organize definitions of play into three categories (or "families"): (1) play as a disposition, in which play is defined by the psychological disposition that occurs during play and distinguishes it from other human behavior; (2) play as observable behavior, in which play is identified by observable types of behaviors; and (3) play as context, in which play is defined by its context.

Play As Disposition

Although play seems to defy definition, there has been convergence among theorists on its dispositional characteristics. Several dimensions of psychological disposition have been identified as distinguishing play from other types of behavior. Rubin and his colleagues (1983) presented six factors that arise from different theoretical perspectives and that seem to be mutually exclusive. Although generally there has been agreement that these characteristics are representative of play, there continues to be disagreement on how they should be used to rule out what is and what is not play. The six factors are:

1. Intrinsic motivation. Play is intrinsically motivated. It is not ruled by compliance with social norms, expectations, or the promise of external rewards (Rubin et al., 1983). In play, an activity is done for its own sake. In the play literature, the term "autotelic" is sometimes used as an adjective to refer to this quality. Intrinsic motivation is the feature of play that seems to be accepted universally across different theories and definitions of play.

2. *Focus on means rather than ends.* Play is characterized by self-imposed goals that can change at the whim of the player. As such, play can be spontaneous. Focus on the means of the behavior rather than its ends demarcates play from other intrinsically motivated behaviors with specific, often externally imposed goals, such as work (Rubin et al., 1983).

3. *Organism-centered rather than object-centered behavior.* This factor is used by some authors to discriminate between exploratory and play behaviors. Exploratory behavior is centered on an unfamiliar or poorly understood object and is guided by the need to gain information about its features. It is guided by the question, "What can this object do?" Play is organism-centered behavior in that it is guided by the question, "What can I do with this object?" Play occurs with familiar objects and it is

thought to stimulate and maintain the organism's arousal level. An important implication of the view of play as organism-centered is that play involves an internal locus of control (Rubin et al., 1983).

4. *Relation to instrumental behaviors.* Play is noninstrumental. "Play behaviors are not serious renditions of the activities they resemble: the individual is not really fighting, but is play fighting" (Rubin et al., 1983, p. 699). Objects are treated as if they were something else. There is a pretend quality to play that distinguishes it from other nonpretend behaviors.

5. *Freedom from externally imposed rules.* This factor has been used by some theorists to differentiate play from games. Flexibility has been said to characterize play, but many scholars disagree with this nonoverlapping classification of games and play (Rubin et al., 1983).

6. *Active engagement.* The player is actively engaged in a play activity. This factor discriminates between play and passive states of inactivity and boredom. It begs the question, however, of whether daydreaming is a form of play. Some theorists argue that it is, because in daydreaming one plays with ideas (Rubin et al., 1983).

Play As Observable Behavior

Various taxonomies have been developed that identify discrete types of play (Rubin et al., 1983). For example, Piaget (1962) described three types of play that followed a developmental sequence: (1) practice games, (2) symbolic games, and (3) games with rules. Other theorists have defined "play" in terms of categories of behavior, such as play with language, play with motion and interaction, and play with objects (Garvey, 1990) or categories of social interaction, such as onlooker, solitary independent play, parallel play, associative play, and cooperative play (Parten, 1932). Taxonomies of play are useful because they provide criteria that can be used to observe play behaviors; they lead to the development of narrower categories of play that may be easier to observe, describe, and explain; and they lend themselves to developmental explanations that may be obscured by a focus on psychological dispositions of play (Rubin et al., 1983). However, these taxonomies tend to emphasize observable behaviors; the problem that then arises is that the person's experience is ignored, and, as is well known, what is experienced as play for one person may be experienced as work or even drudgery for another. Further, if categories are narrowed to more easily observed behaviors (such as patterns of manual manipulation or social interaction), there is a risk that the essence of play may be lost, even as the observer gains more detailed knowledge of the particular behaviors examined.

Play As Context

Definitions that portray play in terms of context emphasize the influence of culture upon play. These definitions contain the beliefs held by the adults within a specific culture about the nature of play and the conditions under which it is likely to occur (Rubin et al., 1983). The role of context needs to be addressed because theoretical discussions of play often fail to recognize hidden assumptions made about its context. Definitions of play that emphasize context describe the conditions under which play occurs. These include the provision of a safe, comfortable, and friendly environment; the availability of a variety of interesting objects, materials, people, or activities with which to interact; the freedom of choice to play or not; a time in which the child is not tired, hungry, ill, or otherwise stressed; and the cultural sanction that communicates "This is play" via cues from an adult and/or arrangements of the physical environment.

Is a Definition of Play Always Necessary?

Why has so much effort gone into attempts to define play? Scholars have devoted a great deal of attention to the definitional problem because, when it becomes an object of study, a concept must be defined clearly enough to enable researchers and consumers of research to agree that they are talking about the same thing (Garvey, 1990; Reynolds, 1971). Furthermore, from the viewpoint of traditional science, precise definitions are desirable because they enable precise measurement, which in turn can be used in research to explore the nature of the phenomenon and its relationships with other phenomena (Reynolds, 1971). According to this reasoning, a good definition of play should enable therapists to develop a good test or evaluation of play, which in turn would enable them to do research examining the relationship between play and other capacities or outcomes, such as problem-solving ability or adaptive skills. Despite the many definitions of play that have been generated by scholars over the years, however, no specific definition of play has gained widespread acceptance. As Rubin et al. (1983) point out, no single approach "adequately encompasses the range of plausible perspectives that continue to be germane to an intuitive meaning of play" (Rubin et al., 1983, p. 698).

The inability to settle on a precise definition of play has led some scientists to abandon the quest to study play in favor of more easily defined constructs (Berlyne, 1969). Experts in the field of occupational therapy, however, have not given up play as a topic worthy of study. Intuitively, play seems to be an important aspect of human experience that is deserving of study. Historically, play has been considered to be so significant to the profession of occupational therapy, that it (along with the term "leisure," often used interchangeably with "play") is one of the major categories in taxonomies of occupation or occupational performance that have been generated by occupational therapists (e.g., American Occupational Therapy Association, 1994; Christiansen, 1991; Clark et al., 1991; Kielhofner, 1995; Meyer, 1922; Reilly, 1969; Yerxa et al., 1989). Moreover, from a pragmatic standpoint, play is a powerful concept when applied in clinical practice, and usefulness in the context of practice is crucial in assessing the value of a concept or theory (Hoshmand & Polkinghorne, 1992).

It is interesting to note that Wittgenstein, in his analysis of the problem of definition, asserted that drawing the boundaries of a concept was not necessary for it to be useful in a pragmatic sense: "we can draw a boundary—for a special purpose. Does it take that to make the concept usable? Not at all! (Except for that special purpose.)" (1958, p. 33). This stance leads to the conclusion that, although precise definitions of play may be appropriate for the specific purposes of particular research programs, a concise, all-purpose definition of play to suit the diverse needs of the entire profession may not be necessary, possible, or even desirable.

The complexity of the play concept led Mary Reilly (1974), a prominent occupational therapy theorist, to describe it as a cobweb, an image that evokes Wittgenstein's notion of a "complicated network of similarities overlapping and criss-crossing" (1958, p. 32). Rather than submit to pressures from the scientific community to atomize play into subcomponents that could be easily studied or to compromise its essence by reducing it to an easily operationalized definition, Reilly chose to synthesize a vast terrain of multidisciplinary literature on play to cultivate a full appreciation of its meanings and potential clinical applications. An overview of this literature is presented next to give the reader a background on the diverse theoretical views that have contributed to therapists' understanding of play.

EXPLANATIONS OF PLAY

Many theories of play have been proposed, each contributing its own explanation of play. They generally fall into two groups of theories: classical theories and modern theories (Mellou, 1994). Classical theories originated in the years before World War I, specifically in the late nineteenth and early twentieth centuries (Gilmore, 1971). Modern theories are those that have been developed after 1920 (Mellou, 1994).

Classical Theories of Play

Classical theories of play attempt to provide reasons for the existence of play and to determine its antecedent conditions and its inferred purpose (Gilmore, 1971; Mellou, 1994). Four classical theories have been identified (Gilmore, 1971): (1) the surplus energy theory (Spencer, 1878/1978), (2) the recreation (Lazarus, 1883) or relaxation theory (Patrick, 1916), (3) the preexercise theory (Groos, 1898/1978), and (4) the recapitulation theory (Hall, 1908/1978). After these four theories have been discussed, the reader should try Exercise 2 in Box 1-2.

Surplus Energy Theory. The surplus energy theory (sometimes called the Schiller-Spencer theory) is one of the earliest attempts to explain why play occurs. An early version of this theory was developed by Friedrich von Schiller, an eighteenth century poet and philosopher (Rubin et al., 1983). A more refined version of this theory was developed by Spencer (1878/1978), a nineteenth century psychologist and philosopher. The basic idea behind the surplus energy theory is much older, however; it can be traced back to the Aristotelian concept of catharsis (Mellou, 1994). The surplus energy theory posits that play is a prominent behavior among the young of a species because it is a result of their surplus energy. The main thesis is that any organism has a finite quantity of available energy that must be expended. When it is not needed for self-preservation, it is manifested as non–goal directed behavior, or play (Gilmore, 1971). Since the young of a species are dependent upon caregivers for maintenance and preservation and do not have to expend energy on these functions, they possess an excess of energy that must be expelled; so they play. The surplus energy theory attempts to explain where the energy in children's play originates, but it provides no explanation for why children choose to play in the many different ways that they do (Slobin, 1964).

Recreation or Relaxation Theory. In direct contrast to the surplus energy theory stands the recreation or relaxation theory. This theory postulates that play derives not from a surplus of energy but from a deficit of energy. The purpose of play is to replenish spent energy. Play is most likely to be seen in childhood because fatigue builds up in the child in response to energy expenditures in unfamiliar and relatively new tasks (Gilmore, 1971). Lazarus (1883) viewed play as a recreational activity that restored energy, whereas Patrick (1916) saw play as an opportunity for relaxation (Mellou, 1994). Both proponents of this theory believed that play had no cognitive content or function. Similar to the surplus energy theory of play, the recreation or relaxation theory does not consider the content of play; it simply states that play occurs (Slobin, 1964).

Preexercise Theory. The preexercise theory views play as an instinctive behavior. Play emerges from instincts and exercises these instincts in preparation for their serious use in the future. According to Groos (1898/1978), childhood is a period of immaturity, the purpose of which is to provide the opportunity for instinctive behaviors to be refined into the mature behaviors that are required in adult life. Play is the primary vehicle in which this refinement of instinctive behavior occurs. Groos theorized that the length of the period of immaturity varied according to the complexity of the organism and its place on the phylogenetic scale. As organisms became increasingly complex on an evolutionary scale, longer periods of immaturity were needed for them to practice the complex skills that would be required for survival at maturity. As a result, play is a more prominent behavior among the young of the more complex species. Thus, Groos believed that play serves an adaptive purpose in the evolutionary process.

Groos's ideas continue to be very influential among contemporary play theorists. For example, Vandenberg (1978) has continued Groos's line of thinking about the evolutionary function of play. His view is that, with increased complexity along the phylogenetic scale, the young of the species are not born with the skills that will be necessary to survive and flourish in adulthood. Instead, they need to construct the adaptive skills that they will require throughout life, and they accomplish this in play. Vandenberg (1978) used the term "constructive adaptation" to explain how phylogenetically higher species construct the skills they need to adapt to the environment. Both Groos and Vandenberg suggested that play was the product of an evolutionary biological process that linked play in childhood to the learning of behaviors critical to adaptation in adulthood.

Recapitulation Theory. The recapitulation theory of play also views play as a product of an evolutionary biological process (Mellou, 1994). This theory differs from the preexercise theory in that it posits that play functions "to rid the organism of primitive and unnecessary instinctual skills carried over by heredity" (Gilmore, 1971, p. 313). The word "recapitulation" captures the idea that the ontogeny of the child reenacts the phylogeny of the human species. In other words, the development of the individual human being follows the evolutionary development of the entire human species. Thus, children's play passes through developmental stages of the human race in an evolutionary sequence, such as the animal stage when the child climbs and swings on structures and the tribal stage when the child participates in team games (Mellou, 1994; Rubin et al., 1983). In the process, primitive instincts, no longer needed in modern life, become weakened and played out, thereby allowing more complex levels of behavior to develop.

Modern Theories of Play

The classical theories of play have been called "armchair" theories because they are based more on philosophical thought than on empirical research (Ellis, 1973). However,

---

Box 1-2	**EXERCISE 2: EMBEDDED THEORIES**

Reread the first sentence of this chapter, which is part of a quotation from a paper by Norma Alessandrini (1949). The rudiments of at least two different classical theories of play are implicit in this statement. Which two are they? The core ideas of the classical theories of play seem to be part of the "folk wisdom" of our culture and are often embedded in the offhand comments that people (especially parents) make about children's play, for example, "He needs to go outside and blow off some steam." Can you think of another example or two of such comments?

---

they provide a foundation for modern theories of play, which address both the causes of play and the role of play in development. Modern theories may be grouped into the following categories: (1) arousal modulation, (2) psychodynamic, (3) cognitive developmental, and (4) sociocultural theories of play.

Arousal Modulation Theories of Play. Arousal modulation theories of play were initially developed to respond to theoretical weaknesses within the drive theories of learning. According to drive theories, play and exploration were seen as secondary to behaviors that served to reduce basic drives, such as those aimed at reducing hunger, cold, or thirst (Rubin et al., 1983). Research demonstrated, however, that animals would exhibit exploratory or play behaviors in place of drive-reducing behaviors even when the drives were assumed to be strong. For example, rats were observed to explore new features of their environment first before satisfying their hunger (Berlyne, 1966). Findings such as these led researchers to distinguish between external and internal motivation.

Berlyne (1969) developed a theory of intrinsic motivation in which play was associated with exploration and explained in terms of its role in the modulation of arousal states within an organism. In his view, tissue needs, such as hunger, thirst, and sex, lead to externally motivated behavior, but central nervous system functions are responsible for intrinsically motivated behavior (Berlyne, 1960, 1966). These self-motivated behaviors directly affect the level of arousal within the central nervous system. Arousal modulation theories posit that the central nervous system of an organism has an optimal arousal level (Berlyne, 1966; Ellis, 1973). When faced with novelty, discrepancy, or uncertainty, an organism will attempt to reduce its level of arousal through exploration of the source of arousal. The resulting behaviors are called specific exploration (Berlyne, 1966) and are thought to be rewarded by consequent arousal reduction. Diversive exploration occurs when an organism seeks stimuli with novel, discrepant, complex, or ambiguous properties not out of curiosity but out of boredom. In diversive exploration, the stimulus-seeking behaviors are thought to be rewarded by a moderate arousal increment (Berlyne, 1971). Specific exploration occurs when high levels of environmental stimulation are present; diversive exploration occurs with low levels of environmental stimulation. Both high and low levels of stimulation are equally aversive; therefore the organism's behavior is motivated by the need to avoid an aversive state (Rubin et al., 1983).

Ellis (1973) extended Berlyne's work on arousal levels and their connection to play behavior. He discriminated between behaviors that serve stimulus-seeking functions and those that serve stimulus avoidance functions. Stimulus avoidance behaviors reduce the intensity of the organism's internal stimulation. Stimulus-seeking behaviors generally increase the stimulation levels, usually through obtaining external stimulation. Ellis suggested that, in the absence of fatigue and the need to satisfy basic drives, all organisms would demonstrate stimulus-seeking behaviors. Such stimulus-seeking behavior can be serious in that it sustains the organism, which Ellis calls work, or it can be apparently useless, in which case it is called play. He concluded that work could satisfy both types of needs or drives, that is, need reduction drives or stimulus-seeking drives, but that play was purely driven by stimulus-seeking behavior. Based on these conclusions, Ellis defined play as "that behavior that is motivated by the need to elevate the level of arousal towards the optimal" (1973, p. 110).

Arousal modulation theories led to a theoretical distinction between exploratory behaviors and play behaviors (Mellou, 1994). For example, Hutt (1970) differentiated between exploration and play. In her framework, exploration occurs in a novel situation and involves the child's investigating the nature of a new object or setting. It is characterized by serious affect and focused attention to novel aspects of the environment. In exploration, the child asks, "What can this object do?" Play, on the other hand, occurs after the child has achieved a degree of comfort in a familiar situation and involves the child's experimenting with what he or she can do with the familiar object or setting. It is characterized by a relaxed, somewhat nonchalant attitude and positive affect. In play, the child asks, "What can *I* do with this object?" (Hutt, 1970). Although Hutt (1970) advocated a formal conceptual distinction between exploration and play, this distinction is not always clear or meaningful in the ecology of children's everyday activities (Weisler & McCall, 1976); thus its pragmatic usefulness is questionable.

Psychodynamic Theories of Play. Although Freud (1961) did not develop an articulated theory of play, he referred to play many times throughout his work. Later theorists expanded upon his work; therefore his view of play has made a significant impact upon theories of play, especially those that have attempted to explain the role of play in the emotional development of children (Rubin et al., 1983). Freud hypothesized that play served two functions for children: (1) wish fulfillment, that is, the desire to be big, powerful, or simply in someone else's shoes; and (2) mastery of traumatic events, through which children could take an active role in a situation where they were previously passive victims (Gilmore, 1971; Rubin et al., 1983).

Erikson (1963) used the mastery component of Freud's theory of play to address ego development and the coping effects of play for children. In play, children create situations in which they can successfully deal with anxieties and uncertainty, leading to their ability to master reality. Erikson's work on the mastery aspect of play became the foundation for psychodynamically oriented play therapy, which traditionally is conducted by psychologists and psychiatrists. Through repetition of a traumatic event in play therapy, children with emotional difficulties become active agents with feelings of mastery rather than passive victims overwhelmed by anxiety and helplessness. Thus, using Freudian and Eriksonian con-

cepts of mastery through play, children are encouraged in play therapy to "play out" their emotional problems just as adults may "talk out" their problems (Axline, 1969).

Cognitive Developmental Theories of Play. Cognitive developmental theories of play generally describe play as a voluntary activity in which children often interact with objects or toys that are under their control. Play is seen as a cognitive process and is believed to contribute to cognitive development, including problem solving and creativity (Sutton-Smith, 1980). The focus of these theories is usually upon children's formation of and manipulation of concepts and symbols.

Play, creativity, and adaptation. Some cognitive theories of play emphasize its link to development of novelty and flexibility in human behavior (Rubin et al., 1983). Two theorists in particular, Sutton-Smith (1967) and Bruner (1972), have proposed that play provides a safe context in which ideas and behaviors can be combined in new ways. These new combinations may then be used in other contexts outside of play. In this manner, play contributes to the behavioral adaptation of humans (Rubin et al., 1983). As in Groos's preexercise theory, play in childhood is seen as preparatory for the demands of adulthood (Mellou, 1994).

Sutton-Smith (1967) used the term "as if" to describe symbolic play in which the child uses something or someone "as if" it were something different. Children interact and play with sticks "as if" they are guns or with a sibling "as if" she or he is a cat. Through play, they combine ideas into new forms or alternative symbolic constructions (Rubin et al., 1983). Later on, in "serious," nonplay situations requiring problem solving, these alternative symbolic constructions may be called into action and thus contribute to adaptation (Sutton-Smith, 1977). Consequences of the "as if" phenomenon for human development include divergent thinking, thought that breaks free from set and restricted modes; role flexibility and reversals; and feelings of autonomy.

In contrast to Sutton-Smith's focus on the manipulation of ideas within play, Bruner (1972) suggested that play provides an opportunity for new combinations of cognitively guided motor behaviors, particularly the manual and handling skills required for tool use. According to Bruner, play in childhood affords a pressure-free environment within which behavioral subroutines of complex skills required for adulthood may be combined and recombined in novel ways without concern for the result or goal of the actions. Children are free to attend to the means of their behavior, not its ends. This behavioral flexibility in play accounts for both children's and the human species' adaptation and development over time (Bruner, 1972).

Common to both Bruner's and Sutton-Smith's theories is the hypothesis that play develops behavioral innovation and flexibility, leading to enhanced problem solving and adaptation. Active experimentation in play results in formation of a repertoire of skills and behaviors needed for future creative and cognitive tasks. Thus, these theories suggest that play prepares children for adulthood through its opportunity to generate novel and flexible thinking and behaviors (Mellou, 1994).

Cognitive development and play. Some of the most well-known descriptions of play as a manifestation of cognitive development can be found in the work of Piaget (1951/1962). Piaget, however, was focused on the study of the emergence of intelligence, not on play per se. In his formal theory of intellectual development, play at its purest is considered to be an expression of the cognitive process of assimilation, that is, the interpreting of experience in light of existing mental structures. In this view, play is not the origin of novel problem-solving efforts; rather it is a joyful exercising of existing cognitive abilities through action. The nature of play is viewed as different from imitation, in which actions and their underlying mental structures are modified to correspond to new experiences (a process called accommodation). Piaget's limited view of play contrasts with the theoretical orientation of Sutton-Smith (1967), who considers play to be a powerful vehicle for creative problem solving. According to Sutton-Smith, play is an important source of innovation in culture because of its creative potential, but Piaget's strict definition of play leads to the opposite conclusion since innovative problem solving would not originate in play. In a well-known debate, Sutton-Smith (1966) challenged Piaget on this important point.

Piaget (1951/1962) discussed the development of play behavior through his classification of games, which has been very influential in shaping child development research. He described three types of games, corresponding to stages of cognitive development: practice games, symbolic games, and games with rules (Piaget, 1951/1962).

Practice games involve the doing of actions purely for the pleasure of practicing them, without elements of make-believe or socially shared rules. An example would be a child jumping into a puddle of water simply for the pleasure of jumping and experiencing the splash. This type of play dominates the first 2 years of infancy but also occurs throughout childhood, whenever new skills are acquired and practiced (Piaget, 1951/1962). The term "sensorimotor play" is often used to apply to this type of play because it is characterized by exploration of sensations and movements (Fig. 1-1).

Symbolic games have an imaginative element because they involve make-believe or pretend play. An example would be a child feeding a doll with invisible food or with an object that represents food. Piaget felt that symbolic play was a significant milestone in cognitive development because it marked the child's ability to imagine objects and events that were not present, thus laying the groundwork for abstract problem solving and language development. The term "functional play" is sometimes used to refer to presymbolic games, in which the infant uses an object in a functionally appropriate way in relation to his or her own body (Largo & Howard, 1979), for example, raising an empty cup to the lips. This kind of play typically appears around 12 months of age and evolves into pretend actions directed toward a doll (e.g., giving the doll a drink). When pretend play involves an agent other than the self (for example, the doll), the term "representational play" is often used (Largo & Howard, 1979), although this term is sometimes used more broadly to include functional play as well. In true symbolic play, the child uses an unrealistic or invisible object in pretense, as in giving the doll a drink using a coin or using his or her empty hand as if it held a cup. Such symbolic play is typically seen by 24 months of age (Fein, 1981). Symbolic play becomes increasingly complex in the preschool years, with longer sequences of pretend behaviors evolving into dramatic scenarios with peers, a type of play known as "sociodramatic play."

Games with rules predominate in the play of 7 to 11 year olds and continue to be a dominant mode of play throughout life (Piaget, 1951/1962). Piaget referred here to explicit rules that are socially constructed and abided by in the cooperative play of at least two individuals. Games with rules may be handed down, as is the case when children learn to participate in games such as jacks or dodge ball, or they may be invented spontaneously, as when a group of several children make up rules for playing with a new object. Piaget (1951/1962) felt that these types of games were important agents of socialization and that they replaced functional and

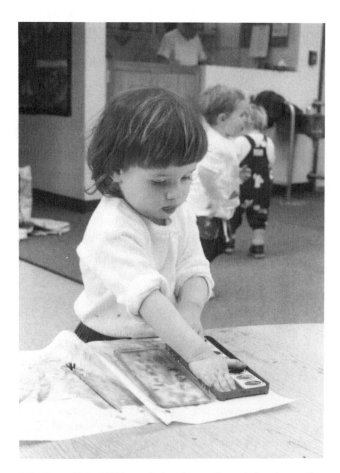

FIG. 1-1 This child is exploring the tactile and visual sensations associated with paint, rather than trying to create a picture. This is usually called sensorimotor play. Piaget would call this activity a practice game, whereas Reilly would call this exploratory behavior. (Courtesy Shay McAtee.)

symbolic games, which essentially disappeared in later childhood. This latter point contrasts with the viewpoints of authors such as Sutton-Smith (1966) and the Singers (Singer & Singer, 1990), who believe that symbolic play, in the form of imagination, does not disappear but goes "underground" in the form of internalized fantasy and plays a critical role in maintaining creativity and emotional health throughout life.

Development of creativity in play. Gardner (1982), like Piaget (1951/1962), has examined childhood play in relation to cognitive development. Instead of focusing on the child's ability to solve problems or comply with rules, however, Gardner (1982) has traced the unfolding of creativity and its expression through the arts.

In the first 2 years of life, children acquire direct knowledge about the physical world and, to some extent, the social world through the use of their senses and the consequences of their actions (Gardner, 1982). Thus their understanding of the world is dependent on their active involvement with the things, people, and space around them. Between the ages of 2 and 7 years, children's knowledge expands to include symbolic forms of information, including speech and language, hand and body gestures, music, numbers, and pictures. Children are now capable of understanding and communicating their experiences through use of the many symbols in their culture (Gardner, 1982). It is at this point in their development that children frequently combine these symbols in unique and striking ways.

Gardner (1982) refers to the preschool years as the "golden age of creativity" (p. 86). Children in this age group exhibit highly imaginative and inventive behaviors. In addition to intricate and fascinating structures designed out of play dough or blocks, preschool aged children create rich, colorful, and beautifully composed drawings and paintings. They sing and dance in a creative fashion. Even their language has a poetic quality (Gardner, 1982). Unfortunately, by elementary school age, children appear to lose this creative approach and their participation in artistic endeavors declines. At this point, children have reached what Gardner calls "the literal stage," a time of conformity and compliance with convention (1982, p. 88). Children at this age want to be like their peers. Their play is dominated by a desire to follow the rules and not to deviate from the norm. Similarly, their symbolic activities are often convention riddled; they have little interest in novelty or experimentation. Drawings become copies rather than creations, and many children do not draw at all. The poetic language of the preschool years declines. Gardner believes that this stage of development is essential for development of artistic creativity because it is a time for mastery of rules. Although children may begin to understand and show an interest in artistic works of others in the literal stage of development, it is not until adolescence that a sensitivity to artistic qualities may reemerge.

Sociocultural Theories of Play. Sociocultural theories of play focus on the relationship of play with culture. Contemporary theorists think of play as having a reciprocal relationship with culture, meaning that it both influences and is influenced by culture (Roopnarine & Johnson, 1994).

First, play influences culture: Play contributes to the socialization and enculturation of children because it is the context for children's learning of social norms, values, roles, and behaviors (Schwartzman, 1978). Furthermore, human collective behavior is organized through play (Sutton-Smith, 1980). The Dutch historian Huizinga (1944/1950) went so far as to assert that play was the germinal element that gave rise to civilization itself.

Second, culture influences play: Culture is expressed or embodied in play (Roopnarine & Johnson, 1994). Play is both a type of communication and an interpretation of society (Sutton-Smith, 1980). As such, play mirrors or, indeed, parodies the socialization process of society (Schwartzman, 1978).

Play as socialization. George Herbert Mead (1934) theorized that children learn social rules and norms through their play in games with other children. As they move between roles within a game, children's perspectives change. To participate in games with rules, each player must understand and be able to take on the perspective of the other players in addition to his or her own role. In so doing, each player is able "to predict what will happen next and adjust his [sic] behavior accordingly" (Slobin, 1964, p. 69). These changes in roles and perspectives lead to the development of a self-identity and of the concept of a "generalized other," that is, the perspective of the collective group. Through the process of developing an awareness of a "generalized other," the player learns social rules and norms that regulate the conduct of members of society (Mead, 1934). Self-identity is formed as the player compares his or her abilities with those of the other players (Slobin, 1964) and as social rules become internalized.

Mead's theory (1934) is an example of what Schwartzman (1978) called the "play as preparation or socialization" school of thought. This school of thought is based on functional analysis, which attempts to explain the stability of a culture or social system in terms of its parts, or structures, which function to preserve the sameness of its whole. Thus, certain structural systems within a society, such as kinship, religious, or economic systems, are thought to function as mechanisms to maintain the status quo. When functional analysis is extended to the play of children, their seemingly purposeless play becomes "transformed into activities functional for the maintenance and perpetuation of the social order" (Schwartzman, 1978, p. 100). For example, children playing house may be interpreted as imitating adults. In this view, the purpose of play is to provide a context within which children can practice and learn socially appropriate adult behaviors or roles. Thus, play, according to functional analysis, serves a socialization function. Some sociocultural theorists have challenged this view of play, suggesting that play may, in fact, be a form of communication (Schwartzman, 1978).

Play as communication. Bateson (1972) was the first theorist to put forth the idea that play is a type of communication (Sutton-Smith, 1980). In the course of exploring the paradoxical and ambiguous nature of communication, he coined the term *metacommunication,* that is, communication about communication, within play. The message "This is play," which is universally signaled by players before beginning to play, is a metacommunication (Bateson, 1972). Wrestling or physical fighting, when preceded by the signal "This is play," does not denote the same thing that it would had the play signal not been communicated. The view of play as communication does not separate play from reality; play and reality are related (Rubin et al., 1983; Sutton-Smith, 1980). In contrast to play as socialization, play is not seen as an agent of socialization, developing skills needed for adulthood. Instead, play itself is the skill required to function within the real world of daily life (Sutton-Smith, 1980). Rather than learning about how to be a parent by taking on the role of a mommy or daddy in play, children are learning about how to frame or reframe roles themselves. Thus "they are not learning about a particular role, but about the concept of roles" (Rubin et al., 1983, p. 712) (Fig. 1-2).

Schwartzman (1978), among others, has elaborated on Bateson's notion of play as communication. Children's play frequently consists of parody, satire, or caricature that inverts or even subverts the current social order (Schwartzman, 1978). Many children's games mock and challenge society's authority and power structures in the form of parents, teachers, or police. Schwartzman suggests that, in their play, children may be questioning the assumptions of existing social roles and systems. Thus play, as a form of communication, reflects and interprets culture as seen through the eyes of a child (Sutton-Smith, 1980).

HISTORICAL PERSPECTIVE ON PLAY IN OCCUPATIONAL THERAPY

Occupational therapy's interest in play reaches back across time to the early years of the profession. Founders of occupational therapy in the United States viewed human beings in terms of their occupational nature, which encompassed a rhythmic temporal pattern and dynamic balance of work, rest, play, and sleep. Adolph Meyer (1922) referred to work, rest, play, and sleep as "the big four" rhythms that helped shape the "whole of human organization" (p. 641) and that needed to be balanced even under difficult circumstances for an individual to adapt to the demands of living in a complex social world. Meyer's philosophy of occupation was influential in the development of early occupational therapy programs for people with physical and psychosocial disabilities (Dunton, 1915; Kidner, 1931; Saunders, 1922; Slagle, 1922; Stevenson, 1932). Writers in the profession spoke of a play spirit that was essential for worthwhile living (Saunders, 1922; Slagle, 1922; Ziegler, 1924). In the eyes of these founders, play was viewed as a human trait that was as important to health as work.

During the founding years of the profession, play was a highly visible aspect of occupational therapy programming, especially in occupational therapy for children. The association of play with occupational therapy was so strong that the occupational therapist (who typically was a woman) might be called the "play lady" by the children with whom she worked (Whittier, 1922). Nevertheless, putting Meyer's philosophy of occupation into practice in the first few decades of the profession was not a straightforward enterprise.

As Granoff (1995) has pointed out, the literature of the early twentieth century indicates that there was a tremendous amount of inconsistency in how play was incorporated into treatment programs. Economic pressures strongly influenced programming. For example, patients who were capable of working often were placed in industrial settings, such as the laundry or book bindery, where they could make an economic contribution to the institution, whereas patients considered unable to work or produce salable goods were often encouraged to participate in recreation programs (Inch, 1936). Furthermore, it became apparent that the experience of the individual influenced whether a given occupation was play or work; this realization complicated the task of planning group work and play programs. It also became apparent that play and work could be viewed as overlapping constructs, rather than distinct entities, and thus could exist simultaneously in a given activity, making it dif-

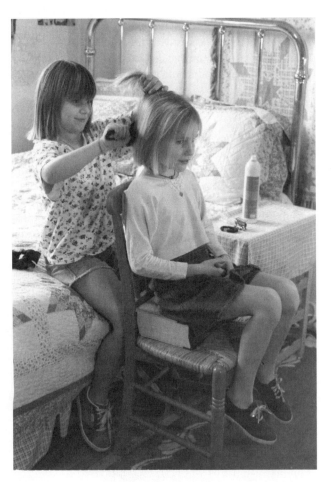

FIG. 1-2 In playing beauty shop, these girls are playing with the concept of roles. (Courtesy Shay McAtee.)

ficult to evaluate and treat the "balance" of work, rest, and play. The therapeutic goals of play or recreational activities also varied from one setting to another. In some settings, recreation was used to render patients more compliant and manageable (Ellis, 1934); in others, it was used as a diversion, simply to make patients' lives more pleasant and to keep them busy (Hohman, 1938); whereas in yet other settings, it was used for specific remedial or curative purposes (Slagle, 1934). These practice dilemmas involving economic pressures, conceptual ambiguity, and therapeutic goals in relation to play still confront contemporary practitioners.

Perhaps these pragmatic difficulties contributed to the fact that, by the midtwentieth century, occupational therapy had drifted away from its original commitment to the occupational nature of its patients. Although the concept of play as occupation still appeared in the profession's literature (Alessandrini, 1949; Smith, 1958), play was eclipsed by more scientifically and technically oriented concerns. In the pediatric occupational therapy literature, discussions of issues such as neuromuscular techniques, handedness, adaptive equipment, specific motor and self-care skills, and sensory–perceptual functions became the dominant topics, with little or no reference to occupation (Abbott, 1950; Ayres, 1958; Derse, 1950; Grayson, 1948; Rood, 1956). This shift in focus, according to Kielhofner and Burke (1977), was the result of external pressures on occupational therapy to become more respectable through adoption of a scientific posture. As occupational therapy became more scientifically oriented the identity of the occupational therapist as "play lady" became an embarrassment and, if still alive at all, was hidden away in the closet.

Mary Reilly is to be credited with bringing the concept of play back into focus as a topic worthy of study in occupational therapy. Her landmark book, *Play As Exploratory Learning* (1974), was the culmination of more than a decade of scholarship that sought to construct a comprehensive conceptual framework for the practice of occupational therapy. This framework was built on a concept called "occupational behavior," which linked play with work in a developmental continuum (Reilly, 1969). Under Reilly's leadership, the play lady was taken out of the closet (Florey, 1971), and a new generation of leaders and scholars in the profession were inspired to reclaim play as a fundamental concept in occupational therapy practice and to make it an object of research. Because her work continues to be very influential in the profession today, her ideas are reviewed in more detail in the following section.

CONTEMPORARY VIEWS OF PLAY IN OCCUPATIONAL THERAPY

The Occupational Behavior Tradition

The occupational behavior frame of reference emerged in the 1960s under the leadership of Mary Reilly (1966, 1969). According to Reilly (1974), play is significant because it is intermeshed with the struggle for mastery within one's environment, particularly the struggle of people with disabilities to develop skills and competency. The theme of the human struggle for mastery and achievement, regardless of individual circumstances, is a central tenet of the occupational behavior frame of reference. Play and work are viewed as the contexts in which mastery, achievement, and adaptation emerge (Reilly, 1969, 1974). Play in childhood is seen as the primary vehicle for the cultivation of skills, abilities, interests, and habits of competition and cooperation needed for competence in adulthood. Thus childhood play "is the antecedent preparation area for work" (Reilly, 1969, p. 302). Play in adulthood, in the form of recreational behavior, is interpreted as a support to adult work patterns. The entire developmental continuum of play and work is called "occupational behavior" (Reilly, 1969).

Reilly noted that clinical experience had indicated that play had "an organizing effect" upon patients who were behaviorally incompetent or disorganized (1974, p. 9). With this clinical legacy in mind, she embarked on a quest to understand why and how play contributes to mastery.

Reilly's Systems Explanation of Play. Reilly (1974) acknowledged that play was complex and could be viewed from the perspective of many different disciplines. To begin to grasp the "cobweb" that was play, she integrated the literature on play from the fields of anthropology, evolutionary biology, psychology, and sociology using a general systems approach. She chose a systems approach because it enabled her to organize isolated disciplinary constructs into a more comprehensive network of interrelated, hierarchically nested processes. For example, rather than interpreting play as purely a regulator of neurophysiological arousal mechanisms (Ellis, 1973) or as a manifestation of cognitive processes (Piaget, 1951/1962), she developed a view of play in which neurologically based arousal systems gave rise to the emergence of cognitive–symbolic systems. She was convinced that play was a multidimensional phenomenon; therefore, she advocated an interdisciplinary account of play as "a bio-social phenomenon" (Reilly, 1974, p. 122).

Rule learning through play. Given her assumption that play had an organizing effect upon behavior, Reilly believed that it must have an adaptive function. To explain how play serves adaptation Reilly (1974) used the concept of rule learning. She hypothesized that play was a dimension of the imagination that culminated out of three hierarchical action systems: the neurological subsystem, the symbolization subsystem, and the language subsystem. At the lowest level of the hierarchy, the central nervous system selectively takes in and organizes information from the environment. At the next level (the symbolization subsystem), sensory data are transformed into meaning in the form of symbols. These symbols provide a sort of shorthand for experiences, leading to the human capacity to think in a complex, yet economical, manner and to generalize from one situation to another. Finally, at the highest level of the hierarchy is the language subsystem. Reilly described the language subsystem as having diverse aspects, one of which dealt with play. Play at this level entails the complex use of symbols derived from action on the environment. These action-related symbols are called "rules." Reilly used the term "rules" to refer to mental representations or symbols for how the world and the self operated. These rules, she hypothesized, were generated in play. Thus, play deals with "reality problems" and is viewed as "processing or mastering reality" (Reilly, 1974, p. 145).

Through play, children learn sensorimotor rules, rules of objects and of people, and rules of thinking. Once rudimentary rules are generated, complex organizations of rules can be consolidated, and these give rise to the skills needed for the competency of the adult individual and the technology of society. Robinson (1977), one of Reilly's students, elaborated on this idea by describing a rule as a map of reality that guided actions. This is to say that a person's understanding of an object determines the way he or she interacts with it. For example, a ball is a thing that is spherical, and people's rules about spherical objects tell them that they can roll, kick, throw, and possibly bounce the ball, but they are not likely to have much success stacking it on top of another ball. Robinson called these simple rule-driven actions "subroutines," and further posited that subroutines are gradually linked together in a flexible series to form skills that are responsive to changing environmental conditions. Consider a child learning to play soccer. First, the child would need to know the rules about how balls work, as well as rules about how her or his body works. These would enable the child to generate subroutines of kicking and stopping the ball with her or his foot. Then, the child would combine these subroutines in a sequence and integrate them with other subroutines, for example, running and kicking at the same time. When the child begins to practice and combine these subroutines while playing with friends, she or he needs to integrate them with subroutines derived from rules of people, particularly those related to reciprocity and communication. Finally, the child would refine the skills of kicking, running and kicking, and stopping the ball while playing under varying conditions, such as with different team members or on different playing surfaces.

Reilly's developmental stages of play. Drawing from Berlyne's work on arousal (Berlyne, 1960), Reilly (1974) linked play with an exploratory drive of curiosity and conflict. As a child interacts with the environment, conflict between the expected and the unexpected and between the known and the unknown arises. This conflict generates curiosity, which serves to energize and motivate play as the child searches for rules to understand how objects, people, ideas, and events work. Building on this idea, Robinson (1977) noted that the optimal situation for learning rules is a safe environment for play in which there is neither too much nor too little challenge: "The right challenge or conflict is necessary for the state of curiosity to exist that will support the individual's play and thus the generating of rules" (pp. 251-252).

According to Reilly, the exploratory drive of curiosity is expressed in three hierarchical stages of play development through which competencies emerge. The three stages occur progressively during childhood. The stages are (1) exploratory behavior, (2) competency behavior, and (3) achievement behavior.

Exploratory behavior occurs in infancy and early childhood play or in novel, unfamiliar situations. It arises from an interest in the environment and its focus is on the means of behavior, not its ends (Reilly, 1974). Engagement in this behavior is intrinsically motivated. The emphasis is on sensory experience as children test the limits of reality in their search for rules. When children engage in exploratory behavior in a safe environment, hope and trust are generated.

Competency behavior is characterized by effectance motivation (Reilly, 1974), which is an inborn urge toward competence (White, 1959). Competence may be defined as the ability to meet adequately the demands of a particular situation (White, 1971). Effectance motivation produces feelings of efficacy and "joy in being a cause" (White, 1971, p. 273). Children's play in the form of competency behavior is driven by their need to interact with the environment, to have an effect on it, and to receive feedback from their actions on it (Reilly, 1974). The attitude of children engaged in this behavior is one of "I want to do it myself." They display intense concentration and persistence while involved in the activity. Through practice, mastery is achieved and self-confidence and self-reliance are generated (Reilly, 1974).

Achievement behavior is the third stage of play development and incorporates the learning of the first two stages. The concept of achievement is associated with expectations of success or failure and with criteria of winning or losing (Reilly, 1974). Performance is compared to some standard of excellence; achievement behavior is therefore seen as more extrinsically motivated than exploratory and competency behaviors. There is a competitive element here; children compete either with themselves or with others. Engagement in achievement behavior involves risk taking and strategizing with skills. During this stage, the hope, trust, self-confidence, and self-reliance generated in the first stages are transformed into courage (Reilly, 1974).

Occupational Role of Player. "Occupational role" is a central organizing concept in the occupational behavior frame of reference. *Role* is conceived as "the expected pattern of behavior associated with occupancy of a distinctive position in society," whereas *occupational role* is the "activity in an individual's life that contributes to society, and thereby, defines the person's societal worth" (Heard, 1977, p. 244). These concepts, imported from the field of social psychology, tie occupational behavior to the individual's capacity to perform services to society and thus to survive economically in a technically complex world (Heard, 1977; Reilly, 1966). Occupations, from this perspective, are activities that fill economically based niches in society. Occupational roles change across the lifespan: An individual is transformed from player and preschooler to student; then to worker or homemaker; and finally to retiree. Each occupational role involves a set of expectations for behavior (Heard, 1977).

The primary occupational role of the infant and young child is that of player (Heard, 1977). The player role, like other occupational roles, comes with a set of expectations, for example, playing in the manner that is expected by caregivers at home or at preschool. Being a player is deemed a legitimate occupational role because it is through play that essential rules, skills, and habits are acquired for competence in later occupational roles (Burke, 1993; Heard, 1977; Robinson, 1977). The term "habit" refers here to skills that have become so routinized that they are performed automatically, enabling the individual to attend to the novel demands of a task. Skills and habits generated in childhood play lay the groundwork for the individual's decisions regarding occupational choice in late adolescence or early adulthood (Shannon, 1974) and provide essential ingredients for success as an adult worker (Heard, 1977). Skills of decision making and risk taking are thought of as particularly important outcomes of play that will contribute to later occupational choice and work performance (Shannon, 1974). (At this point, the reader should try the exercise in Box 1-3.)

The child's occupational role as player is a focal point in the work of influential contemporary writers in occupational therapy. For example, Burke, Heard-Igi, and Kielhofner, all students of Reilly during the 1970s, collaborated to produce the first published version of the Model of Human Occupation, a frame of reference that is built upon occupational behavior concepts and has gained considerable attention in the occupational therapy profession internationally (Kielhofner & Burke, 1980; Kielhofner et al., 1980; Kielhofner, 1995). Occupational role is a guiding concept in the Model of Human Occupation, and the young child's major occupational roles are identified as player and family member (Kielhofner, 1995). Janice Burke (1993) describes the occupational role of player as a key construct in the application of occupational therapy assessment and treatment methods in early intervention. This view is elaborated in Chapter 5 of this volume, in which Burke collaborates with Roseann Schaaf to show how family narratives can be used by the therapist to construct a story of the child as player.

Box 1-3

EXERCISE 3: DEVELOPING SKILLS THROUGH PLAY

Write down two activities that were favorite play occupations for you when you were a child. These may be the two occupations that you listed in Exercise 1 in this chapter. What skills did you develop in the course of practicing those play occupations? In what ways do you use those skills today in your work occupations?

A Cadre of Scholars on Play. Reilly guided many of her graduate students at the University of Southern California during the late 1960s and 1970s to explore the topic of play in search of insights to guide occupational therapy practice. Thus, she systematically developed a cadre of scholars who grappled with play as a form of occupational behavior. Many of these scholars wrote papers that became classic pieces in the occupational behavior literature, and many of their ideas continue to be influential in contemporary practice.

Linda Florey (1971), for example, proposed that the concept of intrinsic motivation be used as an organizing construct for the study of play. She noted that play was a learning process that occurred throughout every child's day; therefore occupational therapists needed to attend to children's play outside, as well as inside, the boundaries of treatment programs. Florey (1971) also expressed concern for the potentially aversive effects of illness or disability on children's play: "a child with a reading disability may also have a 'playground disability' or a 'cub scout disability'" (p. 277). She urged occupational therapists to attend to these often overlooked, yet important, aspects of a child's play life. Over the years she has developed an impressive store of pragmatic knowledge regarding how to translate these ideas into practice. In Chapter 8 of this volume, she collaborates with her colleague, Sandra Greene, to describe the reasoning processes behind the use of play in treatment programs for very challenging children with psychiatric diagnoses.

Grounded in the assumption that play progresses in a predictable developmental fashion, Takata (1974) constructed a taxonomy of six developmental phases of childhood play, which she called "play epochs". These are described in Table 1-1. Takata's taxonomy differs from Reilly's stages of play in that it describes changes in the observable structure of children's play instead of changes in the underlying dynamics of play (Fig. 1-3). Using her play epochs as a guide, Takata constructed a Play History instrument to be used as an assessment tool by occupational therapists. This tool was designed to help therapists develop a play diagnosis and play prescription for children with dysfunction. An updated perspective on the Play History is discussed by Kimberly Bryze in Chapter 2 of this volume.

Another play assessment instrument, the Play Scale, was developed by Susan Knox (1974) under Reilly's guidance. The Play Scale has been widely used as a research and clinical tool. Knox reviews the literature on this instrument and proposes a new revision of it in Chapter 3 of this volume.

Others who were schooled in the occupational behavior perspective also developed instruments for assessing play. Readers interested in exploring these may find it useful to start with the integrative review provided by Florey (1981). Many of these occupational behavior–based instruments were critiqued by Kielhofner and Barris (1984), who also included instruments generated outside of occupational therapy in their review of methods available for the assessment of play.

TABLE 1-1 Takata's Play Epochs

Epoch	Age	Description
Sensorimotor	0-2	Purely autotelic play with sensations and motion in first 18 months: peek-a-boo, pat-a-cake, hide and chase, and imitation with caregivers; dropping objects; container play; exploration of object properties; practice of new motor skills; simple problem solving.
Symbolic and simple constructive	2-4	Symbolic play: beginning make-believe and pretend play; experiences represented in play. Shift from solitary play to parallel play. Builds simple constructions that represent another object or situation. Climbing and running are honed.
Dramatic, complex constructive, and pregame	4-7	Expansion of social participation: shift from parallel to associative play; dramatic role play enacting child's daily experiences, social roles, and fairy tales and myths. Skill in activities requiring hand dexterity. Daredevil activities involving strength and skill outdoors. Constructions are realistic, complex. Verbal humor, creates rhymes.
Game	7-12	Games with rules: fascination with rules; masters established rules and makes up new ones; risk taking in games; concern with peer status; friendship groups important; interest in sports and formal groups (e.g., scouts); cooperative play. Interest in how things work, nature, crafts.
Recreational	12-16	Formal peer group orientation: teamwork and cooperation; respect for rules; games that challenge skills; competitive sports; service clubs. Realistic constructive projects and complex manual skills.

*Adapted from Takata (1974). Play as a prescription. In M. Reilly (Ed.), *Play as exploratory learning* (pp. 209-243). Beverly Hills, CA: Sage Publications. Ages are in years, and are approximate. The terms "solitary," "parallel," "associative," and "cooperative" are from Parten (1932). Solitary, no peer interaction; parallel, side by side with peer but little or no interaction; associative, participates in group play with shared activity; cooperative, cooperates extensively with peers in highly organized activity.

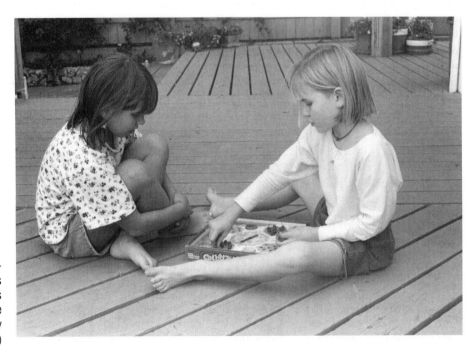

FIG. 1-3 These girls are on the threshold of Takata's game epoch, which is dominated by what Piaget called games with rules. They are absorbed in the process of learning to abide by socially agreed upon rules. (Courtesy Shay McAtee.)

Integration of Play into Specialty Practice Arenas

As the occupational behavior frame of reference gained prominence in the profession, play reemerged as a legitimate and promising topic for study and clinical application, and therapists became intrigued by its potential for enriching and transforming practice in areas of clinical specialization. This trend has been particularly evident in the specialty area of sensory integration. A compatibility between sensory integration and occupational behavior tenets was first pointed out by Lindquist, Mack, and Parham (1982), who suggested that sensory integration influenced play and that play experiences, in turn, influenced the development of sensory integration. Building on this proposition, Schaaf and her colleagues used a sensory integrative approach in an occupational therapy treatment program for preschoolers and then documented treatment effectiveness using measurement of play behaviors (Schaaf, 1990; Schaaf, et al., 1987). The relationship between sensory integration and play was deemed interesting and important enough to devote two special issues of the *Sensory Integration Special Interest Section Newsletter* of the American Occupational Therapy Association to it (Schaaf & Burke, 1992). In Chapter 7 of this volume, Zoe Mailloux and Janice Burke discuss play in relation to sensory integrative development, as well as the role of play in classical sensory integration treatment.

The putative relationship between sensory integration and play suggests that children with poor sensory integration are likely also to have compromised play skills. Research by Bundy and Clifford indicates that this is often but not always so (Bundy, 1989; Clifford & Bundy, 1989). Using Knox's Play Scale, Bundy (1989) found that groups of preschool aged boys with and without sensory integrative dysfunction did indeed differ significantly, on the average, in level of play development, with lower play scores characterizing the dysfunctional children. However, about one third of the group of boys with sensory integrative dysfunction had play skills within normal expectations. Furthermore, most preschoolers with sensory integrative dysfunction, like those without dysfunction, were found to express strong preferences for the types of play in which their play skills were strongest (Clifford & Bundy, 1989). In other words, most children seemed to have matched their play preferences with their abilities (Bundy, 1991). This strategy might be adaptive in the short run in that it preserves self-esteem and minimizes disruption to play skills. On the other hand, it is possible that there may be long-range negative effects if the child continues to avoid certain types of play, thereby missing out on some of the opportunities to develop motor and social skills that are available to most children. More research is needed to clarify issues such as these. From this line of research, Bundy (1991) concluded that sensory integration clearly might influence the child's ability to play but was only one of many complex foundations of play. Based on her research and clinical experience, she suggested that assessment of

sensory integration alone did not provide an adequate assessment of play and, further, that improving an individual's sensory integrative functioning might not automatically improve his or her play.

Questions regarding how to incorporate play into other specialty areas of practice are just beginning to be addressed in the profession. For example, very little attention has been given to play as a viable intervention technique for children with cerebral palsy, even though there is some evidence that play-based intervention can produce measurable developmental gains in preschoolers with this condition (Sparling et al., 1984). Issues surrounding play in occupational therapy for children with cerebral palsy are discussed in depth by Erna Blanche in Chapter 13 of this volume. Other chapters address a number of other specialty areas. For example, in Chapter 11, Elise Holloway discusses parent–infant play interactions in the context of the neonatal intensive care unit. A model program incorporating play into school-based practice is described in Chapter 9 by Ann Neville-Jan, Linda Fazio, Bonnie Kennedy, and Carolyn Snyder. And in Chapter 15, Linda Fazio describes the use of storytelling as a play modality in child psychiatry.

Emerging Themes on Play as Occupation

Play as occupation is a theme upon which divergent theorists and clinicians in occupational therapy are converging. Play is valued as a major class of occupations in which people engage throughout the course of their lives (Christiansen, 1991; Kielhofner, 1995; Primeau et al., 1989; Yerxa et al., 1989).

Most contemporary writers on play as occupation adopt, for the most part, the traditional occupational behavior stance, placing emphasis on the child's occupational role as player. However, two emerging bodies of work are pointing toward new ways of looking at play and applying it in clinical practice: the work in occupational science and the work on Bundy's model of playfulness.

Occupational Science. Occupational science is an emerging academic discipline that has been designed to provide a knowledge base for the practice of occupational therapy (Clark et al., 1991). This discipline is intended not only to provide a knowledge base for existing practice but also to lead to innovative clinical practice. By illuminating the nature of occupation and how it influences health, occupational science is expected to stimulate new ideas for intervention (Yerxa et al., 1989).

It is important to note that occupation is the central construct for study in occupational science. A promising strategy for studying occupation is to make it the primary unit of analysis in research (Parham, 1995). In other words, if therapists want to understand play as occupation, they need to study play directly. This approach differs from previous research that has sought to understand occupation by studying component abilities, such as cognitive, motor, or social skills, in hopes that by putting the pieces together eventually therapists will come to understand occupation.

Detecting patterns of play. Because play is a major category of occupation, it is an important area for research within occupational science. In the research that has been done and that currently is in process, play is studied by observing it as it occurs in natural environments and by garnering information from people regarding their experiences and perceptions of play, so as to provide a description of naturally occurring patterns of play. This, in turn, is expected to lead to new insights that have the potential to restructure clinical practice.

An example from the first generation of emerging occupational science studies on play at the University of Southern California may help the reader to appreciate how this research may lead to new insights about play as occupation. Loree Primeau (1995) studied the orchestration of parent–child play within the context of daily routines in the home. To identify patterns of parent–child play, she spent extensive amounts of time observing 10 families with preschool children in their homes and conducting intensive interviews of the parents involved. Her occupational science orientation led her to identify some patterns of parent–child play that had not previously been documented in the play literature. Specifically, she found two main types of strategies used by parents to incorporate play into daily routines at home: strategies of segregation and strategies of inclusion. In strategies of segregation, the child's play takes place as an entirely separate activity from parental household work, as when parents take a break from work to play with the child or when they work while the child plays independently. In strategies of inclusion, the child's play is embedded in the parent's work, as when the parent participates in household work and plays with the child at the same time or when the parent allows the child to participate playfully in the adult work task.

Primeau (1995) found that when a child participated in adult chores, often the parents would structure and support the activity so that the child could perform as much of it as possible; thus, the situation becomes one in which the child develops skills under the adult's guidance. For example, the parent may modify the physical environment, provide verbal suggestions, or eliminate unnecessary steps to allow the child to participate maximally. Primeau called this process "occupational scaffolding" because the adult's guidance became a scaffold on which the child learned to perform the task (Fig. 1-4). Interestingly, she found that children were highly motivated and enthusiastic during situations that involved occupational scaffolding and that most parents interpreted their children's involvement in the task as play, even though conventionally the task itself was thought of as household work. Parents interpreted their own experiences as simultaneously work and play during occupational scaffolding situations. Primeau (1995) suggested that occupational scaffold-

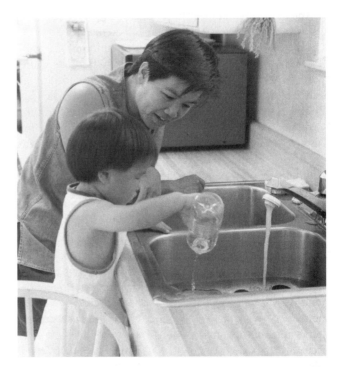

FIG. 1-4 This is an example of occupational scaffolding. The child is being allowed to participate in a cleanup task, and his mother is structuring the activity by providing verbal cues and a chair at the right height, so that he can do his part of the task successfully. This is play for the child and may be experienced by the mother as both play and work. (Courtesy Shay McAtee.)

ing may be an important process through which participation in childhood occupations fosters competence in adulthood.

There are several implications of this research for the fields of occupational science and occupational therapy. First, it identifies occupational scaffolding as the possible dynamic through which children learn skills for doing household work occupations; it thus addresses the important question of how childhood occupations shape adulthood accomplishments (Primeau, 1995; Primeau et al., 1989). Second, it calls attention to the fact that work and play are not always separate experiences; it thus calls for a rethinking of the notion of a balance of work, rest, and play (Primeau, 1995). Finally, it is a source of new ideas for intervention. It tells therapists that parents employ a variety of strategies to manage their children's play in the context of daily household routines. This knowledge can be the source of suggestions that therapists can share with families who are struggling to meet the demands of household management, work outside the home, and child care, while at the same time valuing opportunities to play with their children. Families who have children with disabilities may be especially appreciative of hearing about different strategies that other families have found useful for managing their complex daily occupations.

Another occupational scientist, Doris Pierce, is conducting a longitudinal study of infant play interactions with the physical environment. Her past research on infant play with objects (Pierce, 1991) and her preliminary findings in the current study are already influencing the way she practices in early intervention. She presents a detailed discussion of her unique approach to infant play with the spatial and temporal dimensions of the physical environment in Chapter 6 of this volume.

Movement away from role theory. As noted earlier, the child's role as player has been emphasized by most writers in occupational therapy who are concerned with play (Burke, 1993; Christiansen, 1991; Kielhofner, 1995; Reilly, 1969; Yerxa et al., 1989). Within the occupational science community of scholars at the University of Southern California, however, a move away from role theory is taking place. This move was instigated by Jeanne Jackson (1995).

Jackson (1995) has proposed that the concept of occupational role is not necessary to occupational science and, furthermore, that reliance on occupational role actually may be detrimental to some individuals served by the profession of occupational therapy. A serious problem with the concept of role is that, because it implies a given set of social expectations, it perpetuates an illusion that there is a proper or appropriate way to behave within a given role. The concept of occupational role minimizes the diverse and creative ways in which people organize their occupations and downplays the influence of subjective experiences, unique circumstances, and personal values on people's choices regarding what, when, where, and how to perform these occupations. Perhaps most worrisome is the potential of role theory to marginalize people who do not fit dominant roles because of factors such as gender, age, sexual orientation, or ethnicity. Thus role theory may lead practitioners unconsciously to penalize individuals who do not fit a dominant stereotype regarding appropriate role behaviors or to try to shape individuals to fit dominant roles regardless of personal circumstances.

This critique of role theory questions whether the potential harm in retaining role theory outweighs it usefulness. Jackson (1995) suggests that, instead of relying on role theory, occupational science should place occupation at the center of analysis. This would entail an appreciation of the interplay between personal visions of the individual and the environmental contingencies faced by that individual (Jackson, 1995). Occupational therapy, then, would aim to help the individual negotiate the personal and social–environmental issues that bear on his or her daily occupations, rather than simply relying on dominant stereotypes of how occupations should be performed.

As occupational science shifts away from role theory, the concept of the occupational role of player fades as a central organizing construct. Instead, the focus shifts to play as occupation: its features and how it is supported, or not supported, by intrapersonal and environmental factors (Fig. 1-5).

Valuing of play for its own sake. In the occupational behavior tradition, play in childhood is deemed important because it prepares the child for the student role and, ultimately, for the adult worker role. In adulthood, leisure or recreation is important because it refreshes or prepares the person to return to work (Reilly, 1966). This position is what Parham (1996) has called a functionalist view: that play is important because it is an effective way to develop other functions, such as sensory integrative, motor, social, cognitive, self-care, or work skills. In other words, play is justifiable only because it is a means to an end.

An alternative view that seems to be gaining momentum is that play is a legitimate end in itself because it is a critical element of the human experience. As Bundy has eloquently put it, "because we freely choose them, our play and leisure activities may be some of the purest expressions of who we are as persons" (1993, p. 217). Play, therefore, may be understood as a vehicle of meaning; it reveals what makes life worth living for an individual (Parham, 1996). Thus from this perspective, play becomes a quality of life issue in the here and now. Play is health promoting not only because it prepares for work at some later time (Reilly, 1969) but also because it is an active ingredient of a healthy lifestyle in the present (Ornstein & Sobel, 1989; Parham, 1996). The exer-

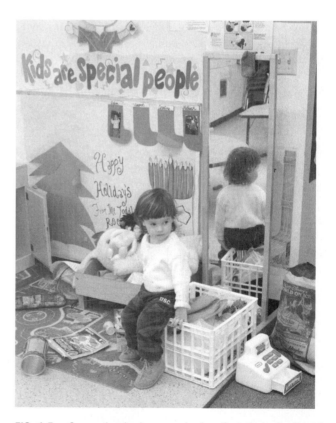

FIG. 1-5 Occupational science emphasizes the unique situation of the individual child, addressing intrapersonal characteristics such as temperament as well as how the environment supports and shapes play. (Courtesy Shay McAtee.)

cise in Box 1-4 may help the reader to appreciate this aspect of play.

The valuing of play for its own sake does not preclude adopting a functionalist position; both stances make powerful contributions to clinical practice. It is likely that the functionalist view dominates occupational therapy practice because, by linking play to accepted school- and work-related outcomes, it may make play in therapy easier to justify in today's economically oriented mindset. However, acknowledgment that play is important in its own right opens the door to intervention that makes enhancement of the child's play life the goal. This may prove to be just as effective in promoting health and well being as always making play a servant of other functions. It is plausible that it may be the most efficient way to influence health in some circumstances.

Part III of this book is devoted to occupational therapy intervention that aims to enhance play. For example, in Chapter 10, Jim Hinojosa and Paula Kramer describe an approach to family-centered intervention that is highly original in that it makes quality family play a goal of occupational therapy. A pilot group program designed by Julie Ewald to improve play experiences of preschoolers with prenatal drug exposure is described in Chapter 12. And a review of how technological aids can be used to promote play for children with a variety of physical and developmental disabilities is presented by Jean Deitz and Yvonne Swinth in Chapter 14.

Knowledge of the nature of play and of how play may be facilitated is crucial to developing sound programs that aim to facilitate play. For example, an occupational science study being conducted by Knox aims to describe play styles of preschoolers and identify the situations in daily life that af-

fect the expression of play style. A pilot study she conducted indicated that environmental and caregiver characteristics were highly influential on the playfulness of a child (Knox, 1996). The characteristics that she identifies in her current study have the potential to become organizing concepts in intervention programs. The work of Bundy, reviewed in the following section, also has tremendous potential to contribute to our knowledge of how to facilitate play and playfulness.

Bundy's Model of Playfulness. Anita Bundy (1993) has proposed that occupational therapists are unique in their perspective of play as an occupation. They use play as a tool to create therapeutic situations in which their clients can try out new behaviors and skills with fewer risks and consequences for failure than would normally exist in their daily lives. Thus, occupational therapists "make a living by creating 'play' and by enabling others to play" (Bundy, 1991, p. 48). She concluded that occupational therapists must form a precise definition of play simply because it is an important tool of intervention; play must be distinguished from nonplay. If occupational therapists truly believe that conceptualization of play as an occupation makes a valuable contribution to play theory and research as well as to their clients' lives, then they "must take play seriously" (Bundy, 1993, p. 221). Reliable and valid assessments of play must be developed, the process of integrating elements of play into interventions must be examined, and play must be promoted as an explicit and distinct goal of occupational therapy (Bundy, 1993).

With these objectives in mind, Bundy developed a model of playfulness (Bundy, 1991) and designed an ingenious assessment tool, the Test of Playfulness (ToP). These are discussed in Chapter 4 of this volume. In her chapter, Bundy provides illustrations of how the ToP can be used in clinical practice to assess a child's playfulness.

Bundy's concepts of play and playfulness potentially are useful not only in assessment, but also in planning intervention. Morrison, Metzger, and Pratt (Morrison et al., 1996) have provided an excellent discussion of how assessment and intervention can be designed to facilitate play, drawing from work by Bundy and her colleagues. One intervention approach may be to treat the underlying component skills, such as fine or gross motor skills, that interfere with the child's play. Another approach may be to examine the match or mismatch between play preference and play skills (Clifford & Bundy, 1989). An example of a mismatch is when the child is motivated to play a sport that is popular among his peers but does not have the skills to do so competently. Morrison et al. (1996) consider this sort of mismatch to constitute a play deficit. Intervention for a child with such a play deficit may involve (1) treatment of the underlying skill deficiencies in hopes that it will improve ability to participate in the preferred play activities; (2) exposure of the child to other types of play for which he or she has adequate skills to be successful, in hopes the child

---

Box 1-4	**EXERCISE 4: PLAY FOR QUALITY OF LIFE**

Again reflect on the two favorite childhood play activities that you analyzed in Exercise 3. This time, consider what it was that you enjoyed about them. For example, did they put you outdoors in touch with nature? Did they give you special quiet time alone? Did they provide fun times with friends? Search your memories for clues as to why these occupations were important to you.

After you have identified the qualities that have been meaningful to you in these childhood play occupations, consider the occupations that you engage in now. Are there any that provide you with the same qualities that you enjoyed in your favorite childhood play occupations? If so, what are they? They need not be play or leisure activities. If not, do you miss having occupations with those qualities you enjoyed as a child, or do you prefer entirely different experiences now?

will alter his or her preferences; and (3) alteration of the environment to facilitate the child's preferred type of play, for example, adapting the equipment or materials involved to facilitate success.

Morrison et al. (1996) consider another type of play deficit to be one in which the child is not playful. Playfulness is understood here as a quality of a child's play that involves flexibility and spontaneity (Knox, 1996) rather than simply the child's skill in performing specific play activities. The ToP may be particularly useful in identifying this kind of play deficit (see Chapter 4). Morrison et al. (1996) suggest that a number of therapeutic strategies be used when a child demonstrates a low level of playfulness: (1) setting the environment to facilitate the child's sense of control over the situation, (2) building trust and providing just the right challenges (Ayres, 1979), and (3) integrating a playful attitude into other aspects of intervention, such as working on underlying skill components.

CONCLUSION

Play is a complex phenomenon that has been examined by many different academic disciplines, from evolutionary biology to anthropology and sociology. Occupational therapists have acknowledged that play is a multidimensional, biopsychosocial phenomenon and in recent years have begun to generate research that builds on their long history of concern with play as an integral part of a healthy lifestyle. Furthermore, systematic applications of play principles in practice are being developed in the profession, as is demonstrated by the remaining chapters in this book.

The topic of play is usually addressed in occupational therapy in relation to children, but concepts of play are likely to be relevant throughout the lifespan, and play applications to adults need to be explored. For example, questions arise as to the concept of playfulness and whether it contributes to flexibility, and therefore adaptation, in adulthood. How can playfulness be encouraged in adults and how may it contribute to intervention? How does play fit into the lives of adults at various life stages? Is it meaningful to separate play from other occupations, such as self-care and work, or may it be more useful to consider it an attitude that can permeate any occupation? Can health-related effects of play be demonstrated, for example, through changes in the immune system? It is hoped that occupational therapists in the next decade will take play seriously enough to investigate the ways in which play concepts may be applied to benefit all people, regardless of age.

REVIEW QUESTIONS

1. Why has so much attention been given to the definition of play? Why is it so difficult to define play?
2. Describe the elements of definitions that address play as disposition, play as observable behavior, and play as context.
3. Compare and contrast the four classical theories of play.
4. Explain arousal modulation theories of play.
5. Describe psychodynamic theories of play.
6. Contrast Sutton-Smith's with Piaget's view of play.
7. Outline and describe the content of the following taxonomies of play development: Piaget's classification of games, Reilly's stages of play development, Takata's play epochs.
8. Discuss sociocultural theories of play.
9. How did play fit into Meyer's philosophy of occupation?
10. What is the significance of rule learning in the occupational behavior framework?
11. What is an occupational role? Why is the player role considered to be a legitimate occupational role?
12. Discuss the major themes in occupational science that address play.
13. Describe the strategies used by parents to incorporate play into daily routines in the home. What is occupational scaffolding, and how may it contribute to competence in adulthood?
14. What are two types of play deficit identified by Morrison et al. (1996)? What intervention strategies do these authors suggest to facilitate play and playfulness in children with these play deficits?

REFERENCES

Abbott, M. (1950). Present day trends in cerebral palsy. *American Journal of Occupational Therapy, 4,* 53-55.

Alessandrini, N. A. (1949). Play—A child's world. *American Journal of Occupational Therapy, 3,* 9-12.

American Occupational Therapy Association (1994). Uniform terminology for occupational therapy: Third edition. *American Journal of Occupational Therapy, 48,* 1047-1054.

Axline, V. (1969). *Play therapy.* New York: Ballantine Books.

Ayres, A. J. (1958). The visual-motor function. *American Journal of Occupational Therapy, 12,* 130-138.

Ayres, A. J. (1979). *Sensory integration and the child.* Los Angeles: Western Psychological Services.

Bateson, G. (1972). *Steps to an ecology of mind.* New York: Ballantine Books.

Berlyne, D. E. (1960). *Conflict, arousal, and curiosity.* New York: McGraw-Hill.

Berlyne, D. E. (1966). Curiosity and exploration. *Science, 153,* 25-33.

Berlyne, D. E. (1969). Laughter, humor, and play. In G. Lindzey & E. Aronson (Eds.). *The handbook of social psychology* (Vol. 3, pp. 795-852). Reading, MA: Addison-Wesley.

Berlyne, D. E. (1971). *Aesthetics and psychobiology.* New York: Meredith.

Bruner, J. S. (1972). Nature and uses of immaturity. *American Psychologist, 27,* 687-708.

Bundy, A. C. (1989). A comparison of the play skills of normal boys and boys with sensory integrative dysfunction. *Occupational Therapy Journal of Research, 9,* 84-100.

Bundy, A. C. (1991). Play theory and sensory integration. In A. G. Fisher, E. A. Murray, & A. C. Bundy (Eds.). *Sensory integration: Theory and practice* (pp. 46-68). Philadelphia: F. A. Davis.

Bundy, A. C. (1993). Assessment of play and leisure: Delineation of the problem. *American Journal of Occupational Therapy, 47,* 217-222.

Burke, J. P. (1993). Play: The life role of the infant and young child. In J. Case-Smith (Ed.). *Pediatric occupational therapy and early intervention* (pp. 198-224). Boston: Andover Medical Publications.

Christiansen, C. (1991). Occupational therapy: Intervention for life performance. In C. Christiansen & C. Baum, (Eds.). *Occupational therapy: Overcoming human performance deficits.* Thorofare, NJ: Slack.

Clark, F. A., Parham, L. D., Carlson, M. E., Frank, G., Jackson, J., Pierce, D., Wolfe, R., & Zemke, R. (1991). Occupational science: Academic innovation in the service of occupational therapy's future. *American Journal of Occupational Therapy, 45,* 300-310.

Clifford, J. M., & Bundy, A. C. (1989). Play preference and play performance in normal boys and boys with sensory integrative dysfunction. *Occupational Therapy Journal of Research, 9,* 202-217.

Derse, P. (1950). The emotional problems of behavior in the spastic, athetoid, and ataxic type of cerebral palsied child. *American Journal of Occupational Therapy, 4,* 252-259.

Dunton, W. R. (1915). *Occupational therapy: A manual for nurses.* Philadelphia: W. B. Saunders.

Ellis, M. J. (1973). *Why people play.* Englewood Cliffs, NJ: Prentice-Hall.

Ellis, W. J. (1934). The importance of occupational therapy in institutional management. *Occupational Therapy and Rehabilitation, 13,* 1-11.

Erikson, E. H. (1963). *Childhood and society.* New York: W. W. Norton.

Fein, G. G. (1981). Pretend play in childhood: An integrative review. *Child Development, 52,* 1095-1118.

Florey, L. L. (1971). An approach to play and play development. *American Journal of Occupational Therapy, 25,* 275-280.

Florey, L. L. (1981). Studies of play: Implications for growth, development, and for clinical practice. *American Journal of Occupational Therapy, 35,* 519-524.

Freud, S. (1961). *Beyond the pleasure principle.* New York: W. W. Norton.

Gardner, H. (1982). *Art, mind, and brain: A cognitive approach to creativity.* New York: Basic Books.

Garvey, D. (1990). *Play.* Cambridge, MA: Harvard University Press.

Gilmore, J. B. (1971). Play: A special behavior. In R. E. Herron & B. Sutton-Smith (Eds.). *Child's play* (pp. 311-325). New York: John Wiley and Sons.

Granoff, N. (1995). *The evolution and operationalization of the concept of play in early occupational therapy.* Unpublished manuscript, University of Southern California, Los Angeles.

Grayson, E. S. (1948). Handedness testing for cerebral palsied children. *American Journal of Occupational Therapy, 2,* 91-94.

Groos, K. (1978). The value of play for practice and self-realization. In D. Muller-Schwarze (Ed.). *Evolution of play behavior* (pp. 16-23). Stroudsburg, PA: Dowden, Hutchinson, & Ross. (Reprinted from The play of animals, pp. 72-81, by K. Groos, trans. by E. L. Baldwin, 1898, D. Appleton & Company.)

Hall, G. S. (1978). Growth of motor power and function. In D. Muller-Schwarze, (Ed.). *Evolution of play behavior* (pp. 24-29). Stroudsburg, PA: Dowden, Hutchinson, & Ross. (Reprinted from *Adolescence, its psychology and its relations to physiology, anthropology, sex, crime, religion and education,* Vol. 1, pp. 202-217, by G. S. Hall, 1908, D. Appleton & Company.)

Heard, C. (1977). Occupational role acquisition: A perspective on the chronically disabled. *American Journal of Occupational Therapy, 31,* 243-247.

Hohman, L. B. (1938). Difficult children and work habits. *Occupational Therapy and Rehabilitation, 17,* 1-9.

Hoshmand, L. T., & Polkinghorne, D. E. (1992). Redefining the science-practice relationship and professional training. *American Psychologist, 47,* 55-66.

Huizinga, J. (1950). *Homo ludens.* Boston: Beacon Press. (Original work published in 1944 in German, trans. unknown.)

Hutt, C. (1970). Specific and diversive exploration. *Advances in Child Development and Behavior, 5,* 119-180.

Inch, C. F. (1936). Therapeutic placement of mental plays in state hospital industries. *Occupational Therapy and Rehabilitation, 15,* 241-248.

Jackson, J. (1995). *Is there a place for role theory in occupational science?* Unpublished manuscript, University of Southern California, Los Angeles.

Kidner, T. B. (1931). Occupational therapy: Its diagnosis, scope, and possibilities. *Archives of Occupational Therapy, 10,* 1-11.

Kielhofner, G. (1995). (Ed.), *A model of human occupation* (2nd ed.). Baltimore: Williams and Wilkins.

Kielhofner, G., & Barris, R. (1984). Collecting data on play: A critique of available methods. *Occupational Therapy Journal of Research, 4,* 150-180.

Kielhofner, G., & Burke, J. P. (1977). Occupational therapy after 60 years: An account of changing identity and knowledge. *American Journal of Occupational Therapy, 31,* 675-689.

Kielhofner, G., & Burke, J. P. (1980). A model of human occupation, Part 1. Conceptual framework and content. *American Journal of Occupational Therapy, 34,* 572-581.

Kielhofner, G., & Burke, J. P., & Igi, C. H. (1980). A model of human occupation, Part 4. Assessment and intervention. *American Journal of Occupational Therapy, 34,* 777-788.

Knox, S. (1974). A play scale. In M. Reilly (Ed.). *Play as exploratory learning* (pp. 247-266). Beverly Hills, CA: Sage Publications.

Knox, S. (1996). Play and playfulness in preschool children. In R. Zemke, & F. Clark (Eds.). *Occupational science: The evolving discipline.* Philadelphia: F. A. Davis.

Largo, R. H., & Howard, J. A. (1979). Developmental progression in play behavior of children between nine and thirty months. I: Spontaneous play and imitation. *Developmental Medicine and Child Neurology, 21,* 299-310.

Lazarus, M. (1883). *Die reize des spiels.* Berlin: Ferd, Dummlers Verlagsbuchhandlung.

Lindquist, J. E., Mack, W., & Parham, L. D. (1982). A synthesis of occupational behavior and sensory integration concepts in theory and practice, Part 2: Clinical applications. *American Journal of Occupational Therapy, 36,* 433-437.

Mead, G. H. (1934). *Mind, self, and society.* Chicago: University of Chicago Press.

Mellou, E. (1994). Play theories: A contemporary review. *Early Child Development and Care, 102,* 91-100.

Meyer, A. (1922). The philosophy of occupation therapy. *Archives of Occupational Therapy, 1,* 1-10.

Merriam-Webster's collegiate dictionary (10th Ed.). (1994). Springfield, MA: Merriam-Webster.

Morrison, C. D., Metzger, P., & Pratt, P. N. (1996). Play. In J. Case-Smith, A. S. Allen, & P. N. Pratt (Eds.). *Occupational therapy for children* (pp. 504-523). St. Louis: Mosby.

Ornstein, R., & Sobel, D. (1989). *Healthy pleasures.* Reading, MA: Addison-Wesley.

Parham, L. D. (1995, April). *The proper domain of occupational therapy research is the study of occupation and its applications to health care.* Paper presented at the Research Colloquium of the American Occupational Therapy Foundation, Denver, CO.

Parham, L. D. (1996). Perspectives on play. In R. Zemke, & F. Clark, (Eds.). *Occupational science: The evolving discipline.* Philadelphia: F. A. Davis.

Parten, M.B. (1932). Social participation among preschool children. *Journal of Abnormal Psychology, 27,* 243-269.

Patrick, G. T. (1916). *The psychology of relaxation.* Boston: Houghton-Mifflin.

Piaget, J. (1962). *Play, dreams, and imitation in childhood.* (C. Gattegno & F. M. Hodgson, Trans.). New York: W. W. Norton. (Original work published in 1951.)

Pierce, D. E. (1991). Early object rule acquisition. *American Journal of Occupational Therapy, 45,* 438-449.

Primeau, L. A. (1995). *Orchestration of work and play within families.* Unpublished dissertation, University of Southern California, Los Angeles.

Primeau, L. A., Clark, F., & Pierce, D. (1989). Occupational therapy alone has looked upon occupation: Future applications of occupational science to pediatric occupational therapy. *Occupational Therapy in Health Care, 6,* 19-32.

Reilly, M. (1966). A psychiatric occupational therapy program as a teaching model. *American Journal of Occupational Therapy, 20,* 61-67.

Reilly, M. (1969). The educational process. *American Journal of Occupational Therapy, 23,* 299-307.

Reilly, M. (Ed.). (1974). *Play as exploratory learning.* Beverly Hills, CA: Sage Publications.

Reynolds, P. D. (1971). *A primer in theory construction.* Indianapolis: Bobbs-Merrill Educational Publishing.

Robinson, A. L. (1977). Play: The arena for acquisition of rules for competent behavior. *American Journal of Occupational Therapy, 31,* 248-253.

Rood, M. S. (1956). Neurophysiological mechanisms utilized in the treatment of neuromuscular dysfunction. *American Journal of Occupational Therapy, 10,* 220-224.

Roopnarine, J. L. & Johnson, J. E. (1994). The need to look at play in diverse cultural settings. In Roopnarine, J. L., Johnson, J. E. & Hooper, F. H. (Eds.). *Children's play in diverse cultures* (pp. 1-8). Albany, NY: State University of New York Press.

Rubin, K. H., Fein, G. G. & Vandenberg, B. (1983). Play. In Mussen, P. H. (Series Ed.). *Handbook of child psychology (Vol. 4).* E. M. Hetherington (Vol. Ed.). *Socialization, personality, and social development* (pp. 693-774). (4th ed.). New York: John Wiley.

Saracho, O. N. (1991). Educational play in early childhood education. *Early Child Development and Care, 66,* 45-64.

Saunders, E. B. (1922). Psychiatry and occupational therapy. *Archives of Occupational Therapy, 1,* 99-114.

Schaaf, R. C. (1990). Play behavior and occupational therapy. *American Journal of Occupational Therapy, 44,* 68-75.

Schaaf, R. C., & Burke, J. P. (Eds.). (1992). From the guest editors. Special issue on sensory integration and play—part 1. *Sensory Integration Special Interest Section Newsletter, 15* (1), 1.

Schaaf, R. C., Merrill, S. C., & Kinsella, N. (1987). Sensory integration and play behavior: A case study of the effectiveness of occupational therapy using sensory integrative techniques. *Occupational Therapy in Health Care, 4,* 61-75.

Schwartzman, H. B. (1978). *Transformations: The anthropology of children's play.* New York: Plenum Press.

Shannon, P. D. (1974). Occupational choice: Decision making play. In M. Reilly (Ed.). *Play as exploratory learning* (pp. 285-314). Beverly Hills: Sage Publications.

Singer, D. G., & Singer, J. L. (1990). *The house of make-believe.* Cambridge, MA: Harvard University Press.

Slagle, E. C. (1922). Training aides for mental patients. *Archives of Occupational Therapy, 1,* 11-17.

Slagle, E. C. (1934). Occupational therapy: Recent methods and advances in the United States. *Occupational Therapy and Rehabilitation, 13,* 289-298.

Slobin, D. (1964). The fruits of the first season: A discussion of the role of play in childhood. *Journal of Humanistic Psychology, 4,* 59-79.

Smith, N. (1958). Occupational therapy in a pediatric section. *American Journal of Occupational Therapy, 12,* 306-313.

Sparling, J. W., Walker, D. F., & Singdahlsen, J. (1984). Play techniques with neurologically impaired preschoolers. *American Journal of Occupational Therapy, 38,* 603-612.

Spencer, H. (1978). Aesthetic sentiments. In D. Muller-Schwarze, (Ed.). Evolution of play behavior (pp. 10-15). Stroudsburg, PA: Dowden, Hutchinson, & Ross. (Reprinted from *The principles of psychology.* Vol. 2, pp. 627-632. by H. Spencer, 1878, Appleton & Company.)

Stevenson, G. H. (1932). The healing influence of work and play in a mental hospital. *Archives of Occupational Therapy, 11,* 85-89.

Sutton-Smith, B. (1966). Piaget on play: A critique. *Psychological Review, 73,* 104-110.

Sutton-Smith, B. (1967). The role of play in cognitive development. *Young Children, 22,* 361-370.

Sutton-Smith, B. (1977). Play as adaptive potentiation. In P. Stevens, (Ed.). *Studies in the anthropology of play.* Cornwall, NY: Leisure Press.

Sutton-Smith, B. (1980). Children's play: Some sources of play theorizing. In K. H. Rubin (Ed.). *New directions for child development: No. 9. Children's play* (pp. 1-16). San Francisco: Jossey-Bass.

Takata, N. (1974). Play as a prescription. In M. Reilly (Ed.). *Play as exploratory learning* (pp. 209-246). Beverly Hills, CA: Sage Publications.

Vandenberg, B. (1978). Play and development from an ethological perspective. *American Psychologist, 33,* 724-738.

Weisler, A., & McCall, R. B. (1976). Exploration and play: Resume and redirection. *American Psychologist, 31,* 492-508.

White, R. W. (1959). Motivation reconsidered: The concept of competence. *Psychological Review, 66,* 297-333.

White, R. W. (1971). The urge towards competence. *American Journal of Occupational Therapy, 25,* 271-274.

Whittier, I. L. (1922). Occupation for children in hospitals. *Occupational Therapy and Rehabilitation, 1,* 41-47.

Wittgenstein, L. (1958). *Philosophical investigations* (3rd ed.) (G. E. M. Anscombe, Trans.). New York: MacMillan. (Original work published in 1953.)

Yerxa, E. J., Clark, F. A., Frank, G., Jackson, J., Parham, D., Pierce, D., Stein, C., & Zemke, R. (1989). An introduction to occupational science, a foundation for occupational therapy in the 21st century. *Occupational Therapy in Health Care, 6,* 1-17.

Ziegler, L. H. (1924). Some observations on recreations. *Archives of Occupational Therapy, 3,* 255-265.

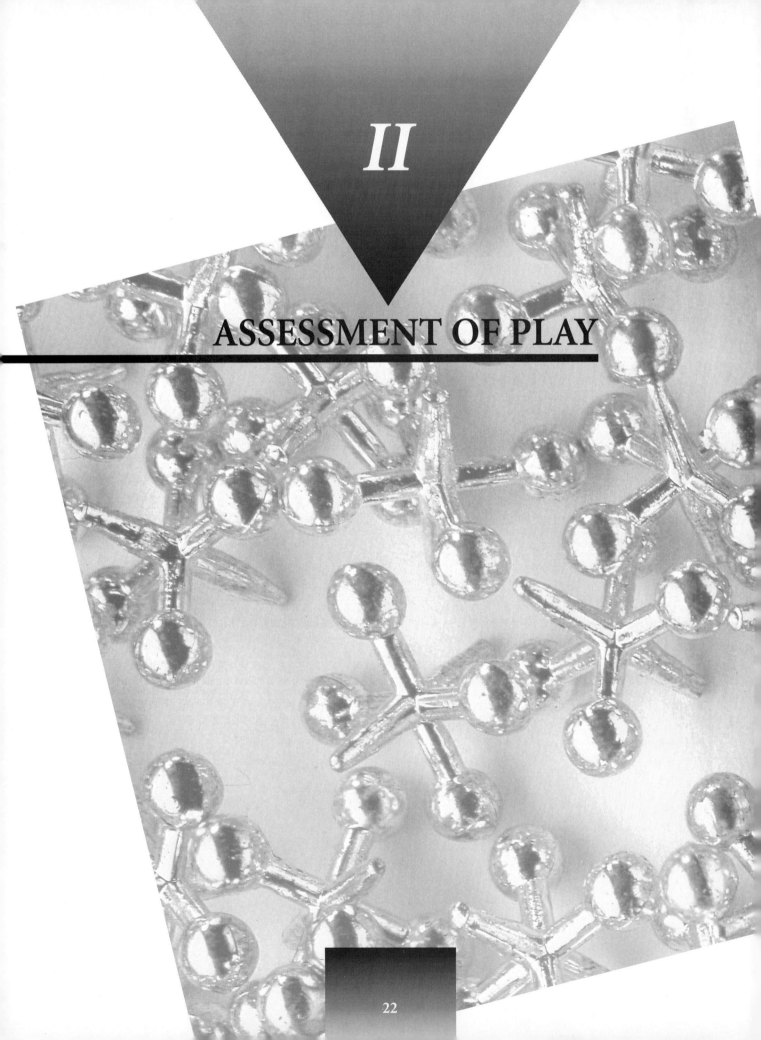

II

ASSESSMENT OF PLAY

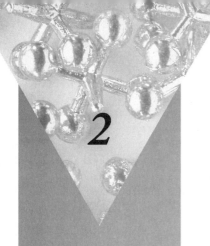

2

NARRATIVE CONTRIBUTIONS TO THE PLAY HISTORY

Kimberly Bryze

KEY TERMS

play history
interview
life story
narrative
narrative methods

T he opportunity to assess a child provides the occupational therapist with a unique glimpse into the child's life in progress. Each child has a past history, is living the present, and is moving toward his or her individual future. The child's past, complete with achievements and struggles, is foundational to who the child is at this present moment. It is the present into which the occupational therapist is invited, to learn, to assess, to influence. It is through a narrative process that the structure of a child's life can begin to be understood. Through a narrative process, the therapist can begin to understand the child's present in light of his or her past and to imagine the child's future story. The child's life, the life of play, is an unfolding story; the occupational therapist's role is to become one episode, or a chapter, in the ongoing story of the child's life. Specifically, the child's life of play is already in process; occupational therapists are allowed into the child's life because of the unique contributions they can offer to the child's present and future stories.

Most likely, the child has been referred to occupational therapy because of concerns about the appropriateness or the quality of his or her ability to perform occupations, of which play is one of the most important. Occupational therapists have traditionally assessed the child's play through observation and administration of various play scales. Inferences have then been made regarding the impact of delayed skill performance on the child's play, and occupational therapists have reasoned that by improving the skills which support play, this overarching occupation of the child will, in turn, improve. These skill-based methods of assessing play provide therapists with information about the child's current play abilities. However, these tools do not provide a historical perspective of how the child has developed into the player he or she is at present. The Play History (Takata, 1974) is one instrument that has been designed to provide a mechanism by which occupational therapists can assess the child's present abilities in light of his or her past play experiences.

This chapter addresses some conceptual and practical concerns about play and the use of the Play History to assess children. The unique contributions of the narrative approach for collecting information about a child's past and present play is offered. Guidelines for utilizing a narrative approach to supplement information obtained by more formal means are also offered.

THE STUDY OF PLAY AND OCCUPATIONAL THERAPY

Occupational therapists have struggled to define clearly what they mean by "play." Therapists have collected together an extensive body of knowledge about play from such disciplines as education, anthropology, and psychology, but relatively little has been done to develop an occupational therapy theory of play. The related bodies of knowledge have contributed to occupational therapists' learning "about play," but this learning has been limited to the interpretations reflective of each discipline. For example, because of their interest in development, researchers in psychology have studied early stages of play as transitions to higher levels of social interaction or pretend play. Occupational therapists have approached the study of play by developing taxonomies for describing play behavior in children. Again, these taxonomies usually reflect other disciplines' knowledge base about play. However, occupational therapists cannot derive all of the information they need about play, and fully understand how play contributes to and supports occupational behavior, from other disciplines' literature.

Further, the interpretations of play vary within occupational therapy itself. This variation may result from the influences of theory or frames of reference from which individual therapists practice (Burke, 1993). For example, therapists with perspectives in practice models such as sensory integration or neurodevelopmental treatment may relate the child's play to an outcome of the ability to process and use sensory input for the production of an adaptive response or as a reflection of neuromotor output.

M. Brewster Smith (1974) asserted that the developmental roots of competence lie in the human capacity for play. Play begins the developmental process of occupational behavior and promotes competency, achievement, and acquisition of occupational roles. The child who adequately learns the skills of occupational behavior through play can transform these skills into the habits and roles of daily life.

Play is also one way children can learn how they "fit" within an environment: how they can affect the environment and, conversely, how they are affected by it. Play is one process by which children adapt to the environment or adapt the environment to themselves. Play is an interactional relationship with the environment, a transaction between the child and the environment that is intrinsically motivated, internally controlled, and not bound by objective reality (Neumann, 1971). Moreover, play is seen as a way to derive meaning from environmental interactions; play is traced as a persistent strategy individuals use to apprehend the unknown (Reilly, 1974). Play may assume various forms of interaction (e.g., sensorimotor, social–emotional, linguistic, or cognitive) and may be realized through various methods of playing, such as qualities of exploration, repetition, replication, or transformation. Play may be directed toward people, toward objects, or for specific functions (e.g., information seeking, social learning, sensorimotor activity, emotional or creative expression). The relationship of the child in dynamic interaction within an environmental context is a continual process that results in the child's learning about her or himself and the social and physical environment(s). This relationship is dependent on the cognitive, creative, and interactional abilities of the child. The quality of a child's play is related to the range of these characteristics as they influence action within and on the environment (Takata, 1974).

Play can be an internal phenomenon or an external event. As such, it may be considered to be a continuum of behaviors that are more or less observable, depending on the degree to which the child is internally controlled, intrinsically motivated, and able to suspend reality (Bundy, 1991; Neumann, 1971). Further, any activity can be playful if the player so wishes; playfulness depends more on process than on the outcome, or product, of play. In similar fashion, play is also a mastery process in which activity is related to capacity; the outcome is skill (Reilly, 1974).

Each stage of development reflects a stepping stone toward maturity through play and its contribution to the acquisition of occupational behavior. If specific skills do not develop within appropriate developmental stages, a child may be at a disadvantage in progressing toward a subsequent stage. Moreover, if the requisite opportunities for activity and interaction are lacking at a critical period, particular skills may not appear, may be delayed in their appearance, or may be deficient. In this way, the processes of development and play parallel each other (Takata, 1974). Moreover, when the physical or human–social environment does not support play, the potential for developing those skills and behaviors may also be reduced. When medical, physical, or cognitive limitations exist, the possibility of learning those skills and behaviors that typically are direct consequences of playful experiences may be affected (Burke, 1993; Reilly, 1974). A child with physical or cognitive disabilities may lack both the abilities and opportunities for successful play experiences and may be vulnerable to limitations posed by cultural and environmental constraints (Reilly, 1974). Moreover, there is always the risk that the child will not develop the quality of play reflective of his or her stage of maturity. It is most important therefore that inadequate play habits be detected and treated (Behnke & Fetkovich, 1984).

AN OVERVIEW OF THE PLAY HISTORY

The Play History (Takata, 1974) was developed on the premise that play and development are intertwined and that assessment of, and intervention for, play dysfunction is vital to the continued development of the child (Takata, 1974; Behnke & Fetkovich, 1984). Since development is viewed as a process that takes place over time, it is important to look at the past as well as the present play behaviors of the child. Therefore occupational therapists' assessments of play should reflect the premise that play reflects development and thus increases in complexity over time (Behnke & Fetkovich, 1984).

The Play History (Takata, 1974) was developed to serve as a guide to address important concerns regarding the extent to which the past and the present environments support, guide, and elicit growth and development of competence and skills for competence in life (Behnke & Fetkovich, 1984). The gathering of the child's unique history is believed to be important in the total process of occupational therapy assessment. Development proceeds in an orderly manner with predictability as well as increasing complexity from one step to the next. Therefore a historical perspective can provide important information pertaining to the child's development and competence in play, which may be used in the planning and implementing of treatment.

This instrument consists of an interview schedule designed to elicit information related to identifying a child's play experiences, interactions, environments, and opportunities across the time progression of his or her life. The Play History is designed to relate information about the quality and quantity of a child's play to each of five developmental phases or epochs: (a) sensorimotor, (b) symbolic and simple constructive, (c) dramatic and complex constructive, (d) games, and (e) recreational. (See Chapter 1 for a summary of these epochs.) These epochs provide the taxonomy for an analysis of the play phenomenon, and in each of these epochs, the following four categories are analyzed: (a) materials (with what does the child play?), (b) action (how does the child play?), (c) people (how does the child play with others?), and (d) setting (where and when does the child play?). These epochs and categories strongly reflect the work of Piaget (1951/1962), Gesell (1945), and other authors in the field of developmental psychology, as well as other occupational therapists working from an occupational behavior perspective (Florey, 1971; Reilly, 1974).

As it was originally designed, the Play History is semistructured, qualitative, and open ended in format (Takata, 1974). It includes a basic set of questions that the interviewer may ask in a meaningful order, depending on the progression of the interview and the content, or depth, of the information provided by the child's parent(s) or primary caregiver(s). Examples of some of the questions include: With what does the child play? How does the child play? How does the child use tools and materials? What type of play is avoided or liked the least? With whom does the child play? How does the child play with others? The entire Play History is shown in Box 2-1.

The answers to these questions may be given in a descriptive manner, rather than by simply saying "yes" or "no." The therapist is required to identify whether the particular criterion under each question has been answered with support-ing "evidence," "no evidence," or "no opportunity" in each of the categories within each epoch. The therapist then interprets the results of the interview using a taxonomy of play (see Table 2-1). The taxonomy is based on the play epochs outlined by Takata (1974) and has been designed to allow the child's play to be analyzed in comparison to the typical development of play (Behnke & Fetkovich, 1984; Burke, 1993; Takata, 1974).

As previously mentioned, the questions and content areas of this tool are used to assess the past as well as the present play behaviors. The content of the Play History is seen as important for the clinical purposes of both diagnosis and planning and implementation of treatment (Takata, 1974).

One study (Behnke & Fetkovich, 1984) provided evidence for the reliability and validity of therapists' judgments regarding play development using the Play History. The researchers developed an ordinal scale to quantify information obtained through interview using the Play History and found high interrater reliability on overall play scores. Test–retest coefficients fell in a moderate range, perhaps reflecting inconsistency in the details recalled by parents from one interview to the next, or increased sensitivity to particular aspects of their children's play as a result of the first interview. Total Play History scores were significantly associated with subscale scores on the *Minnesota Child Developmental Inventory*. This finding indicates that the Play History yields valid information regarding the child's developmental level.

Behnke and Fetkovich (1984) provide encouraging evidence that the Play History is a reliable and valid measure of general developmental trends in play. However, the numerical scores they use in their study do not capture the rich qualitative information that is produced in an interview. In an interview, themes emerge that reflect a child's early and current dominant play behaviors or schemas. Because the emerging themes and specific play patterns paint a unique portrait of the child being assessed, they provide essential information for planning treatment. Therefore the interpretation of interview material is critical in the assessment process. The actual interpretation, or reconstruction, of a child's play history constitutes a difficult yet important step, the basis for which is the depth and quality of the information obtained from the interview.

Although this assessment tool is designed to be an open-ended interview, its application may be limited by problems inherent in all interviews. The purpose of interviews is to obtain information about certain aspects of behavior or experience. In their form and their function, interviews are to be distinguished from more casual or everyday conversations. In casual or friendly conversations, each participant takes turns and shares responsibility for keeping the conversation going. In interviews, the interviewer and the informant take turns, but there is a clear differentiation between who asks the questions and who provides information regarding his or her individual experience; the interviewer asks most of the questions and

---

▼ **Box 2-1** **THE PLAY HISTORY**

(1) GENERAL INFORMATION

Name: Birthdate: Sex:

Date: Informant(s):

Presenting Problem:

(2) PREVIOUS PLAY EXPERIENCES

A. Solitary play

B. Play with others:

 mother   father   sisters   brothers   playmates

 other family members   pets

C. Play with toys and materials (earliest preferences)

D. Gross physical play

E. Pretend and make-believe play

F. Sports and games: group collaboration   group competition

G. Creative interests: arts   crafts

H. Hobbies, collections, other leisure time activities

I. Recreation/social activities

(3) ACTUAL PLAY EXAMINATION

A. *With what* does the child play?

 toys   materials   pets

B. *How* does the child play with toys and other materials?

C. What type of play is *avoided* or liked least?

D. *With whom* does the child play?

 self   parents   brothers   sisters   peers   others

E. *How* does the child play with others?

F. *What body postures* does the child use during play?

G. *How long* does the child play with objects?   with people?

H. *Where* does the child play?

 home: indoors   outdoors

 community: park   school   church   other areas

I. *When* does the child play?

 daily schedule for weekday and weekend

(4) PLAY DESCRIPTION

(5) PLAY PRESCRIPTION

From Takata, N. (1974). Play as prescription. In M. Reilly (Ed.), *Play as exploratory learning.* Beverly Hills, CA: Sage Publications. Reprinted with permission from the publisher.

the informant offers responses to the questions (Spradley, 1979). Moreover, because the interviewer seeks specific types of information, there may be an overriding concern for the informant to provide the "right" answer; this may interfere with the process of the interview and may affect the quality of the results of the overall assessment. Although the questions on the Play History may be arranged and reframed so as to be most meaningful for the infor-mant regarding content and order, the interviewer may be inclined to ask the questions in the same order or in the same phrases in which they have been written and thereby limit the meaningfulness and breadth of the information obtained by the interview process. Given these concerns, it is suggested that the use of a narrative approach contributes greater depth and validity to the assessment process.

TABLE 2-1 Chart: The Use of a Play Milieu and Taxonomy for Diagnosis*

Epochs	Elements	Description	
Sensorimotor, 0 to 2 years	*Materials:* Toys, objects for sensory experiences—see, mouth, touch, hear, smell—rattles, ball, nesting blocks, straddle toys, chimes, simple pictures, color cones, large blocks *Action:* Gross—stand/fall, walk, pull, sit on, climb, open/close Fine—touch, mouth, hold, throw/pick up, bang, shake, carry Motoric imitation of domestic actions *People:* Parents and immediate family *Setting:* Home—crib, playpen, floor, yard, immediate surroundings EMPHASIS: INDEPENDENT PLAY W/EXPLORATION HABITS EXPRESSED IN TRIAL AND ERROR.	Evidence: No Evidence:	Encouraged: Discouraged:
Symbolic and simple constructive, 2 to 4 years	*Materials:* Toys, objects, raw materials (water, sand, clay, paints, crayons) for fine motor manipulation and simple combining and taking apart; Wheeled vehicles and adventure toys to practice gross motor actions. *Action:* Gross—climb, run, jump, balance, drag, dump, throw Fine—empty/fill; scribble/draw; squeeze/pull; combine/take apart; arrange in spatial dimensions Imagination w/storytelling, fantasy; objects represent events/things *People:* Parents, peers, other adults *Setting:* Outdoors—playground; play equipment immediate neighborhood Indoors—home, "nursery" EMPHASIS: PARALLEL AND BEGINNING TO SHARE; SYMBOLIC PLAY EXPRESSED IN SIMPLE PRETENSE AND SIMPLE CONSTRUCTIONAL USE OF MATERIALS	Evidence: No Evidence:	Encouraged: Discouraged:
Dramatic and complex constructive and pregame, 4–7 years	*Materials:* Objects, toys, raw materials for fine motor actions and role playing; large adventure toys for refining gross actions for speed and coordination; pets; nonselective collections *Action:* Gross—"daredevil" feats of hopping, skipping, turning somersaults; dance Fine—combining materials and making products to do well, to use tools, to copy reality Dramatic role playing—imitating reality in part/whole costumes, storytelling *People:* Peer group (2 to 5 members) "imaginary friends" Parents, immediate family, other adults *Setting:* School, neighborhood and extended surroundings (excursions); upper space and off the ground EMPHASIS: COOPERATIVE PLAY WITH PURPOSEFUL USE OF MATERIALS FOR CONSTRUCTIONS, DRAMATIZATION OF REALITY AND BUILDING HABITS OF SKILL AND TOOL USE.	Evidence: No Evidence:	Encouraged: Discouraged:

Continued.

TABLE 2-1 Chart: The Use of a Play Milieu and Taxonomy for Diagnosis*—cont'd

Epochs	Elements	Description		
Games, 7-12 years	*Materials:* Games played w/rules (dominoes, checkers, table card games, Ping-Pong); raw materials and tools for making complex products (weaving, woodwork, carving, needlework)		Evidence:	Encouraged:
	Gross muscle sports—hopscotch, kite flying, skating, basketball			
	Books—puzzles, "things to do" biography, adventure, sports			
	Selective collection or hobby			
	Pet			
	Action: Gross—refining and combining skills of jumping, hopping, running			
	Fine—precision in using variety of tools, finer object manipulation and construction		No Evidence:	Discouraged:
	Making, following, breaking rules; competition and compromise w/peers			
	People: Peer group of same sex; organized groups, e.g., scouts, parents, other adults			
	Setting: Neighborhood, playground, school, home			
	EMPHASIS: ENHANCEMENT OF CONSTRUCTIONAL AND SPORTS SKILLS AS EXPRESSED IN RULE-BOUND BEHAVIOR, COMPETITION, AND APPRECIATION OF PROCESS COOPERATIVE PLAY.			
Recreation, 12 to 16 years	*Materials:* Team games and sports and special interest groups for music, dancing, singing, discussing. Collections and hobbies; parties, books, table games		Evidence:	Encouraged:
	Action: Gross—team sports and individual precision sports (tennis, golf)			
	Fine—applying and practicing fine manipulative skills to develop craftsmanship, special talents		No Evidence:	Discouraged:
	Organized group work			
	People: Peer group of same and opposite sex; parents and other adults			
	Setting: School; neighborhood, and extended community; home			
	EMPHASIS: TEAM PARTICIPATION AND INDEPENDENT ACTION EXPRESSED IN ORGANIZED SPORTS, INTEREST GROUPS AND HOBBIES DURING LEISURE TIME.			
Overall status	High risk			
	Acceptable			

From Takata, N. (1974). Play as prescription. In M. Reilly (Ed.), *Play as exploratory learning*. Beverly Hills, CA: Sage Publications. Reprinted with permission from the publisher.

THE CONCEPTUAL BASES OF THE NARRATIVE APPROACH

Narrative is a natural means of communication between persons regarding daily life situations and events. Narratives are the stories people relate regarding those everyday occurrences that shape people's days and life (Helfrich, Kielhofner, & Mattingly, 1994). For example, the following is a story related by a parent to her child's occupational therapist:

(*Mrs. Thompson and 14-month-old Amy arrive at the clinic for their occupational therapy appointment. Nancy, the therapist, greets them at the waiting room door*):

Nancy: Good morning Amy, Mrs. Thompson. My, what a bruise you have, Amy! How did that happen? (*to Mrs. Thompson*)

Mrs. Thompson: You wouldn't believe the week we've had. You know, Amy is getting so active, she's getting to be quite a handful. Well, two days ago Amy was playing in the living room. I had taken the couch cushions off the couch so Amy could play and crawl on them—you know, from the couch to the cushions on the floor and back up to the couch? That's her "mountain climbing," we call it. Well, Amy was having a great time, crawling around. The phone rang, so I went to get it. It's in the hallway near the kitchen. It was my sister calling to say she was coming for dinner that night. After I hung up the phone, I walked back into the living room just as Amy was toppling off the arm of the couch. She apparently had crawled up to the couch and up to the arm. Well, even though I ran as fast as I could, I couldn't catch her real good. She fell and bumped her head here, see? (*shows Nancy the bruise on her forehead*). I felt so bad. She cried a little bit, but calmed down with some milk and a quiet rock in the rocking chair with me.

Nancy: That must have been scary for you *and* for Amy! I'm glad she's O.K.

Mrs. Thompson: You wouldn't believe how scared I was. The funny part was after she stopped crying and had her bottle of milk, believe it or not, she went back to climbing her "mountain," as if nothing had happened. Up to the couch and back down to the cushions. She did stay away from the arms of the couch, but, boy, does she like to play that rough stuff! I suppose that's normal, huh? What do you think?

Narrative methodology has been described as being a natural means by which to obtain information about an individual's unique life experiences. Narrative methods are modeled after a normal conversation rather than a formal question and answer exchange. In the hearing and interpretation of the shared narratives, the therapist seeks to understand the other person's frame of reference, to see things from the other person's point of view (Mattingly & Fleming, 1994). The therapist regards what the informant says and does as a product of how the informant defines his or her own world.

Mattingly and Fleming (1994) have written that stories place events within a temporal context and that a historical sense is needed to help link people with the past and with some anticipated future. Persons organize their knowledge of the past and the future aspects of their lives through narratives. From this perspective, it is important to learn how the child and the family experience life and therefore how they are inclined to experience meaning in their daily lives. Persons narratively structure their understandings of themselves and their respective lives. Because the parents of children who come to occupational therapy for assessment are the best sources of information concerning their particular child's play, therapists need to listen intently to their stories, to how they experience meaning and view the future (Fig. 2-1).

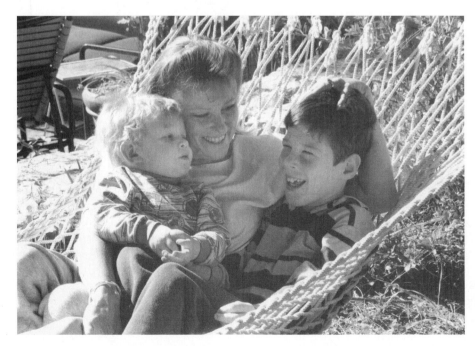

FIG. 2-1 Because parents are the best sources of information concerning their child's play, therapists need to listen intently to their stories. (Courtesy Shay McAtee.)

Moreover, as therapists listen to and understand the parents' stories of their child and his or her play, the therapist can begin to comprehend the family's world into which therapy may be inserted. The therapist and the family often begin to see the child's play life as an integrated whole, or as a picture, and not as a composite list of deficits or needs and problems to be changed.

The therapist is able to listen to the shared stories as chapters of the yet unfolding story of the child's play life. This foundation of narratives helps create a more complete picture of the child and his play. As these stories are organized in temporal fashion, the therapist will have a sense of development over time, making the views and goals for the future more relevant and meaningful for the child and his family. Further, by listening carefully to the kinds of questions and stories the families have about their children, the therapist may also learn what kinds of information are important to them as they engage in the assessment process or therapy (Burke, 1993). Their interests will also be reflected in the meaningfulness of their narrative stories. For example:

Mrs. Perez: Stephen is such a good boy. Maybe he is almost too good, though. Does that go along with his Down syndrome? I mean, maybe because he doesn't move around and explore so much, maybe he really can't get into trouble like the other boys. I kind of miss that.

Actually, last week he did something completely unexpected, and it was great! I was cleaning the kitchen and bathroom areas, and was pretty intent on getting the place spic and span before my husband got home. Stephen was playing with his Tonka trucks on the kitchen floor. Well, I went into the bathroom to scrub the tub, and I wasn't in there too very long, but when I got out of the bathroom was I surprised! Stephen had gotten into the pantry cupboard we have—it's a tall cabinet with floor to ceiling shelves. We keep crackers and baking stuff in there. The cupboard door must not have been closed all the way. Guess what happened?

Stephen got into the crackers and cereal boxes and he dumped about five of them over his head! He was sitting in a huge pile of crackers and cereal and was covered. He had tossed it all over, and he had such a big smile on his face. At first I was pretty angry, then I realized he didn't understand why I was frustrated. It's the first kind of naughty thing he ever did, and he looked awfully proud of himself. I even took a picture of him in all his mess. Wanna see it? Here it is.

Narrative is one way in which therapists can incorporate many fragments of past experience into a coherent whole to be understood. Narratives provide powerful experiences of successfully met challenges, where the child has developed increasing confidence and inner drive to take on challenges as development progresses (Mattingly & Fleming, 1994). The exploration of the child's past play, through the parents'

stories, is one way to connect together a series of early experiences that occur over the child's years; these stories give events and actions meaning and context (Helfrich et al., 1994). In this way, a child's play strengths and play needs can be viewed in light of a coherent life story, and the goals for the future may be interpreted and realized with the foundation of a meaningful past.

The goal of learning about a child's play history through narrative is not achieving correctness in its detail, but in coming to understand the child within the integrity of his or her life story of play (Helfrich et al., 1994). As the parent relays the child's play history, the story lines may evolve and change as the child's developmental progress is conveyed. The meaning of actions or events across stories may change as the parent tells the story and as the child's play and family worlds come to be understood. Specific to the example of Stephen, above, what has once been labeled as being "too good" may now be seen as a paucity of exploratory play; what has once been identified as "naughty" may now be seen within the context of fun, or even typical and "normal." Preliminary interpretations may be modified to adapt to the reality of developmental challenge or progress (Helfrich et al., 1994).

Using narrative can be empowering for the parents as they tell their child's stories, but listening carefully to their narratives is crucial for the therapist because their narratives provide insight into their perceptions of their shared life. Narratives offer a meaningful structure to a child's life across time and illustrate how the child and his or her play change over time (Mattingly & Fleming, 1994).

Clark (1993) has noted that meaningful therapy helps persons to create and continue their life stories into the future. Therapists can only help transform a child's life if the persons involved see meaning and relevance to their life stories; therapy is viewed as an event or as a chapter in the life of the child and family.

CONSIDERATIONS FOR ELICITING NARRATIVES

Utilizing narrative as a means by which to obtain information about the child's play history may be likened to an art. There are guidelines that can be followed, but there are not strict rules under which these methodological guidelines fall. The methods by which the therapist conducts an interview can influence how narratively rich the parent's responses are. Ideally, the narrative interview is a collaborative process in which the therapist and family work together to find a shared meaning of the child's play. In this process, the therapist wants to establish an atmosphere of partnership rather than an expert–patient relationship. The therapist attempts to construct a situation that resembles those in which people naturally talk to each other about important things. The interview should be relaxed and conversational, as people usually interact. The therapist relates to the parents on a more personal level. The therapist is wise to accept whatever hesitant ideas the parent says without making judgments, and to accept the parent as a conversational equal (Taylor & Bogdan, 1984).

It is during the early parts of an interview that the therapist sets the tone of the relationship with the parent. The therapist's initial goal is to establish rapport with the parent. The therapist should convey an attitude of someone who is willing to learn from the informants. In a narrative interview approach, there is a danger of appearing to know all there is about how children "should" play. If the therapist maintains the affect and behavior of one who is just searching for meaningful information about the child within the context of his or her particular family, the parent will be much less guarded or fearful of giving the "wrong" answer about this most precious child. The therapist must create an atmosphere in which the parent feels comfortable to talk freely and openly about his or her child's past and present play.

To see the child's play world, a therapist must carefully pay close attention to what is said throughout the interview process. Although this sounds commonplace, a therapist may need to overcome years of selective attention to the "stories" parents tell him or her about their children's lives. Watching, listening, and concentrating involve the hard work that is needed to uncover the meanings embedded in the story lines (Taylor & Bogdan, 1984).

A narrative approach to interviewing is flexible and dynamic. It can be described as being nondirective, unstructured, nonstandardized, and open ended in nature. Narrative approaches may be used in a one-session interview or over the course of several sessions directed toward understanding parents' perspectives on their child's abilities, experiences, or situations as expressed in their own words. An in-depth, narrative-oriented interview is modeled after a conversation between equals, rather than a formal question and answer exchange. The purpose is not to merely obtain answers, but to learn about meaningful contexts in which the child has played throughout development. Whereas the initial interview may reflect a structured format (i.e., the therapist asks the questions and the parent answers the questions), the methods by which the parent is interviewed may become less formal and more open or informal. A narrative approach to gathering information may be facilitated by the therapist's allowing the informant to guide the direction the interview takes, rather than rigidly sticking to an agenda of particular questions that need to be answered (Taylor & Bogdan, 1984). The therapist will want to ask questions or seek elaboration of information in a way that expresses interest in the child and the parent or family while following the parent's lead in the line of questioning. The therapist seeks the child's and the parents' perspective, and how the parents perceive the child's play, and finds ways of encouraging the parents to begin talking about these perspectives and experiences without structuring the conversation and defining what "should" be said.

It may be helpful for the therapist to use an interview guide to make sure the key topics are explored. This guide is not a structured series of questions or protocol; instead, it is a list of general areas to cover with a parent. For example, consistent with the categories within the Play History, the interview guide may include the following descriptors as cues: (1) previous play experiences; (2) play with others; (3) nature of play with toys and materials in early childhood; (4) nature of gross motor physical play; (5) pretend and make-believe play; (6) participation in sports and games; (7) pursuit of creative interests; (8) pursuit of hobbies, collections, or other leisure-time activities; and (9) participation in recreation and social activities. The interview guide presupposes the therapist's knowledge of the development of play and understanding of various ages and stages through a child's maturation. In the interview situation the therapist decides how to phrase questions and when to ask them; the interview guide serves solely to remind the therapist to ask about certain things.

Early in the interview, the therapist will ask nondirective and nonjudgmental questions. As the therapist acquires knowledge and understanding of how the parent conveys information about his or her child, questioning may become more focused and directive. As themes and perspectives emerge, the therapist may need to seek clarification of the stories for depth and accuracy of the interpretation. This offers the interview process a rich, natural quality as more complete information is gathered. An example of how a therapist might begin the interview process follows:

Therapist: As an occupational therapist, I am interested in how children perform everyday activities in different environments. One of the areas I am very interested in is how children play. In particular, I would like to get an idea of how Susie has played as she has grown and how she plays now. One of the best ways for me to learn about this is by listening to you—the expert on Susie—tell me a story about Susie playing. Can you tell me of one memorable incident of Susie playing, either by herself or with other children that occurred within the past year or so? Tell me about Susie playing.

One of the best ways to begin an interview is to ask the parent to describe, list, or remember and describe one key event or play experience of their child. Of particular importance is how the therapist asks questions. Questions should be phrased in gentle, caring terms that support the parent's disclosure of personal insights or perceptions of the child and, to some extent, the parent herself or himself. Asking questions as if from the parent's perspective will provide a nonthreatening and open atmosphere in which to explore the child's unique characteristics in play. As the parent begins talking, the therapist can encourage expansion of ideas and detail by utilizing encouraging words, cues, and gestures to indicate interest (Taylor & Bogdan, 1984). If possible, the therapist may encourage the parent to show a personal memento, such as photographs of the child playing or taken during some memorable time of the child's life, which can be used to guide the interview without imposing a structure on the parent (Fig. 2-2).

An important principle in asking descriptive questions is that expanding the length of the question tends to encourage an expanded response from the parent (Mattingly & Fleming, 1994). A therapist might ask, "Could you tell me how Janey plays with her dolls?" and a descriptive answer would be obtained. A broader way of asking for such descriptive information might be, "From what you have said, Janey has many dolls. Could you tell me about what she does when she plays with her dolls, how she plays, what she uses to take care of them? Could you tell me what it is like when Janey plays with her dolls?"

As the parent mentions specific experiences, the therapist can probe for greater detail, and the therapist may take notes of topics of which to return at a later time. Knowing when and how to probe is important. Throughout the interview, the therapist follows up on topics that have been raised by asking specific questions, encourages

the parent to describe experiences in detail, and presses for clarification of particular words or phrases (Taylor & Bogdan, 1984). The therapist will want to probe gently for the details of the child's and parent's experiences and the meanings they attach to them. The therapist is interested in the everyday play events as well as the struggles and successful play experiences in which the child engages. The therapist should be aware that any form of sustained questioning implies evaluation and carries the risk of inadvertently returning to a more formal, distant interview process.

It is important to not interrupt a parent's story, even though the topic may not be interesting to you as a therapist. A therapist can usually use subtle gestures, such as not nodding one's head, gently changing the subject during breaks in the conversation, or not taking notes to redirect the conversation. However, this subtle control by the therapist must be utilized very carefully, so as to not direct the conversation in a way that can prevent important information regarding the child's play history.

Moreover, the therapist should ask for clarification of the informants' remarks by restating what was said and requesting confirmation of the restatement. Therapists must conduct interviews with the premise that words and symbols used in their own worlds may have different meanings in the worlds of their clients. They must be attuned to and explore the meanings of words or phrases with which they are not familiar. It should not be taken for granted that phrases used in the context of a narrative story are always accurately understood. If this issue is not attended to, the essential meaning may be lost. Restating what the parent has said demonstrates a nonjudgmental attitude which contributes to the development of rapport. When the therapist restates what a parent says, a powerful, unstated message is communicated. Consider the following example:

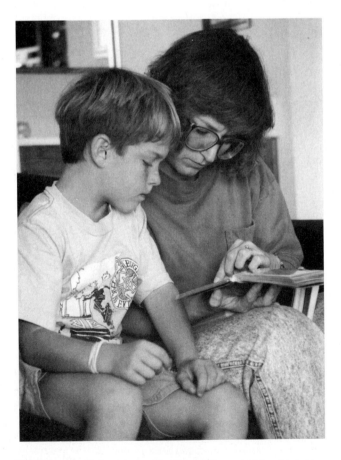

FIG. 2-2   The therapist may encourage the parent to share personal momentos, such as photographs, which then can be used to further shape the interview. (Courtesy Shay McAtee.)

Mrs. Smith: Calvin works so hard at playing. He loves to play basketball and roughhousing. He says he's gonna be Michael Jordan when he grows up, see. I know that ain't gonna happen, but, oh, how he loves to pretend. He says he can fly like Michael Jordan, and he tries to when he shoots baskets. He can play for hours, too. He usually plays by himself, though. He can't keep up with my other kids so good. He's all over the place when he shoots baskets, and usually ends up tripping himself when he try to play. He don't care how he looks when he plays, too. He don't seem to keep it all together, you know what I mean? For instance, when he plays basketball he droops real bad. That drooping, the other kids don't know what to do with him, and they usually leave Calvin be all by hisself. That hurts Calvin real bad, real bad.

Therapist: You said that Calvin droops when he plays. Can you describe what this drooping is? I'm not sure I understand what that means to Calvin.

Mrs. Smith: Calvin droops, you know, when he works real hard at something. His mouth is always open a little, you know, but when he concentrates real bad he droops and his chin gets all wet. Sometimes his shirt gets wet from the drooping, too, he droops so bad. I tells him to swallow, but he forgets right after, and he keeps doing it.

Therapist: I think you mean drooping as I mean drooling. When Calvin plays hard he tends to droop more, and his chin and shirt get wet.

Mrs. Smith: Yeah, that drooping is bad, but Calvin loves to play so. I wish the other kids would play with him more.

The vocabulary used in a setting usually provides important clues to how people define situations and classify their world and thus suggests lines of inquiry and questioning. Certain assumptions may be built into a vocabulary. Therapists must learn to examine vocabularies as a function of the assumptions and purposes of the users, rather than as objective characterizations of the people or objects of reference, even when seemingly common words and phrases are used. The meaning and significance of people's verbal and nonverbal symbols can only be determined in the context of what they actually discuss and how they contextualize their child's play experiences over time. The hallmark of narrative interviewing is learning about what is important in the minds of the parents: their meanings, perspectives, and definitions.

Some aspects of the narrative process mandate caution. With this less structured approach to interviewing, there is a danger of imputing meanings that people do not intend. The therapist is advised to pay attention, which implies an openness or an honoring of the person who is being interviewed.

The therapist should bring an attitude of sensitivity to the interview situation.

Taylor and Bogdan (1984) suggest that therapists look for key words in people's remarks that will enable the therapist to recall the meanings of the parent's remarks. It is sometimes helpful to concentrate on the first and last remarks in each conversation. Conversations usually follow an orderly sequence—a certain question elicits a certain response, one remark provokes another, one topic leads to another related topic for discussion. The temporal flow of the interview offers a continuity for greater understanding for the therapist and the parent.

The therapist actively solicits the parent's remembrance and storytelling about the child's play experiences and constructs the child's play history as the final product. The narrative approach to interviewing is directed toward learning about events and activities that cannot be observed directly. In this type of interviewing the parents act as the therapist's eyes and ears with which to perceive the child's play. The parent's role is not simply to reveal his or her own views but to describe the play situations that have occurred. By asking for clarification, restating ideas, and listening attentively, the therapist supports the parent in becoming a good informant, which will further the process of understanding the child's play.

The quality and the quantity of the information obtained rests with the therapist's knowledge of play and its developmental nature. Furthermore, great skill in listening and interviewing is necessary to extract rich and thorough information that enables the therapist to contribute a salient chapter in a child's developing life story.

REVIEW QUESTIONS

1. Describe the Play History, with respect to development, format, and purpose.
2. Why is the child's life story of concern to the occupational therapist?
3. Define narrative and narrative methodology.
4. How does the narrative approach affect the administration of the Play History?
5. What are the specific strategies a therapist can use to elicit narratives from parents about their child's play?

REFERENCES

Behnke, C. J., & Fetkovich, M. M. (1984). Examining the reliability and validity of the Play History. *American Journal of Occupational Therapy, 38*(2), 94-100.

Brewster-Smith, M. (1974). Foreword. In M. Reilly (Ed.), *Play as exploratory learning.* Beverly Hills, CA: Sage Publications.

Bundy, A. C. (1991). Play theory and sensory integration. In A. G. Fisher, E. A. Murray, & A. C. Bundy (Eds.) *Sensory integration: Theory and practice.* Philadelphia: F. A. Davis.

Burke. J. P. (1993). Play: The life role of the infant and young child. In J. Case-Smith (Ed.), *Pediatric occupational therapy and early intervention.* Boston: Andover Medical Publishers.

Clark, F. (1993). Occupation embedded in a real life: Interweaving occupational science and occupational therapy. *American Journal of Occupational Therapy, 47*(12), 1067-1078.

Florey, L. L. (1971). An approach to play and play development. *American Journal of Occupational Therapy, 25,* 275-280.

Gesell, A. (1945). *The embryology of behavior.* New York: Harper & Bros.

Helfrich, C., Kielhofner, G., & Mattingly, C. (1994). Volition as narrative: Understanding motivation in chronic illness. *American Journal of Occupational Therapy, 48*(4), 311-317.

Mattingly, C., & Fleming, M. H. (1994). *Clinical reasoning: Forms of inquiry in a therapeutic practice.* Philadelphia: F. A. Davis.

Neumann, E. A. (1971). *The elements of play.* New York: MSS Information.

Piaget, J. (1962). Play, dreams, and imitation in childhood. (C. Gattegno & F. M. Hodgson, Trans.). New York: W. W. Norton. (Original work published in 1951).

Reilly, M. (Ed.) (1974). *Play as exploratory learning.* Beverly Hills, CA: Sage Publications.

Spradley, J. P. (1979). *The ethnographic interview.* Fort Worth, TX: Harcourt Brace Jovanovich College Publishers.

Takata, N. (1974). Play as prescription. In M. Reilly (Ed.), *Play as exploratory learning.* Beverly Hills, CA: Sage Publications.

Taylor, S. J., & Bogdan, R. (1984). *Introduction to qualitative research methods: The search for meanings.* New York: John Wiley & Sons.

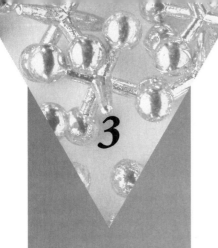

3

DEVELOPMENT AND CURRENT USE OF THE KNOX PRESCHOOL PLAY SCALE

Susan Knox

Susan Knox

KEY TERMS

Preschool Play Scale
Revised Knox
  Preschool Play
    Scale
  space manage-
    ment
  material manage-
    ment
  pretense–
    symbolic
    participation

Play in young children is an automatic, integral part of their lives. All children engage in some form of play and it is through play that they develop an understanding of the world and competence in interacting with it. The way children play reveals physical and cognitive abilities, social participation, imagination, independence, and coping mechanisms (Bergen, 1988; Brown & Gottfried, 1985; Bruner et al., 1976; Garvey, 1977; Hartley & Goldenson, 1963).

From the 1930s through the 1960s, developmental theorists began to describe aspects of play within a normative framework. This work became the precursor to using play diagnostically. Assessment of children's abilities through play became popular in the last two decades. In the 1970s and 1980s, the growing body of literature on play led to the development of a variety of play assessments, based on normative data, that could be used in clinical settings (Schaefer et al., 1991). Play assessments reflect a variety of professional frameworks and examine different aspects of play, such as neurological functioning, cognitive functioning, organization of behavior, playfulness, and dramatic and social play (Bergen, 1988; Hulme & Lunzer, 1966; Kalverboer, 1977; Lieberman, 1977; Rosenblatt, 1977; Smilansky, 1968).

This chapter addresses the use of play in occupational therapy for assessment. Specifically, it focuses on a widely used assessment instrument, the Preschool Play Scale (Knox, 1968, 1974), and traces its development from its inception, through revisions and research applications, to its clinical use. The chapter ends with a proposal for a new Revised Knox Preschool Play Scale.

HISTORICAL PERSPECTIVE ON PLAY ASSESSMENT IN OCCUPATIONAL THERAPY

Play has been described as the child's occupation. Play is characterized as being intrinsic, spontaneous, fun, flexible, totally absorbing, vitalizing, challenging, nonliteral, and an end in and of itself. No single characteristic is common to all kinds of play, but a combination of any of the characteristics is usually seen. Play behavior can be analyzed in relation to cultural and societal roles and the effects of the physical and interpersonal

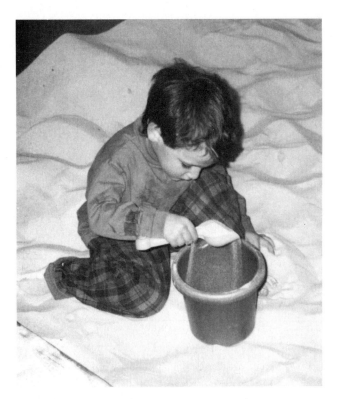

FIG. 3-1   In play, the child becomes totally absorbed.

environment (Cohen, 1987; Ellis, 1973; Reilly, 1974; Rubin et al., 1983; Takata, 1971) (Fig. 3-1).

Assessment of play and of the child's abilities as seen through play are necessary to provide the therapist with tools to analyze play and to plan treatment. Analysis of how children play gives valuable information regarding their cognitive, motor, and social competencies. Occupational therapy focuses on the whole child functioning within the environment; therefore all aspects of development are considered important.

Although occupational therapists have long valued play as treatment media and have recognized the value of play as a reflection of child development, formal assessment of play in occupational therapy did not occur until the 1960s. It was during this time that the theory of occupational behavior was developed by Mary Reilly (1974), having particular relevance to the study of play. Occupational behavior was described as the continuum between play and work, and play was considered one of the child's primary occupations. Reilly (1974) defined play as a multidimensional system for adaptation to the environment. Reilly believed that the exploratory drive of curiosity underlay play behavior. This curiosity drive had three hierarchical stages: exploration, competency, and achievement. Exploratory behavior was seen primarily in early childhood and was fueled by intrinsic motivation. Competency behavior was fueled by effectance motivation, identified by White (1959), and was characterized by experimentation and practice to achieve mastery. The third stage, achievement, was linked to goal expectancies and was fueled by a desire to achieve excellence (Reilly, 1974) (Fig. 3-2, *A* and *B*).

A

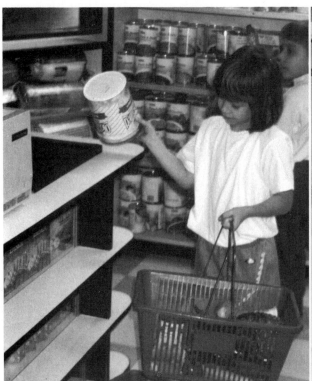

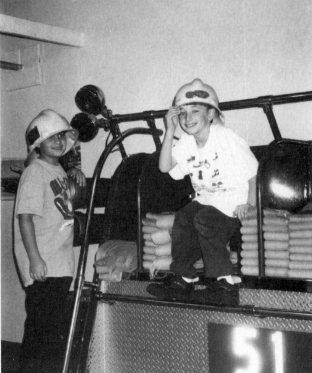

B

FIG. 3-2   **A** and **B**, Children's play reflects their interest in adult roles.

Students working under Reilly developed clinical tools to assess various aspects of occupational behavior. Interviews examining a person's work or play history were developed (Moorehead, 1969; Takata, 1969, 1974). An interest inventory was developed to assess leisure in adults (Matsutsuyu, 1969). Developmental assessments of play were developed (Florey, 1971, 1981; Knox, 1968, 1974), and specific aspects of play were examined, such as intrinsic motivation (Florey, 1969) and the acquisition of rules (Robinson, 1977).

PRESCHOOL PLAY SCALE

The Preschool Play Scale (originally named the Play Scale) was developed in 1968 (Knox, 1968) and it was later published in *Play as Exploratory Learning* (Reilly, 1974). Play was defined for the purposes of the Preschool Play Scale as "the medium through which the child learns about himself and the world around him. It is that spontaneous activity through which he rehearses, experiences, experiments and orients himself to the actual world" (Knox, 1968, p. 5).

The assessment was pilot tested on a population of children with mental retardation and correlated with the children's developmental ages (Knox, 1968). However, at that time no normative data were collected, nor were systematic reliability and validity studies conducted. The Play Scale was revised and renamed the Preschool Play Scale (PPS) by Bledsoe and Shepherd (1982). They collected normative data on 90 children and conducted reliability and validity studies. Reliability and validity data were also gathered on a population with disabilities by Harrison and Kielhofner (1986). Since its development and revision, the PPS has been used to demonstrate differences in the play behavior of different populations (Bundy, 1989; Clifford & Bundy, 1989; Howard 1986; Kielhofner et al., 1983). It has been used to

assess pretreatment and posttreatment status (Schaaf & Mulrooney, 1989) and to assess effects of postural facilitation on free play (Germain & Dwyre, 1988). The PPS has also been used clinically for assessment and as a guide to the developmental nature of play.

In the remainder of this chapter, the content of the Preschool Play Scale is described and studies examining its reliability and validity are discussed. Clinical use of the PPS is described through case examples. A critical examination of the strengths and weaknesses of the PPS is provided. Finally, revisions to the PPS are presented to increase its usefulness as a clinical assessment today.

Description

The Play Scale (Knox, 1968, 1974) is an observational assessment designed to give a developmental description of typical play behavior through the ages 0 to 6 years. Play is described in terms of yearly increments and in terms of four dimensions: (1) space management, (2) material management, (3) imitation, and (4) participation. Each dimension contains a number of factors. The first dimension, space management, describes the way children learn to manage their bodies and the space around them. This is achieved through the processes of experimentation and exploration. Space management contains the factors of gross motor activity, territory or area used in play, and exploration. The second dimension, material management, is the manner in which children handle materials and the purposes for which materials are used. Through material management, children learn control and use of material surroundings. Material management contains the factors of manipulation, construction, interest or attention to specific types of activities, purpose or goal, and attention span (Fig. 3-3).

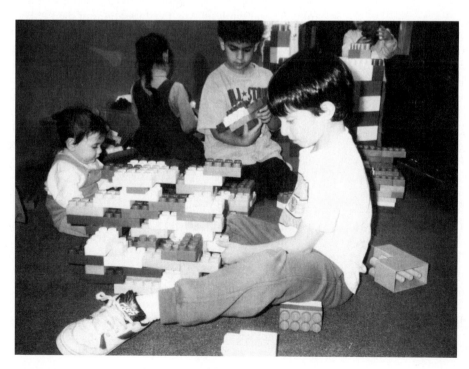

FIG. 3-3   The way children handle materials parallels developmental progress.

The third dimension, imitation, is the way children gain an understanding of the social world. Factors included in this dimension are imitation, imagination, dramatization, music, and books. The last dimension, participation, describes the amount and manner of interaction with persons in the environment and the degree of independence and cooperation demonstrated in play activities. Participation contains the factors of type or level of social interaction, cooperation with others, and language. Table 3-1 depicts the PPS as it is used today (Bledsoe & Shepherd, 1982).

Factors (behavioral descriptions) under each dimension were determined through a review of existing developmental and play scales (Knox, 1968) and were written as actions that the child performed. In this way, children could be assessed in a variety of settings with available playthings, instead of in standard settings with required playthings. The scale was pilot tested on a population of 12 preschool children with diagnoses of mental retardation. The children were observed indoors and outdoors in a preschool setting and rated on all of the factors in the four dimensions. Scoring consisted of marking each factor with either a + when the behavior was present or a − when the behavior was absent. If there was no opportunity to observe a factor, NA was marked. Items of special interest were underlined. A score on a particular dimension was determined by the age level containing the majority of factor pluses. An overall play age was determined by taking the means of the dimension scores and computing an overall mean. The author found that play ages correlated significantly with developmental ages of the children (Knox, 1968).

STUDIES USING THE PRESCHOOL PLAY SCALE

Reliability and Validity Studies

Two studies examined the validity and reliability of the PPS. Bledsoe and Shepherd (1982) conducted validity and reliability studies on the Play Scale and renamed it the *Preschool Play Scale*. They slightly modified some items on the scale for three reasons: "to make all items mutually exclusive, to maintain consistency between categories and age levels, and to update the scale to reflect recent developmental studies on play" (p. 784). Each subject was observed and rated for three $\frac{1}{2}$ hour sessions over a period of 7 days. Subjects were observed in day-care centers and nursery schools during free play periods. All observations were done indoors in settings that had a wide variety of toys and adequate space. Interrater and test–retest reliability studies were significant at the .0001 level. Validity studies correlated the PPS with Lunzer's Scale of Organization of Play Behavior, Parten's Social Play Hierarchy, and chronological age (CA). The Lunzer's Scale of Organization of Play Behavior (Hulme & Lunzer, 1966) measures cognitive development in play and is correlated in this study with the dimensions of material management and imitation. Parten's Social Play Hier-

archy (Parten, 1933) measures social participation in play and is correlated with the participation dimensions of the PPS. All the validity studies were significant at the .0001 level. The authors concluded that "the scale measured play on a developmental continuum of increasing complexity including physical, cognitive and social components" (Bledsoe & Shepherd, 1982, p. 787). Difficulties encountered during the study were limited opportunities to observe the factors of territory, exploration, music, and books.

Harrison and Kielhofner (1986) conducted reliability and validity studies on the PPS with a group of 60 preschool children with disabilities, including cerebral palsy, mental retardation, and developmental delay. They observed free play in classrooms or medical settings for two 15-minute sessions. They collected data with the PPS, the Parten Social Play Hierarchy, and the Lunzer Scale of Organization of Behavior. Their results also showed statistically significant reliability and validity of the PPS for the population with disabilities. However, they found that there were factors on the PPS that were infrequently observed with this population, such as those related to territory, imitation, imagination, cooperation, music, and books. Limitations of their study included the fact that all the observations took place indoors.

Both studies found infrequent observations of territory, exploration, music, and books. In addition, the study of the children with disabilities also found infrequent observations of imitation, imagination, and cooperation. Analysis of the reasons that this occurred pinpointed some of the limitations of both the studies and the PPS. In both studies, the observations were done for limited time spans, and all were done indoors. Outdoor observations would have yielded more information on territory, exploration, and space management. Longer observations would also have yielded more information because children's individual play episodes can be prolonged and a short period of observation may not tap into different kinds of play. Two limitations of the PPS were made evident by these studies. The descriptors of territory do not appear to be adequate in that they require information additional to what can be obtained by observation alone. For example, whether play takes place in the home versus the neighborhood would require prolonged observation in the home or would require questioning caretakers. Music and books, in retrospect, probably rely more on adult presence or facilitation than other factors. Available music and books are not always present in many play settings. These limitations are addressed later in this chapter.

Table 3-2 summarizes the two validity and reliability studies. In summary, they both show that the PPS is a valid and reliable tool with which to assess the developmental aspects of play.

Studies Using Different Populations

Seven studies have examined scores on the PPS and other measures for different diagnostic or socioeconomic groups. These studies contribute to the validity of the PPS by exam-

TABLE 3-1   Preschool Play Scale*

Child Number: _____
Session Number: _____
Observer's Initials: _____

	0 to 1 Year	1 to 2 Years	2 to 3 Years
Space management			
	Gross motor activity: reaches; plays with hands and feet; touches hands to feet; crawls; sits with balance; pulls to stand; moves to continue pleasant sensation	**Gross motor activity:** stands unsupported; sits down; bends and recovers balance; walks and runs—wide stance; climbs low objects; broad movements involving large muscle groups; rides kiddie car	**Gross motor activity:** beginning integration of entire body in activities—concentrates on complex movements (i.e., throwing, jumping, climbing); pedals tricycle
	Territory: crib; playpen; house	**Territory:** home; immediate surrounds	**Territory:** outside; short excursions
	Exploration: of self and objects within reach	**Exploration:** of all unfamiliar things; oblivious to hazards	**Exploration:** Increased exploration of all unfamiliar objects; very curious
	Comments:	Comments:	Comments:
Material management			
	Manipulation: predominant—handles, mouths toys; brings two objects together; picks up; hits; bangs; shakes	**Manipulation:** predominant—throws; inserts; pushes; pulls; carries; pounds	**Manipulation:** remains predominant—feels; pats; dumps; squeezes; fills
	Construction: not evident	**Construction:** little attempt to make product; relates two objects appropriately (i.e., lid on pot); stacks; takes apart; puts together	**Construction:** manipulation predominates; scribbles; strings beads; puzzles 4 to 5 pieces
	Interest: people; gazes at faces; follows movements; attends to voices and sounds	**Interest:** movement of self—explores various kinesthetic and proprioceptive sensations; moving objects (i.e., balls, trucks, pull toys)	**Interest:** explores new movement patterns (i.e., jumping); toys with moving parts (i.e., dumptrucks, jointed dolls); makes messes
	Purpose: sensation or function—uses materials to see, touch, hear, smell, mouth (i.e., rattles, teething rings, colored objects)	**Purpose:** experiments in movement—practices basic movement patterns (i.e., rock, walk, run); process important	**Purpose:** process important—less interest in finished product (ie., scribbles, squeezes play dough); repetition of gross motor skills
	Attention: follows moving objects with eyes	**Attention:** rapid shifts	**Attention:** intense interest; quiet play up to 15 minutes; plays with single object or theme 5 to 10 min
	Comments:	Comments:	Comments:
Imitation			
	Imitation: of observed facial expressions and physical movement (i.e., smiling, pat-a-cake); emotions (hugs toys)	**Imitation:** of simple actions; present events and adults—self-related mimicry (i.e., feeds self with spoon)	**Imitation:** of adult routines with toy-related mimicry (i.e., child feeding doll); toys as agents (i.e., doll feeds self)
	Imagination: not evident	**Imagination:** imaginary objects (i.e., pretend food on spoon)	**Imagination:** personifies dolls, stuffed animals; starts having imaginary friends (i.e., animals, persons)
	Dramatization: not evident	**Dramatization:** not evident	**Dramatization:** portrays single character
	Music: attends to sounds	**Music:** sways; listens	**Music:** responds to music with whole body (i.e., marching, twirling)
	Books: pats; strokes; picks at pictures	**Books:** handles; points to pictures; begins to name pictures	**Books:** likes familiar stories; fills in words and phrases
	Comments:	Comments:	Comments:
Participation			
	Type: solitary play (no effort to interact with other children or choose similar activities)	**Type:** combination of solitary, onlooker play (watches others—speaking but not entering their play)	**Type:** parallel play (plays beside others, play remains independent, but child situates self among others, enjoys their presence)
	Cooperation: demands personal attention; simple give and take interaction with immediate family or caretaker (i.e., tickling, peek-a-boo); 7 to 10 mo—initiates games rather than follows	**Cooperation:** more complex games with a variety of adults (i.e., hide and seek, chasing); offers toys but somewhat possessive; persistent	**Cooperation:** possessive (much snatch and grab, hoarding, no sharing, resists toys being taken away); independent (does not ask for help, initiates own play)
	Language: attends to sounds and voices; babbles; uses razzing sounds	**Language:** jabbers during play—talks to self, often in singsong rhythm; uses gestures and words to communicate wants; labels objects	**Language:** talkative—very little jabber; begins to use words to communicate ideas, information
	Comments:	Comments:	Comments:

Continued.

TABLE 3-1 Preschool Play Scale*—cont'd

The following to be filled in after observations are recorded: Mean ages for dimensions:

Space management: _____ Imitation: _____
Material management: _____ Participation: ____
Play age (mean of all dimensions): _____

3 to 4 Years	4 to 5 Years	5 to 6 Years
Space management		
Gross motor activity: more coordinated body movements, smoother walking, jumping, climbing, running (accelerates, decelerates)	**Gross motor activity:** increased activity level; can concentrate on goal instead of movement; ease of gross motor ability allows stunts, tests of strength, exaggerated movements; clambers	**Gross motor activity:** more sedate; good muscle control and balance; hops on one foot; skips; somersaults; skates; lifts self off ground
Territory: home; immediate neighborhood	**Territory:** neighborhood	**Territory:** likes to be up off ground
Exploration: interest in new experiences, places, animals, nature	**Exploration:** anticipates trips, likes change of pace	**Exploration:** plans and enjoys excursions and trips
Comments:	Comments:	Comments:
Material management		
Manipulation: small muscle activity—hammers, sorts, inserts small objects (i.e., peg boards); cuts	**Manipulation:** Increasing fine motor control allows quick movements, force, pulling	**Manipulation:** uses tools to make things (i.e., cuts more precisely); copies; traces; combines various types of material
Construction: makes simple products (i.e., blocks, crayons, clay); combines play materials; takes apart; arranges in spatial dimension—design is evident	**Construction:** predominates—makes products, specific designs evident, builds complex structures; puzzles 10 pieces	**Construction:** predominates—makes recognizable products; likes small construction, attends to detail (i.e., eyes, nose, fingers apparent in drawings); uses products in play
Interest: anything new; fine motor manipulation of play materials	**Interest:** takes pride in work (i.e., shows and talks about products, compares with friends, likes pictures displayed); complex ideas	**Interest:** in reality—manipulation of real-life situations (i.e., miniature things); making something useful—props for play; permanence of products; toys that "really work"
Purpose: beginning to show interest in result or finished product	**Purpose:** product very important—use to express self; exaggerates	**Purpose:** replicate reality
Attention: longer span—around 30 min; plays with single object or theme 5 to 10 min	**Attention:** amuses self up to 1 hr; plays with single object or theme 10 to 15 min	**Attention:** concentration for long period of time; plays with single object or theme 10 to 15 min
Comments:	Comments:	Comments:
Imitation		
Imitation: more complex imitation of real world—part of dramatization	**Imitation:** more complex imitation of real world as part of dramatization	**Imitation:** more complex imitation of real world as part of dramatization
Imagination: assumes familiar roles—domestic themes, past experiences	**Imagination:** prominent—able to use familiar knowledge to construct a novel situation (i.e., expanding on the theme of a story or TV show)	**Imagination:** prominent—continues to construct new themes but emphasis on reality—reconstruction of real world
Dramatization: imitates simple action and reaction episodes—mirrors experience, emphasis on domestic and animals; portrays multiple characters with feelings (mostly anger and crying); little interest in costumes	**Dramatization:** role playing for or with others; portrays more complex emotions; sequences stories—themes from domestic to magic; enjoys dressups	**Dramatization:** sequences stories—emphasis on copying what occurs in real world; costumes important; props; puppets
Music: sings simple songs—not necessarily on pitch; plays instruments	**Music:** sings whole songs on pitch; musical games (i.e., Farmer in the Dell); good rhythm	**Music:** meaning of songs important; enjoys catchy tunes, songs that tell stories; dances reflect interpretation of music
Books: new or information books; pictures important; relates own experiences to story	**Books:** listens better—doesn't need physical contact with book; looks at books independently—repeats familiar stories	**Books:** looks at books independently or with peer; describes picture to tell story; must be credible
Comments:	Comments:	Comments:
Participation		
Type: associative play (similar activities with groups of 2 to 3, no organization to reach a common goal, more interest in peers than activity)	**Type:** cooperative (groups of 2 to 3 organized to achieve a goal, i.e., assigns roles for pretend play)	**Type:** cooperative (groups of 2 to 5, organization of more complex games and dramatic play)
Cooperation: limited—some turn taking; asks for things rather than grabbing; little attempt to control others	**Cooperation:** takes turns; attempts to control the activities of others (often self-centered, bossy)	**Cooperation:** social give and take evident (i.e., compromises to facilitate group play); rivalry seen in competitive games
Language: uses words to communicate with peers, interest in new words (repeats them, asks their meaning)	**Language:** very talkative—plays with words; fabricates—capable of long narratives; questions persistently; communicates with peers to organize activities	**Language:** very prominent in sociodramatic play (uses words as part of play as well as to organize play); interest in present; relevant how, what for questions
Comments:	Comments:	Comments:

*Modified from Knox, S. (1974). A Play Scale. In M. Reilly (Ed.), *Play as Exploratory Learning*, Beverly Hills, CA: Sage Publications. Reprinted from Bledsoe, N., and Shepherd, J. (1982). A study of reliability and validity of a preschool play scale. *American Journal of Occupational Therapy, 36,* 783-788, with permission from the publisher.

TABLE 3-2 **Reliability and Validity Studies of the Preschool Play Scale (PPS)**					
Authors	*n*	**Ages**	**Categories**	**Measures**	**Results**

Bledsoe and Shepherd (1982)	90	4 mo to 6 yr	Normal	PPS Lunzer's Scale of Organization of Play Behavior Parten's Social Play Hierarchy	Reliability
					  Interrater $r = .996$; $p = .0001$
					  Test–retest $r = .965$; $p = .0001$
					Validity
					  PPS and CA $r = .955$; $p = .0001$
					  PPS and Parten $r = .614$; $p = .0001$
					  PPS and Lunzer $r = .640$; $p = .0001$

Harrison and Kielhofner (1986)	60	2 mo to 5 yr, 11 mo	Multiple handicaps	PPS Lunzer's Scale of Organization of Play Behavior Parten's Social Play Hierarchy	Reliability
					  Interrater $r = .88$; $p = .0001$
					  Test–retest $r = .91$; $p = .0001$
					Validity
					  PPS and CA $r = .74$; $p = .0001$
					  PPS and Parten $r = .60$ to $.64$; $p = .0001$
					  PPS and Lunzer $r = .59$; $p = .0001$

Note: CA = chronological age.

ining how children with identified disabilities from different social classes or reared under different circumstances show differing play patterns.

Kielhofner et al. (1983) studied playfulness as well as the level of play development of three 2-year-old children who had been hospitalized most of their lives and three 2-year-old children living at home. Playfulness was measured by a modified version of Lieberman's Playfulness Scale (Lieberman, 1977). Level of play development was measured by a modified version of the PPS. The children were observed in three different environments: (1) the child's familiar environment with caretaker present and participating, (2) a standardized play environment with the caretaker present but passive, and (3) a standard play environment with the caretaker present and participating. They found statistically significant differences in the developmental level of play and in playfulness between the two groups. They also analyzed differences based on the environments and found the play ages were lower for both groups in the second environment (standard environment, passive caretaker). Playfulness was not statistically significant across environmental groups. Limitations of this study included a very small sample size and medical complications affecting certain areas of play, such as tracheostomies that limited speech and social interaction. An important addition in this study was the use of a measure of playfulness, as this aspect of play is not covered by the PPS. Also important was the finding of the differences in play in familiar environments versus a standard environment. It points out the importance of observing play naturalistically.

Howard (1986) compared developmental play ages as measured by the PPS of two groups of children, of whom 12 were physically abused and 12 were not abused. Children were from 1 to 5 years of age and were paired by age and family income. Children were observed for 40 minutes, independent of the mother, but with at least one other child present. Mothers were also given a questionnaire asking three questions related to the amount of time spent with the child in play and the amount of time the child spent watching television. Statistically significant deficits in the overall developmental play age and in the play imitation category, and a trend toward lower participation, were found in the abused group. These children interacted less imaginatively and were less socially interactive. The abused group also showed a statistically significant difference in the amount of television watched, averaging 1½ hours more per day than the unabused group. This study used a more prolonged observation period and also ensured that peers were available, helping to create a more natural environment conducive to play.

Bundy (1989) compared play behavior of a group of 31 boys with sensory integrative dysfunction with that of 30 boys without sensory integration problems, ages 4 to 6 years. She found significant differences between the mean scores of the two groups on the PPS and its four dimensions. On discriminative analysis of the four play dimensions, space management was the best single predictor of group membership. However, as individuals, many of the boys with sensory integrative dysfunction had age-appropriate skills in one or more areas of play. Bundy recommended that, with this population, observations of playfulness and quality of movement should accompany use of the PPS.

Clifford and Bundy (1989), as part of the same study, studied 31 preschool boys with sensory integrative dysfunction and 35 without dysfunction. They examined play preference, as measured by the Preschool Play Materials Preference Inventory (Wolfgang & Phelps, 1983); play performance, as measured by the PPS; and verbal receptive language, as measured on the Revised Peabody Picture Vocabulary Test (Dunn & Dunn, 1981). The boys were observed both indoors and outdoors. They found that there was no significant difference in the means on the play materials preference scores between the groups because both groups preferred toys representing sensorimotor play over construction and symbolic toys. However, there was a difference with respect to how the two groups used toys and how well they played with them as measured on the PPS. The mean scores on this scale and three of its dimensions (space management, material management, and participation) were significantly lower for the boys with sensory integrative dysfunction. Two types of play deficits were defined. The first type was seen in boys who were unsuccessful at engaging in preferred activities. The second type was seen in boys who showed poor skills but altered their play preferences to compensate. This study is important in that it evaluated play preferences as well as performance.

Von Zuben, Crist, and Mayberry (1991) explored play behavior and its relation to socioeconomic status. They modified the PPS into a teacher rating scale that was administered to 41 middle–socioeconomic status children and 43 low–socioeconomic status children, ages 4 and 5, attending the same school. No significant differences were found for play age, dimensions, or categories. The authors discussed a number of study limitations. The schools were socioeconomically integrated, contained a variety of educational play resources, and were staffed by trained teachers. These factors may have affected the children's experience level and peer interaction. Modification of the PPS into a check list may have additionally altered findings. The teachers were not blind to the socioeconomic status and no interrater reliability studies were conducted. On the other hand, the teachers had opportunities to observe the children in a variety of play settings and over time. These are important limitations that may have significantly altered the findings. It would have been interesting to have observed the children both at school and in their homes or neighborhoods to determine whether the school environment fostered different levels of play.

Morrison, Bundy, and Fisher (1991) examined the contribution of playfulness and motor skills to play performance in children without disabilities and in those with juvenile rheumatoid arthritis (JRA). They defined playfulness in terms of the child's feelings of internal control over the environment, as measured on the Preschool and Primary Internal–External Locus of Control Scale (Norwicki & Duke, 1974), and ability to be creative or imaginative, as measured by tests of associative fluency from the Walloch and Koogan Scale, revised by Ward (Ward, 1968). Motor proficiency was measured by the Bruininks-Oseretsky Test of Motor Proficiency (Bruininks, 1978). Play was measured by the PPS.

Two groups of children, 15 without disabilities and 14 with JRA, ranging in age from 4 years, 6 months to 6 years, 6 months, were tested. The authors set a significance level of $p \leq .10$. They found that there were no significant differences in the two groups on the PPS, the internal locus of control test, the tests of associative fluency, total Bruininks, or fine motor Bruininks. There were significant differences, however, on the gross motor section of the Bruininks. The authors correlated the dimensions of the PPS with the other scales for both groups. For the group without disabilities, associative fluency correlated with material management and space management, internal locus of control correlated with material management, and the gross motor and fine motor Bruininks correlated with participation. For the group with JRA, the fine motor Bruininks correlated with the total PPS, and the gross motor Bruininks correlated with the dimension of space management.

The authors concluded that minor dysfunction did not always result in play deficits and that some children with disabilities could compensate for areas of dysfunction and play normally. A limitation of this study was that the authors were not able to observe the children in their usual play environments with familiar peers. The children with JRA were tested during clinic visits and the nondisabled children in preschools. This would affect overall play as well as participation specifically.

Restall and Magill-Evans (1994) studied the play of preschool children with autism. The purposes of their study were to "compare the play of children with autism with the play of children without dysfunction in their homes" and to "examine the relationship between children's play preferences and their communication, social, and motor abilities" (p. 113). Nine children with a diagnosis of autism and nine children with typical development were studied. Children were between the ages of 3 and 6 years and were matched for gender, age (chronological age for those without dysfunction and mental age for those with autism), and socioeconomic status. The children were observed under two conditions: unstructured play and a structured setting with specific toys and the parents available to the child. Children were rated on the PPS, the Vineland Adaptive Behavior Scales (Sparrow et al., 1984), and types of play materials chosen.

The results showed a statistically significant difference between the two groups on the total PPS score and on the participation dimension. There was no difference between groups on the play materials chosen. The group with autism showed significantly lower Vineland scores. The PPS was significantly correlated with the Vineland for both groups and the total PPS score was correlated with the communication variable of the Vineland for the autistic group and on the socialization variable for the nonautistic group. This study lends support for naturalistic observations in familiar settings. Limitations included limited opportunities for peer social interaction and limited opportunities to observe a variety of play within the time periods designated.

Table 3-3 summarizes the studies using the PPS with different categories of children. In summary, the autistic, physically abused, and prolonged hospitalization groups all showed statistically significant differences in total play ages from their normally developing counterparts. The children with autism had the most difficulty in social participation, the children with physical abuse showed problems in imitation, and those with sensory integrative dysfunction showed

TABLE 3-3 Studies Using the Preschool Play Scale (PPS) with Different Populations

Authors	n	Ages (yr)	Categories	Measures	Results
Kielhofner et al. (1983)	3/3	2	Hospitalized Nonhospitalized	PPS Playfulness Scale Three Environments	Significant difference in total PPS between groups Significant difference in playfulness score No difference in playfulness for three environments Significant difference in PPS for both groups in standard environment with passive caretaker
Howard (1986)	12/12	1 to 5	Abused Nonabused	PPS Parent Questionnaire	Significant difference in total PPS between groups Significant difference in imitation Questionnaire: significant difference in number of hours of TV—abused watched $1\frac{1}{2}$ hr more/day
Bundy (1989)	31/30	4 to 6	SI dysfunction No dysfunction	PPS	Significant difference in total PPS and in all four dimensions
Clifford and Bundy (1989)	31/35	4 to 6	SI dysfunction No dysfunction	PPS Peabody Picture Vocabulary Preschool Play Materials Preference	No difference in play materials preference Significant difference in total PPS and the dimensions of space and material management and participation
Von Zuben, Crist, and Mayberry (1991)	41/43 15/14 9/9	4 to 5	Middle socio-economic Low socio-economic	Modified PPS	No difference in total PPS, dimensions, or categories between groups
Morrison, Bundy, and Fisher (1991)		$4\frac{1}{2}$ to $6\frac{1}{2}$	nondisabled JRA	PPS Bruininks - Oseretsky Internal–External Locus of Control Association fluency	No difference in total PPS between groups No difference in total Bruininks-Oseretsky, Internal–External, or association fluency between groups Significant difference in ($p \leq .10$) in gross motor on Bruininks-Oseretsky
Restall and Magill-Evans (1994)		3 to 6	Autistic nonautistic	PPS Vineland Types play materials	Significant difference in total PPS between groups Significant difference in participation dimension No difference in play materials PPS not correlated with MA or CA Significant correlation of PPS and Vineland for both groups Significant correlation of total PPS with communication for autistic Significant correlation of total PPS with socialization for normals

Note: CA = chronological age; MA = mental age; JRA = juvenile rheumatoid arthritis; SI = sensory integrative.

problems with space management. There were no differences in the studies of children with juvenile rheumatoid arthritis (JRA) or with socioeconomic differences. These studies show the usefulness of the PPS in differentiating developmental play abilities in a variety of populations but also point out the individual nature of play and the children's ability to overcome some disabilities and develop typical play skills. The studies also point out the need for additional measures of play, such as play style or playfulness and play material preference, to tap into some of the more qualitative aspects of play.

Studies of Treatment Effects

Two studies have used the PPS as a measure of treatment effects. Schaaf and Mulrooney (1989) used the PPS along with an unpublished Parent/Teacher Play Questionnaire and the Peabody Developmental Motor Scales (Folio & Fewell, 1984) to assess the effectiveness of specific occupational therapy intervention on five subjects enrolled in an early intervention program. All subjects had developmental delay and were scheduled to receive occupational therapy. They collected data during a 4-week baseline period and a 10-week intervention period. The PPS was administered twice during the baseline period and four to five times during intervention. Teachers filled out the questionnaire weekly, and the Peabody was administered before and after intervention. Intervention consisted of direct and consultative occupational therapy with an emphasis on the facilitation of play behaviors. The authors found the Preschool Play Scale helpful in determining change; however, because of their small sample size and other limitations, they recommended more extensive exploration.

Germain and Dwyre (1988) used the PPS to determine effectiveness of occupational therapy intervention on play behavior. Six physically handicapped children were observed under each of two conditions: (1) handled, in which the therapist facilitated postural responses while the child was playing, and (2) unhandled, in which the child engaged in free play. They found that the children displayed greater play skills, as demonstrated on the PPS, in the unhandled condition, which was contrary to their expectations. The study raised the question as to the effects of therapist's handling on child performance. As the authors pointed out, there is a delicate balance between giving a child enough support or assistance to facilitate play and giving too much, so that the child becomes dependent on the therapist, thus decreasing self-initiated behaviors.

In summary, the studies utilizing the PPS have shown good reliability and validity with populations of normal children as well as those with disabilities. The PPS has also proved useful in differentiating developmental play abilities in a variety of populations with handicaps. In addition, it has been helpful in assessing the effectiveness of various treatment techniques.

CLINICAL USE

Clinically, the PPS has been useful in assessment in a variety of ways, which will be illustrated by case studies. It should be noted that clinically, overall play level is usually not as important as looking at the profile of play skills, determining strengths and weaknesses, and determining interest areas.

The PPS has been especially helpful when a child is not testable on standardized tests. For example, young children with autism often do not respond to direction and refuse standard test items. Because the PPS correlates significantly with developmental age, it is often possible to estimate developmental levels by observing free play.

CASE EXAMPLE 1: ANDREW

Andrew was a 3-year-old boy with a diagnosis of autism. When attempts were made to do standardized testing, he refused to sit in the chair, threw or pushed aside all test items, and tried to leave the room; therefore the therapist decided to assess him during free play with the PPS. She took him into a large clinic room equipped with swings, trampoline, bolsters and other climbing equipment, sandbox, toys for manipulation, and toys that provided sensory input. Andrew was allowed to choose his activities, and the therapist provided assistance if necessary. At times, the therapist offered various types of toys to observe his response.

On the PPS, he was observed to be most interested in gross motor activity, choosing swings, trampoline, and climbing apparatus. Gross motor activity was characterized by the use of his entire body, throwing, jumping, and climbing. He was very curious about the unfamiliar objects in the room and explored them. Movements were coordinated and he was able to accelerate, decelerate, and change course. On the space management dimension, he showed play skills at the 3- to 4-year level. (Fig. 3-4)

In material management, however, his play was at the 1- to 2-year level. Manipulation consisted of throwing, pounding, squeezing, and mouthing objects with unusual textures. Primary interest was in sensation and movement. There were no aversive responses to textures, except to shaving cream. His mother reported that he did not play with toys at home.

On the dimension of imitation, skills were also at the 1- to 2-year level. No imitation was observed in the clinic; however, his mother reported that he had learned most of his activities of daily living by observation and imitation.

Participation skills were also at the 1- to 2-year level. Play was generally solitary in nature. He occasionally watched others in the room but did not imitate them or enter into their play. In language he hummed to himself and primarily used gestures to communicate his desires.

The most striking findings with Andrew were the discrepancies between space management and the other dimensions. Although he showed coordinated gross motor movements, he avoided manipulative activity or played with toys and objects for their sensory qualities alone. Imitation was severely limited and participation with peers was nonexistent. Analysis of these discrepancies assisted in treatment planning. Goals in therapy included improving purposeful play with toys and imitation of and interaction with adults and peers in play.

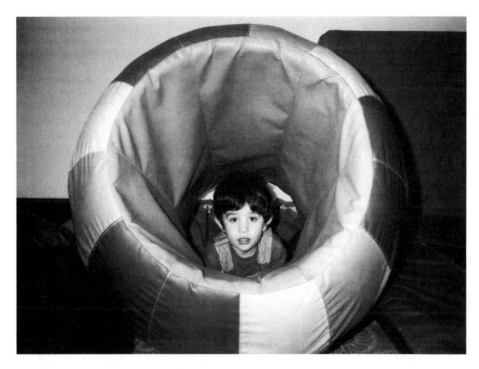

FIG. 3-4 Andrew's play preferences were for gross motor activity.

Another example of the usefulness of the PPS is with children who, because of their disability, may need adult intervention, such as in a testing situation, but in free play settings do not show the same skills. An illustration of this is the case example of Jane. This case also illustrates the use of the PPS to assess progress.

CASE EXAMPLE 2: JANE

Jane was a twin born at 26 weeks of age. She had an atrial septal defect repaired at 15 months of age, as well as severe visual problems caused by retrolental fibroplasia. She also had a history of seizures and was receiving medication. Jane experienced feeding difficulties that interfered with the transition from the bottle to the cup and from liquid to solid foods. Her twin was developing typically. Jane was referred to occupational therapy at 20 months of chronological age (corrected age of 16 months), after she had stabilized from surgery to repair the heart defect. Jane's parents stated that before the surgery, they had been told she was "too fragile" to be handled much, so most of the time, she was in her crib or propped in a corner of the couch with pillows around her.

When Jane was seen initially, a complete developmental and feeding evaluation as well as observations of free play were conducted. Results of the full evaluation are not presented at this time except for those facts that relate to the results on the PPS. Jane showed a strong aversive response to touch stimulation on her hands and face. As a result, she avoided holding, handling, or mouthing toys. She enjoyed being swung, bounced, and moved. She responded to auditory input, but her only visual response was slight turning toward strong light.

On the PPS, all dimensions were scored at the lowest level. In space management, she played with her hands and feet in the supine position, and she moved to continue pleasant sensations, such as shaking her head from side to side. She made no attempt to explore her environment with hands or body and stayed in the position in which she was placed.

to explore her environment with hands or body and stayed in the position in which she was placed.

In material management, manipulation could not even be scored because she avoided holding or handling any toys or objects. When given a toy, she would hold it only for a few seconds, then drop it. She made no attempt to find toys with her hands once they were dropped. She attended to voices and sounds, but could not see persons or objects in her environment. In imitation, she attended to sounds and made some imitative noises. After adult intervention, she imitated pat-a-cake.

In participation, she demanded personal attention by crying, fussing, or smiling when she heard familiar voices. She babbled to herself when alone in the crib. She attended to sounds and turned toward them. She didn't initiate any social games with caretakers but seemed to enjoy them, when engaged. There was no effort to interact with her twin sister. Evident throughout the PPS was Jane's extreme dependence on adult intervention for almost all sensory and social input because of her visual impairment and extreme tactile defensiveness. Self-initiated play was virtually nonexistent. Again, the results on the PPS helped define goals for occupational therapy intervention.

She was treated by the occupational therapist twice weekly in the home until she was 2½, when treatment changed to a center-based program. At the time of the change, she was again assessed on the PPS. Although she was still primarily dependent on adults to facilitate her play, she actively manipulated toys with a variety of textures. She was beginning to reach for dropped toys and for those that made noise. She also could operate a push pad to activate a fan or sound toy. She transferred toys at midline and actively manipulated or explored them. She banged a piano and drum with her hands and was interested in cause and effect toys that made noise. In space management, she could transition from prone to sitting and back and was beginning to crawl toward sounds. In imitation, she really enjoyed songs and simple hand play initiated by adults. Participation was still primarily with adults, but she was more aware of her siblings and smiled and vocalized when they played with her.

In Jane's case, significant changes were seen on the PPS during the 10 months of treatment, primarily in terms of factor descriptors but also in a higher age level in the material management dimension.

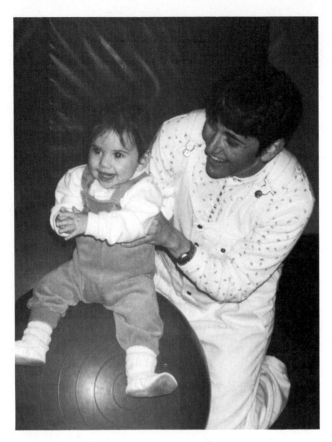

FIG. 3-5   Suggestions can be given to parents for appropriate and fun play activities.

A limitation to using the PPS to denote progress has been that the yearly age increments have been too large to see changes. This will be addressed in the revisions.

Another way in which the PPS has been useful clinically is as a guide to the developmental aspects of play. Here, therapists can use the descriptions to help parents understand typically developing play and encourage appropriate play skills (Figure 3-5).

STRENGTHS AND WEAKNESSES OF THE PRESCHOOL PLAY SCALE

It has been rewarding to this author, as the original creator of the PPS, to see how much the scale has been used and to see its value clinically. However, the studies discussed here and this author's clinical experience have revealed both strengths and weaknesses in the PPS. One of the advantages is that it covers all areas of development and reflects developmental status, as demonstrated in the validity studies. Thus if a child cannot be evaluated on a standardized developmental assessment, that child can be observed during free play and assessed on the PPS, and the therapist can feel fairly confident that play levels approximate developmental level.

Another big advantage is that the PPS does not require specialized toys or equipment and assesses the child in natural settings. In addition, it assesses natural behaviors rather than requested ones. This is particularly important to occupational therapists because their concerns are with children's occupational role behaviors within their everyday environments.

Some of the disadvantages of the PPS are described and are further addressed in suggested revisions. One disadvantage is that the measurement is in yearly increments, rather than more frequent intervals. This can be a problem, particularly when looking at progress, because the child may make significant changes but may not change levels, as demonstrated in the case of Jane. However, there may be changes within the factor descriptors that may denote progress, so clinically it still is helpful.

Some of the major disadvantages relate to descriptions of the dimensions and factors. Some factors may not be seen without adult involvement, such as books and music; and some factors are difficult to assess without additional information from caretakers, such as territory. These factors probably should not be required in the observation process, but information about them could be garnered through parental interview. The imitation dimension, as well as its factors, has been confusing because both the dimension and a factor share the same name (imitation). Also some of the behaviors reflecting imitation (imitation, imagination, and dramatization) may reflect a common underlying process of symbolic ability. In analyzing what is addressed primarily in this dimension, the underlying concept is the child's development of symbolism and pretense. For this reason, a change in the dimension name to pretense–symbolic is proposed, with some of the factors combined.

Many new assessments of various aspects of play are currently available that reveal additional factors which can be more precisely measured. These will also be considered in revising factor descriptors.

There has also been a lack of clarity about methodology (i.e., length and locale of observations) and confusion regarding scoring. Recommendations for improving scoring are to be addressed. Finally, the PPS looks only at developmental aspects of play and does not consider affect, emotions, or other qualities of play that might be considered under play style or playfulness. The PPS should be used in conjunction with other measures of play such as style, playfulness, or toy preference and with other measures of development.

NEW REVISION OF THE KNOX PRESCHOOL PLAY SCALE

After review of the usefulness of the Preschool Play Scale, as well as its limitations, it has been decided to revise the PPS. This section addresses the new revision, item descriptions, scoring, and administration. Table 3-4 depicts the Revised Knox Preschool Play Scale. Additions and changes in the factor descriptions are based on current research in developmental play (Bergen, 1988; Linder, 1990; Rubin et al., 1983).

TABLE 3-4 Revised Knox Preschool Play Scale*		
0 to 6 Months	**6 to 12 Months**	**12 to 18 Months**
Space management		
Gross motor: swipes, reaches, plays with hands and feet, moves to continue pleasant sensations	**Gross motor:** reaches in prone, crawls, sits with balance, able to play with toy while sitting, pulls to stand, cruises	**Gross motor:** stands unsupported, sits down, bends and recovers balance, walks with wide stance, broad movements involving large muscle groups, throws ball
Interest: people, gazes at faces, follows movements, attends to voices and sounds, explores self and objects within reach	**Interest:** follows objects as they disappear, anticipates movement, goal-directed movement	**Interest:** practices basic movement patterns, experiments in movement, explores various kinesthetic and proprioceptive sensations, moving objects (i.e., balls, trucks, pull toys)
Material management		
Manipulation: handles, mouths toys, bangs, shakes, hits	**Manipulation:** pulls, turns, pokes, tears, rakes, drops, picks up small object	**Manipulation:** throws, inserts, pushes, pulls, carries, turns, opens, shuts
Construction: brings two objects together	**Construction:** combines related objects, puts object in container	**Construction:** stacks, takes apart, puts together, little attempt to make product, relates two objects appropriately (i.e., lid on pot)
Purpose: sensation—uses materials to see, touch, hear, smell, mouth	**Purpose:** action to produce effect, cause and effect toys	**Purpose:** variety of schemas, process important, trial and error, relational play
Attention: follows moving objects with eyes, 3 to 5 sec attention	**Attention:** 15 sec for detailed object, 30 sec for visual and auditory toy	**Attention:** rapid shifts
Pretense/symbolic		
Imitation: of observed facial expressions and physical movement (i.e., smiling, pat-a-cake), imitates vocalizations	**Imitation:** imitates observed actions, emotions, sounds and gestures not part of repertoire, patterns of familiar activities	**Imitation:** of simple actions, present events and adults, imitates novel movements, links simple schemas (i.e., puts person in car and pushes it)
Dramatization: not evident	**Dramatization:** not evident	**Dramatization:** beginning pretend using self (i.e., feeds self with spoon), pretend on animated and inanimated objects
Participation		
Type: solitary, no effort to interact with other children, enjoys being picked up, swung	**Type:** infant to infant interaction, responds differently to children and adults	**Type:** combination of solitary and onlooker, beginning interaction with peers
Cooperation: demands personal attention, simple give and take interaction with caretaker (tickling, peek-a-boo)	**Cooperation:** initiates games rather than follows, shows and gives objects	**Cooperation:** seeks attention to self, demands toys, points, shows, offers toys but somewhat possessive, persistent
Humor: smiles	**Humor:** smiles, laughs at physical games and in anticipation	**Humor:** laughs at incongruous events
Language: attends to sounds and voices, babbles, uses razzing sounds	**Language:** gestures intention to communicate, responds to familiar words and facial expressions, responds to questions	**Language:** jabbers to self during play, uses gestures and words to communicate wants, labels objects, greets others, responds to simple requests, teases, exclaims, protests, combines words and gestures

Continued.

TABLE 3-4	Revised Knox Preschool Play Scale*—cont'd	
18 to 24 months	**24 to 30 months**	**30 to 36 months**
Space management		
Gross motor: runs, squats, climbs on and off chairs, walks up and down stairs (step to gait), kicks ball, rides kiddy car	**Gross motor:** beginning integration of entire body in activities—concentrates on complex movements, jumps off floor, stands on one foot briefly, throws ball in stance without falling	**Gross motor:** runs around obstacles, turns corners, climbs nursery apparatus, walks up and down stairs (alternating feet), catches ball by trapping it, stands on tiptoe
Interest: means–end, multipart tasks	**Interest:** explores new movement patterns (i.e., jumping), makes messes	**Interest:** rough and tumble play
Material management		
Manipulation: operates mechanical toy, pulls apart pop beads, strings beads	**Manipulation:** feels, pats, dumps, squeezes, fills	**Manipulation:** matches, compares
Construction: uses tools	**Construction:** scribbles, strings beads, puzzles 4 to 5 pieces, builds horizontally and vertically	**Construction:** multischeme combinations
Purpose: foresight before acting	**Purpose:** process important—less interested in finished product (i.e., scribbles, squeezes), plans actions	**Purpose:** toys with moving parts (i.e., dumptrucks, jointed dolls)
Attention: quiet play 5 to 10 min; play with single object 5 min	**Attention:** intense interest, quiet play up to 15 min, plays with single object or theme 5-10 min	**Attention:** 15 to 30 min
Pretense/symbolic		
Imitation: representational, recognizes ways to activate toys in imitation, deferred imitation	**Imitation:** of adult routines with toy-related mimicry (i.e., child feeding doll); imitates peers, representational play	**Imitation:** toys as agents (i.e., doll feeds self) more abstract representation of objects, multischeme combinations (i.e., feed doll, pat it, put to bed)
Dramatization: acts on doll (i.e., dresses, brushes hair), pretend actions on more than one object or person, combines two or more actions in pretend, imaginary objects	**Dramatization:** personifies dolls, stuffed animals, imaginary friends, portrays single character elaborates daily events with details	**Dramatization:** evolving episodic sequences (i.e., mixes cake, bakes it, serves it)
Participation		
Type: onlooker, simple actions and contingent responses between peers	**Type:** parallel (plays beside others but play remains independent), enjoys the presence of others, shy with strangers	**Type:** parallel, beginning associative, plays with 2 to 3 children, plays in company 1 to 2 hr
Cooperation: more complex games with a variety of adults (hide and seek, chasing), commands others to carry out actions	**Cooperation:** possessive, much snatch and grab, hoarding, no sharing, resists toys being taken away, independent, initiates own play	**Cooperation:** understands needs of others
Humor: laughs at incongruous labeling of objects or events	**Humor:** laughs at simple combinations of incongruous events and use of words	**Humor:** laughs at complex combinations of incongruous events and words
Language: comprehends action words, requests information, refers to persons and objects not present, combines words together	**Language:** talkative, very little jabber, begins to use words to communicate ideas, information, questions, comments on activity	**Language:** asks wh- questions, relates temporal sequences

TABLE 3-4 Revised Knox Preschool Play Scale*—cont'd		
36 to 48 Months	**48 to 60 Months**	**60 to 72 Months**
Space management		
Gross motor: more coordinated body movement, smoother walking, jumping, climbing, running, accelerates, decelerates, hops on one foot 3 to 5 times, skips on one foot, catches ball, throws ball using shoulder and elbow, jumps distances	**Gross motor:** increased activity level, can concentrate on goal instead of movement, ease of gross motor ability, stunts, tests of strength, exaggerated movement, clambers, gallops, climbs ladder, catches ball with elbows at side	**Gross motor:** more sedate, good muscle control and balance, hops on one foot 5 + times, hops in a straight line, bounces and catches ball, skips, somersaults, skates, lifts self off ground
Interest: anything new, fine motor manipulation of play materials, challenges self with difficult tasks	**Interest:** takes pride in work (i.e., shows and talks about products, compares with friends, likes pictures displayed), complex ideas, rough and tumble play	**Interest:** in reality—manipulation of real-life situations, making something useful, permanence of products, toys that "really work"
Material management		
Manipulation: small muscle activity—hammers, sorts, inserts small objects, cuts	**Manipulation:** increased fine motor control, quick movements, force, pulling, yanks	**Manipulation:** uses tools to make things, copies, traces, combines materials
Construction: makes simple products, combines play materials, takes apart, three-dimensional, design evident	**Construction:** makes products, specific designs evident, builds complex structures, puzzles 10 pieces	**Construction:** makes recognizable products, likes small construction, attends to detail, uses products in play
Purpose: beginning to show interest in finished product	**Purpose:** product very important and used to express self, exaggerates	**Purpose:** replicates reality
Attention: span around 30 min, plays with single object or them 10 min	**Attention:** amuses self up to 1 hr, plays with single object or theme 10 to 15 min	**Attention:** plays with single object or theme 15 + min
Pretense/symbolic		
Imitation: more complex imitation of real world, emphasis on domestic play and animals, symbolic, past experiences	**Imitation:** pieces together new scripts of adults (i.e., dressup), reality important	**Imitation:** continues to construct new themes with emphasis on reality—reconstruction of real world
Dramatization: complex scripts for pretend sequences in advance, story sequences, pretend with replica toys, uses one toy to represent another, portrays multiple characters with feelings (mostly anger and crying), little interest in costumes, imaginary characters	**Dramatization:** uses familiar knowledge to construct a novel situation (i.e., expanding on theme of a story or TV show), role playing for or with others, portrays more complex emotions, sequences stories, themes from domestic to magic, enjoys dressup, shows off	**Dramatization:** sequences stories, costumes important, props, puppets, directs actions of three dolls—making them interact, organizes other children and props for role play
Participation		
Type: associative play, no organization to reach a common goal, more interest in peers than activity, enjoys companions, beginning cooperative play, group play	**Type:** cooperative, groups of 2 to 3 organized to achieve a goal, prefers playing with others to alone, group games with simple rules	**Type:** cooperative groups of 3 to 6, organization of more complex games and dramatic play, competitive games, understands rules of fair play
Cooperation: limited, some turn taking, asks for things rather than grabbing, little attempt to control others, separates easily, joins others in play	**Cooperation:** takes turns, attempts to control activities of others, bossy, strong sense of family and home, quotes parents as authorities	**Cooperation:** compromises to facilitate group play, rivalry in competitive play, games with rules, collaborative play where roles are coordinated and themes are goal directed
Humor: laughs at nonsense words, rhyming	**Humor:** distortions of the familiar	**Humor:** laughs at multiple meanings of words
Language: uses words to communicate with peers, interest in new words, sings simple songs, uses descriptive vocabulary, changes speech depending on listener	**Language:** plays with words, fabricates, long narratives, questions persistently, communicates with peers to organize activities, brags, threatens, clowns, sings whole songs, uses language to express roles, verbal reasoning	**Language:** prominent in sociodramatic play, uses words as part of play as well as to organize play, interest in present, conversation like adults', uses relational terms, sings and dances to reflect meaning of songs

*Modified from Knox, S., (1974). A Play Scale. In M. Reilly (Ed.), *Play as Exploratory Learning*, Beverly Hills, CA: Sage Publications. Reprinted from Bledsoe, N., & Shepherd, J. (1982). A study of reliability and validity of a preschool play scale. *American Journal of Occupational Therapy, 36*, 783-788, with permission from the publisher.

Dimension Descriptions

The definitions of the new dimensions are as follows:

Space management: The manner in which children manage their bodies and the space around them. It includes the following factors:
  Gross motor activity: play involving the whole body
  Interest: attention to specific types of activity
Material management: The way in which children manage their material surroundings. It consists of the following factors:
  Manipulation: fine motor play
  Construction: combining objects and making products
  Purpose: goals of the activity
  Attention: length of time in independent play
Pretense–symbolic: The way children learn about the world through imitation and the development of the ability to understand and separate reality from make-believe. It contains the following factors:
  Imitation: mirroring aspects of the cultural environment
  Dramatization: pretend, introduction of novelty, and role play
Participation: The amount of and manner of social interaction. It contains the following factors:
  Type: level of social interaction in play
  Cooperation: ability to get along with others in play
  Humor: understanding and expression of humorous or incongruous words or events
  Language: communication with others in play

Age Ranges

Attempts were made further to refine the age ranges so as to be more discrete. This could be done easily from birth to 3 years of age, but after 3 years, the literature descriptions of play behaviors still tended to be in yearly increments. Therefore the Revised Knox Preschool Play Scale is organized in 6-month increments up until age 3 years and in yearly increments from 3 to 6 years of age.

Administration

Settings. Children should be observed both indoors and outdoors in as naturalistic or familiar an environment as possible, with peers present. Indoor and outdoor settings are essential so as to see the variety of behaviors necessary to score the dimension of space management adequately. Peers are necessary to assess participation.

Length of Observation. A minimum of two 30-minute periods, indoors and outdoors should be given. This is important to observing shifts in play episodes and to seeing the differences in play that the two settings afford.

Instructions for Scoring

Within the factors, place a mark above each descriptor each time it is observed. Then rank the factor at the highest level, unless the descriptor is insignificant (i.e., done for less than 1 minute or by chance). Descriptors typical of the child's behavior may be underlined. Each factor is scored at the upper age of the age grouping. For example, the 6- to 12-month level is scored as 12 months; the 30- to 36-month level is scored as 36 months. To score each dimension, the mean of the factor scores is taken. To score an overall play age, the mean of the dimension scores is taken.

Limitations and Future Directions

It is recommended that additional information be gathered at the time of testing from parental interview and also that other measures of play, such as toy preference, playfulness, or play style, be included. It is important to note that the revised Knox Preschool Play Scale still needs standardization, reliability, and validity studies. These are in the planning stage.

SUMMARY

The Preschool Play Scale has been reviewed from its initial development in 1968. Standardization, reliability, and validity studies with children developing normally and those with disabilities have shown that the PPS is a valid and reliable test of the developmental nature of play. Further validity has been demonstrated through a number of studies using different populations.

Two studies have used the PPS to assess effects of treatment. Case studies have been presented to further illustrate clinical use. Strengths and limitations of the PPS have been addressed and revision has been done to make the PPS more useful today. The Revised Knox Preschool Play Scale is presented here and its administration and scoring have been clarified.

REVIEW QUESTIONS

1. Describe the Play Scale. Discuss its history, intention, and methodology.
2. Discuss reliability and validity studies of the PPS. What might be the strengths and limitations of the scale? What are the clinical implications of these strengths and weaknesses?
3. The Revised Knox Preschool Play Scale includes the dimensions of space management, material management, pretense—symbolic, and participation. Describe what is addressed in each of these dimensions.
4. Discuss the developmental changes (from birth to age 5 years) that are outlined within each of the four dimensions of the Knox Preschool Play Scale.
5. Describe how the author suggests that the Revised Knox Preschool Play Scale be administered and scored.

REFERENCES

Bergen, D. (1988). *Play as a Medium for Learning and Development.* Portsmouth, NH: Heinemann Educational Books.

Bledsoe, N., & Shepherd, J. (1982). A study of reliability and validity of a preschool play scale. *American Journal of Occupational Therapy, 36*(12), 783-788.

Brown, C., & Gottfried, A. (Eds.). (1985). *Play Interactions.* Skillman, NJ: Johnson and Johnson Baby Products Co.

Bruininks, R. (1978). *Bruininks-Oseretsky Test of Motor Proficiency.* Circle Pines, MN: American Guidance Service.

Bruner, J. S., Jolly, A., & Sylva, K (Eds.). (1976). *Play—Its Role in Development and Evolution.* New York: Basic Books.

Bundy, A. (1989). A comparison of the play skills of normal boys with sensory integrative dysfunction. *Occupational Therapy Journal of Research, 9*(2), 84-100.

Clifford, J., & Bundy, A. (1989). Play preference and play performance in normal boys and boys with sensory integrative dysfunction. *Occupational Therapy Journal of Research, 9*(4), 202-217.

Cohen, D. (1987). *The Development of Play.* New York: New York University Press.

Dunn, L., & Dunn, L. (1981). *Peabody Picture Vocabulary Test—Revised.* Circle Pines, MN: American Guidance Service.

Ellis, M. (1973). *Why People Play.* Englewood Cliffs, NJ: Prentice-Hall.

Florey, L. (1969). Intrinsic motivation: the dynamics of occupational therapy theory. *American Journal of Occupational Therapy, 23,* 319-322.

Florey, L. (1971). An approach to play and play development. *American Journal of Occupational Therapy, 25,* 275-280.

Florey, L. (1981). Studies of play: Implications for growth, development and for clinical practice. *American Journal of Occupational Therapy, 35*(8), 519-524.

Folio, R., & Fewell, R. (1984). *Peabody Developmental Motor Scales.* Allen, TX: Developmental Learning Materials.

Garvey, C. (1977). *Play.* London: Fontana/Open Books Publishing.

Germain, A., & Dwyre, M. (1988, April). Unpublished paper presented at the annual conference of the American Occupational Therapy Association, April 17-20, 1988 Phoenix AZ.

Harrison, H., & Kielhofner, G. (1986). Examining reliability and validity of the preschool play scale with handicapped children. *American Journal of Occupational Therapy, 40*(3), 167-173.

Hartley, R., & Goldenson, R. (1963). *The Complete Book of Children's Play.* New York: The Cornwall Press.

Howard, A. (1986). Developmental play ages of physically abused and non-abused children. *American Journal of Occupational Therapy, 40*(10), 691-695.

Hulme, I., & Lunzer, E. A. (1966). Play, language and reasoning in subnormal children. *Journal of Child Psychology and Psychiatry, 7,* 107.

Kalverboer, A. (1977). Measurement of play: clinical applications. In Tizard, B., & Harvey, D. (Eds.). *Biology of Play* (pp. 100-122). Philadelphia: J. B. Lippincott.

Kielhofner, G., Barris, R., Bauer, D., Shoestock, B., & Walker, L. (1983). A comparison of play behavior in non-hospitalized and hospitalized children. *American Journal of Occupational Therapy, 37*(5), 305-312.

Knox, S. (1968). *Observation and Assessment of the Everyday Play Behavior of the Mentally Retarded Child.* Unpublished master's thesis, University of Southern California. Copyright.

Knox, S. (1974). A play scale. In Reilly, M. (Ed.). *Play as Exploratory Learning* (pp. 247-266). Beverly Hills, CA: Sage Publications.

Lieberman, J. (1977). *Playfulness: Its Relationship to Imagination and Creativity.* New York: Academic Press.

Linder, T. (1990) *Transdisciplinary Play-Based Assessment.* Baltimore: Paul H. Brooks Publ. Co.

Matsutsuyu, J. (1969). The interest check list. *American Journal of Occupational Therapy, 23,* 323-328.

Moorehead, L. (1969). The occupational history. *American Journal of Occupational Therapy, 23,* 329-334.

Morrison, C., Bundy, A., & Fisher, A. (1991). The contribution of motor skills and playfulness to the play performance of preschoolers. *American Journal of Occupational Therapy, 45*(8), 687-694.

Norwicki, S., & Duke, M. (1974). A preschool and primary internal-external control scale. *Developmental Psychology, 10,* 874-880.

Parten, M. (1933). Social play among pre-school children. *Journal of Abnormal and Social Psychology, 28,* 136-147.

Reilly, M. (1974). *Play as Exploratory Learning.* Beverly Hills, CA: Sage Publications.

Restall, G., & Magill-Evans, J. (1994). Play and preschool children with autism. *American Journal of Occupational Therapy, 48*(2), 113-120.

Robinson, A. (1977). Play: The arena for acquisition of rules of competent behavior. *American Journal of Occupational Therapy, 31,* 248-253.

Rosenblatt, D. (1977). Developmental trends in infant play. In Tizard, B., & Harvey, D. (Eds.). *Biology of Play* (pp. 33-44). Philadelphia: J. B. Lippincott.

Rubin, K., Fein, G., & Vandenberg, B. (1983). Play. In Mussen, P. (Ed.). *Handbook of Child Psychology: Vol 4* (4th ed., pp. 693-774). New York: Wiley.

Schaaf, R., & Mulrooney, L. (1989). Occupational therapy in early intervention: A family centered approach. *American Journal of Occupational Therapy, 43*(11), 745-754.

Schaefer, C., Gitlin, K., & Sandgrund, A. (1991). Introduction. In C. Schaefer, K. Gitlin, & A. Sandgrun (Eds.), *Play Diagnosis and Assessment.* New York: John Wiley and Sons.

Smilansky, S. (1968). *The Effects of Sociodramatic Play on Disadvantaged Preschool Children.* New York: John Wiley and Sons.

Sparrow, S., Balla, D., & Cicchetti, D. (1984). *Vineland Adaptive Behavior Scales.* Circle Pines, MN: American Guidance Service.

Takata, N. (1969). The play history. *American Journal of Occupational Therapy, 23*(4), 314-318.

Takata, N. (1971). The play milieu—a preliminary appraisal. *American Journal of Occupational Therapy, 25,* 281-284.

Takata, N. (1974). Play as a prescription. In Reilly, M. (Ed.). *Play as Exploratory Learning.* (pp. 209-246). Beverly Hills, CA: Sage Publications.

Von Zuben, M., Crist, P., & Mayberry, W. (1991). A pilot study of differences in play behavior between children of low and middle socioeconomic status. *American Journal of Occupational Therapy, 45*(2) 113-118.

Ward, W. C. (1968). Creativity in young children. *Child Development, 39,* 737-754.

White, R. (1959). Motivation reconsidered: The concept of competence. *Psychological Review, 66,* 297-333.

Wolfgang, C., & Phelps, P. (1983). Preschool play materials preference inventory. *Early Child Development and Care. 12,* 127-141.

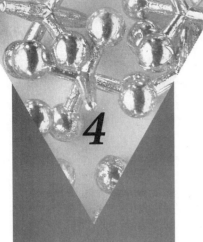

4

PLAY AND PLAYFULNESS:
WHAT TO LOOK FOR

Anita C. Bundy

Play differs from other occupations such as self-care or work by the source of the motivation and the degree of freedom associated with it. Self-care and work are largely obligatory and extrinsically motivated, whereas play is self-chosen and intrinsically motivated.

Although there is some variability in culturally acceptable dress, there is a relatively specific outcome associated with dressing. Further, considerable gain can be derived from dressing fashionably, whereas considerable embarrassment may result from misjudging the expected dress for a particular event. The product of this self-care activity, rather than the process, provides the primary motivation. Similarly, a person's job brings with it expected outcomes. Whereas work may be pleasurable, both a paycheck and recognition from coworkers and supervisors are important extrinsic motivators for most people in their jobs.

By contrast, in play activities the process (doing) rather than the product (outcome) provides the primary source of the reward (Rubin, Fein, & Vandenberg, 1983) (Fig. 4-1). Although it may be desirable to win a particular game, winning is not the primary reason for playing. In fact, the lack of predictability about who will win often increases the motivation to play. When people know unequivocally who will win, they often stop playing. For example, when it is clear who will win a hand of cards, other players usually throw in the hand and begin the next round (Caillois, 1979).

Because play is process rather than product driven, it is not bound by the predictability generally characteristic of self-care and work. Whereas an individual may put on different clothing depending on the occasion or the weather, the actual process of dressing remains much the same. Even work, which for some individuals varies considerably from day to day, retains a certain sameness derived from the expected outcomes.

Play activities, however, vary widely. There is no single correct way to do a particular play activity. In fact, when attempting a new strategy for any activity, an individual may be heard to say, "I was playing with it to see what would happen." (Fig. 4-2).

Like work and self-care, play is an important lifelong occupation (Kielhofner, 1985). Thus their clients' abilities to play should be a chief concern of occupational therapists. However, play has long been a problem for occupational therapists (Bundy, 1993). Even when the clients are children, for whom play is the primary occupation (Bundy, 1992), therapists rarely assess the play (Lawlor & Henderson, 1989; Stone, 1991).

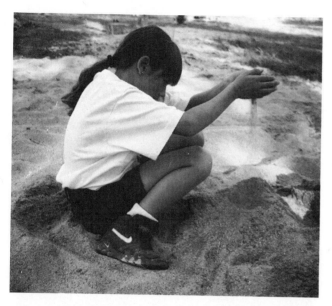

FIG. 4-1   Play involves more attention to process than product. (Courtesy Becca Austin.)

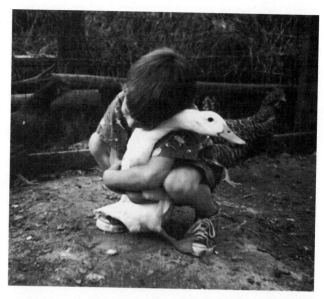

FIG. 4-3   It may matter less what you do in play than how you do it. (Courtesy Becca Austin.)

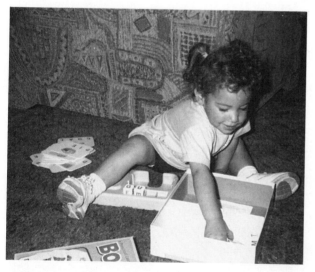

FIG. 4-2   There is no "right way" to play with a game or toy. (Courtesy Becca Austin.)

The failure to include assessments of play in therapists' battery of evaluations may be, in part, because so few true evaluations of play exist in occupational therapy literature. However, the lack of valid play assessments may stem from difficulties with developing such assessments. That is, researchers who have attempted to develop play assessments have failed to recognize that evaluation of the constituent skills used in play (e.g., motor, cognitive) does not constitute an evaluation of play.

Further, unlike work and self-care, the play activities in which individuals engage may matter less than whether the individual approaches those (and other) activities in a playful manner (Bundy, 1993) (Fig. 4-3). It may be playfulness rather than play activities that, when evaluated, provides therapists with the information they seek regarding their

young clients' development. This chapter describes and operationally defines a model of playfulness, discusses the development and preliminary analysis of a test of playfulness, and suggests and illustrates with two case examples a framework for the systematic evaluation of playfulness in young children.

A MODEL OF PLAYFULNESS

Playfulness can be determined within any transaction by evaluating for the presence of three elements: intrinsic motivation, internal control, and the freedom to suspend reality (Bundy, 1991, 1993; Kooij, 1989; Kooij & Vrijhof, 1987; Morrison, et al., 1991; Neumann, 1971). "Intrinsic motivation" refers to some (unnamed) aspect of the activity itself, rather than to an external reward, that provides the impetus for the individual's involvement in the activity (Figs. 4-4 and 4-5). "Internal control" suggests that the individual is largely "in charge" of his or her actions and at least some aspects of the activity's outcome (Figs. 4-6 and 4-7). "Freedom to suspend reality" means that the individual chooses how close to objective reality the transaction will be (Fig. 4-8).

Each of the three elements (intrinsic motivation, internal control, and freedom to suspend reality) can be represented by a continuum. Each continuum can be used to reflect the relative presence of a specified trait in a particular transaction. The summative contribution of the three tips the balance and determines the relative presence of playfulness or nonplayfulness, which also is represented by a continuum (Bundy 1991, 1993; Neumann, 1971) (Fig. 4-9).

It is unlikely, and perhaps not even desirable, for any transaction to be totally intrinsically motivated, internally controlled, or free of the constraints of reality. Thus, this model should be viewed with caution. Nonetheless, the con-

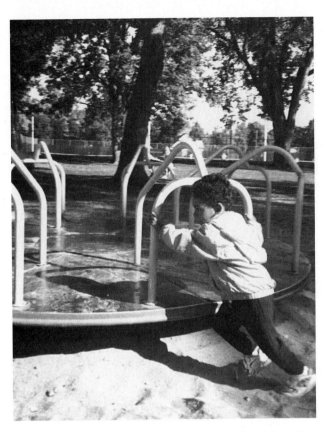

FIG. 4-4 Mastery can be an important source of intrinsic motivation. (Courtesy Becca Austin.)

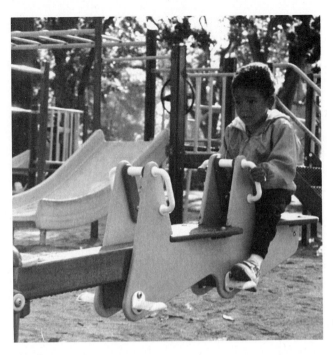

FIG. 4-5 The pure sensation of movement can be an important motivator. (Courtesy Becca Austin.)

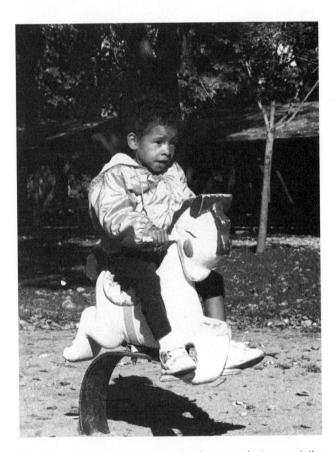

FIG. 4-6 A horse is a horse, but that horse can be transportation or imply a source of sensation—the choice is the player's. (Courtesy Becca Austin.)

cept is useful, particularly for therapists in need of a quick, informal means for evaluating a particular transaction (generally a treatment session).

In addition to the three primary elements of play, Bateson (1971, 1972) described a fourth concept, framing, that seems critical to play and playfulness. Bateson likened the play frame to a picture frame that separates the wallpaper from the picture. He described play as a frame in which the player gives cues to others about how they should act toward him or her. To be a good player, a person must be able to both give and read such cues. Of course, the ability to give and read social cues is a part of many nonplay transactions. However, Bateson argued that in play cues are exaggerated and thus easier to learn. Further, people do not need language to learn about play cues. Thus infant–adult play serves as an excellent early medium for learning to give and read social cues.

If the concept of playfulness as a reflection of the combined presence of intrinsic motivation, internal control, freedom to suspend reality and framing is to be used in a formal manner to evaluate individual children's playfulness, then each trait must be defined in a more operational manner. That is, how will a child act if he or she is intrinsically motivated, internally controlled (Fig. 4-10), free of selected constraints of reality, entering or maintaining the frame? This operationalization of the elements is a vital step in the

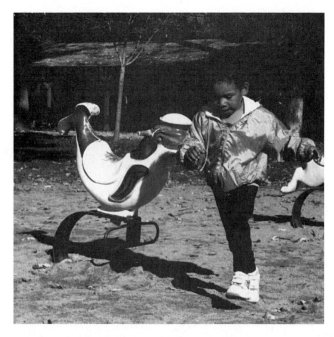

FIG. 4-7 All players must retain enough control to say (verbally or nonverbally), "I'm finished. I want to do something else now." (Courtesy Becca Austin.)

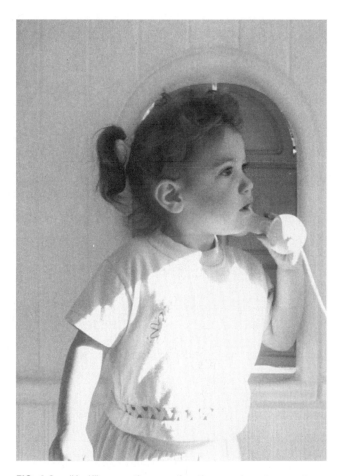

FIG. 4-8 "As if" serves the same function as rules. (Courtesy Becca Austin.)

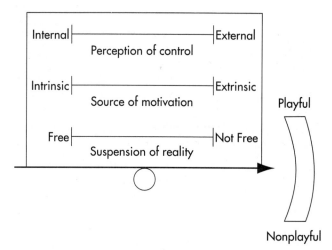

FIG. 4-9 Schematic representation of the elements of playfulness. (Modified from A. Bundy, 1991.)

development of a valid assessment of playfulness—one that may allow therapists to capture the important aspects of play and thus include it routinely in their evaluations of young children. The operationalization of these concepts leads to creation of the actual test items (Bundy, 1993; Fisher, 1993).

Operationalizing the Elements of Playfulness

Many resources yield potential operational definitions of the elements of playfulness. Play literature is a primary source. In fact, the most common means for defining play is by listing the traits that separate it from nonplay (Rubin et al., 1983). Although these traits vary slightly from theorist to theorist, when the various criteria for play are examined two points become clear.

First, many of the commonly cited traits of play actually are operational definitions of an aspect of intrinsic motivation, internal control, and/or the suspension of reality. That is, they appear to be subclassifications of the more encompassing elements of play. They answer one or more questions about how intrinsic motivation, internal control, or the suspension of reality are recognized when they are seen.

Second, intrinsic motivation, internal control, and the suspension of reality are not mutually exclusive. That is, certain behaviors may suggest that more than one of these elements are present. Table 4-1 by no means represents an exhaustive review of play literature. However, it illustrates relationships among various commonly cited traits defining play and intrinsic motivation, internal control, and the suspension of reality.

Framing is somewhat more difficult than the other elements of playfulness to operationalize clearly. There may be a number of reasons for this. First, only Bateson (1971, 1972) wrote about framing explicitly and in the context of play. Second, the giving and receiving of social cues and the ability to maintain a play frame, despite necessary breaks for negotiation or the meeting of other needs, are somewhat elusive skills, often difficult to describe and recognize. Perhaps

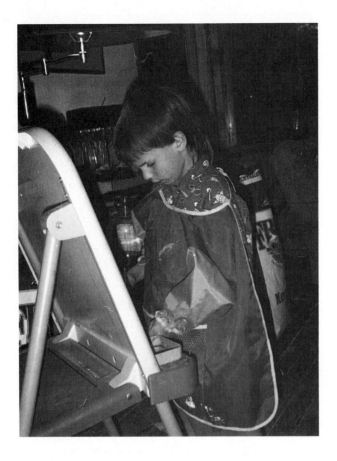

FIG. 4-10 A player who experiences internal control can make material things do whatever his competence allows. (Courtesy Becca Austin.)

the ability to give and read social cues is so much a part of our cultural expectations that knowledge of them is tacit. Only their impairment or absence is obvious.

The Test of Playfulness (ToP)

Drawing heavily on the elucidations of the elements of play cited in play literature, Peggy Metzger, Barbara McNicholas, and this author created a 60-item observational assessment of playfulness called the Test of Playfulness (ToP). The ToP was designed to be scored from videotapes of children engaged in free play.

The initial version of the ToP was examined for evidence of construct validity and interrater reliability with 77 children (68 developing typically, 9 with developmental delays) ranging in age from 22 to 118 months. Data from 12 trained raters were entered into the initial Rasch analysis of the ToP (Metzger, 1993).

This preliminary analysis of the first version of the ToP was very promising. A total of 53 of the 60 items appeared to define a unidimensional construct that reflected playfulness. Further, this construct seemed adequate for describing 95% of the children developing typically. However, the scoring pattern of more than half of the children with special needs differed considerably from that of the children developing typically. Because of the small sample size, it was not possible to determine whether these differences reflected diagnostically useful information. Thus additional research is necessary. However, the goal was to create a scale that could be used across age and diagnostic groups. For several reasons, it was felt that the ToP could be improved by a fairly

TABLE 4-1 **Relationship of Commonly Cited Play Traits to the Three Primary Elements of Play and Playfulness**

Play Element	Play Trait	Theorist
Intrinsic motivation	Play is all absorbing.	Csikszentmihalyi (1975a, 1975b, 1990)
	Play involves more attention to the process than to the product.	Rubin et al., (1983)
	Play is usually thought to be fun although that perception may be clearer after the play has ended than while it is happening.	Csikszentmihalyi (1975a)
	Play is more surprising than predictable.	Caillois (1979)
Internal control	Play is more safe than risky.	Caillois (1979)
	In play, the player reaches beyond him- or herself to meet a challenge.	Csikszentmihalyi (1975a, 1975b, 1990)
Internal control, suspension of reality	In play, the player makes things come out the way he or she wants or acts out his or her worst fears. The player can be whoever he or she desires. The player can control material things and make them do whatever his or her competence allows.	Connor, Williamson, & Seipp (1978)
Suspension of reality	In play, the usual meanings of objects no longer apply.	Rubin et al., (1983)
	"As if" serves the same function as rules. Rules create fiction. No activity in real life corresponds to games with rules.	Caillois (1979)

significant revision of items and scoring. This author undertook that revision in the spring of 1993 together with three colleagues, Peggy Metzger, Christy Morrison, and Cay Reilly.

Some of the items on the initial version of the ToP (e.g., "is physically active in play") seemed to artificially penalize some young children, particularly those with disabilities. This item was drawn originally from the Children's Playfulness Scale (CPS) (Barnett, 1990). The CPS was patterned after a well-known assessment of playfulness developed by Lieberman (1977). Some of the items also were included in the initial version of the ToP.

Being physically active was thought originally to reflect some degree of internal control. If a child felt in control of a situation, he or she might be more active within it. However, in retrospect, there seemed little about level of physical activity that contributed significantly to playfulness. Depending on the context, individuals could be very playful but not very active. Further, children with physical disabilities are often very playful but unable to demonstrate that playfulness with high levels of physical activity. Thus that item was eliminated in the revised version of the ToP because it no longer seemed to contribute to defining the construct of playfulness (Metzger, 1993).

Other items (e.g., "using unconventional objects in play") were difficult to observe reliably since raters did not necessarily agree on what constituted "unconventional." This item, also drawn from the CPS (Barnett, 1990), reflected suspension of reality. In retrospect, however, it seemed to better capture an aspect of that element when it was combined with a similar item, "uses conventional objects in unconventional ways." Thus these items were revised to reflect an improved operational definition of one aspect of the suspension of reality (Metzger, 1993).

In addition to item revision and item generation (to fill holes that became apparent), the scoring procedure for the ToP was also revised. The proportion of time an item could be observed was measured in an "extent" scale; however, through the pilot study it became clear that this was not always the most relevant criterion. For example, with one item, "persists in overcoming obstacles to play," the amount of time that the child persisted seemed less important than the intensity with which the child attempted to overcome the obstacle. Thus an "intensity" scale was created to capture the degree to which some items were present.

For some items (e.g., "enters an existing group"), a relevant criterion seemed to pertain to the skill or the ease with which a child was able to accomplish a task. Thus a third scale, "skillfulness," was created. None of the scales pertains to all the items. However, more than one scale frequently can be applied to a particular item. Scales that do not apply are shaded out in the scoring sheet that appears in Table 4-2.

The revised ToP represents the original conceptualization of playfulness shown in Fig. 4-9. Whereas the elements of play are not mutually exclusive and thus more than one can be reflected in each item, the items seem to be somewhat

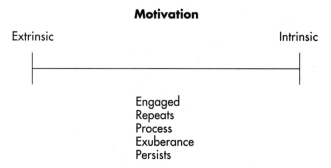

Motivation

FIG. 4-11   Items associated with intrinsic motivation.

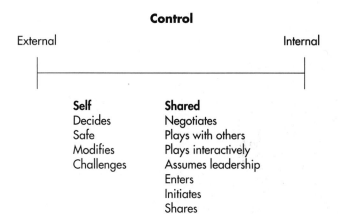

Control

FIG. 4-12   Items associated with internal control.

more strongly associated with one element than the others. These associations are represented graphically in Figs. 4-11 through 4-14. The items are defined in Table 4-3.

The revised ToP is composed of 68 items. Like the initial version, it is designed to be scored by a trained examiner observing a child playing for approximately 15 minutes, both indoors and outdoors. However, the need for evaluation in two settings currently is being examined by Tyler (in preparation).

Although the initial version of the ToP was tested primarily with children 2 to 10 years of age developing typically, additional researchers have examined its use with toddlers and with children who have disabilities. Hutchinson (1995) has found the scale to be valid with children as young as 18 months. Gaik and Rigby (1994) demonstrated preliminary reliability and validity of the scale with children who have physical disabilities. A second study (Harkness, in preparation) will extend Gaik's and Rigby's findings.

USING THE MODEL OF PLAYFULNESS IN ASSESSMENT: CASE EXAMPLES

Because the validity and reliability of the revised ToP currently are being evaluated in a series of studies (Brooks, 1995), meaningful scores cannot yet be derived. However,

TABLE 4-2 ToP Protocol Sheet

TEST OF PLAYFULNESS (ToP)—Adapted

Name: _____

Age: _____

Date: _____

	EXTENT	INTENSITY	SKILLFULNESS
	3 = Almost always	3 = Highly	3 = Highly skilled
	2 = Much of the time	2 = Moderately	2 = Moderately skilled
	1 = Some of the time	1 = Mildly	1 = Slightly skilled
	0 = Rarely or never	0 = Not	0 = Unskilled
	NA = Not Applicable	NA = Not Applicable	NA = Not Applicable

Item	Ext	Int	Skill	Comments
Is actively engaged.				
Appears self-directed. Decides what to do and how to do it.				
Appears to feel safe.				
Demonstrates obvious exuberance, manifest joy.				
Tries to overcome difficulties, barriers, or obstacles to persist with an activity.				
Actively modifies complexity and/or demands of activity.				
Engages in mischief or commits a minor infraction of the implicit or explicit rules.				
Repeats actions, activities; stays with same basic theme.				
Engages in process aspects of activity.				
Pretends.				
Incorporates objects or other people into play in novel, imaginative, creative, unconventional, or variable ways.				
Engages in challenges (motor, cognitive, or social).				
Negotiates with others to have needs or desires met.				
Plays with others.				
Plays interactively with others.				
Assumes leadership role.				
Enters a group already engaged in an activity.				
Initiates play with others.				
Teases or jokes with others (verbal or nonverbal).				
Clowns.				
Shares playthings, play equipment.				
Gives facial, verbal, and body cues appropriate to the situation and that say, "This is how you should act toward me."				
Responds to others' facial or body cues.				
Maintains cohesiveness of play frame.				

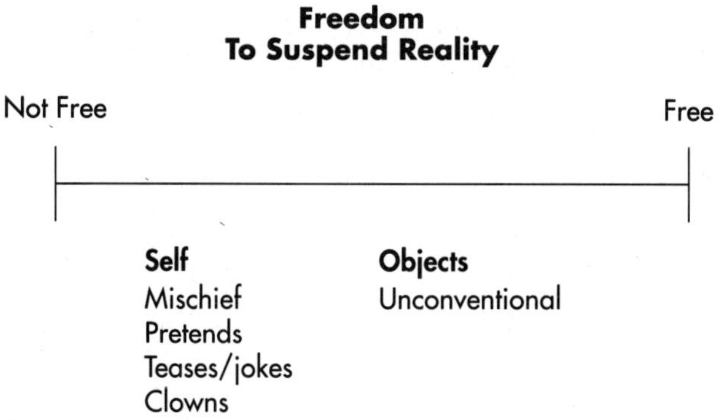

**Freedom
To Suspend Reality**

Not Free   Free

Self   **Objects**
Mischief   Unconventional
Pretends
Teases/jokes
Clowns

FIG. 4-13   Items associated with suspension of reality.

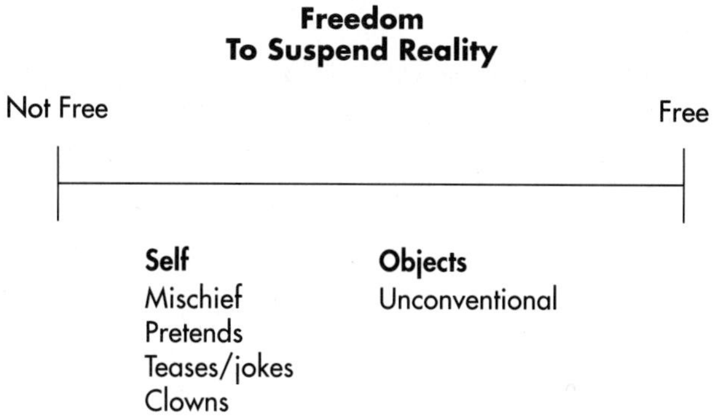

**Freedom
To Suspend Reality**

Not Free   Free

Self   **Objects**
Mischief   Unconventional
Pretends
Teases/jokes
Clowns

FIG. 4-14   Items associated with framing.

TABLE 4-3 Definitions of ToP Items	
Item	**Description**
Is actively engaged.	Extent—Proportion of time the child is involved in activities rather than aimless wandering or other nonfocused or undesirable activity. Intensity—Degree to which the child is concentrating on the activity or playmates).
Appears self-directed. Decides what to do and how to do it.	Extent—Proportion of time during which the child appears to have a purpose and a plan.
Appears to feel safe.	Extent—Proportion of time during which the child seems to feel physically and emotionally safe.
Demonstrates obvious exuberance, manifest joy.	Extent—Proportion of time during which the child exhibits outward and obvious signs of having fun, being gleeful.
Tries to overcome difficulties, barriers, or obstacles to persist with an activity.	Intensity—Degree to which the child perseveres in order to overcome obstacles to continuing the activity.
Actively modifies complexity and/or demands of activity.	Skill—Ease with which the child actively changes the requirements or complexity of the task in order to vary the challenge or degree of novelty.
Engages in mischief; commits a minor infraction of the implicit or explicit rules.	Extent—Proportion of time during which the child is involved in minor infractions of the implicit or explicit rules. The mischief is not done out of a spirit of meanness. Intensity—The level of infraction committed. Note.The action should not cross the boundaries into "meanness" or excessively poor judgment resulting in someone's getting hurt. Skill—The adeptness with which the child creates and carries out the mischief.
Repeats actions or activities; stays with same basic theme.	Extent—Proportion of time the child stays with same basic action or theme even if the objects used vary.
Engages in process aspects of activity.	Extent—Proportion of time during which the child seems more interested in how something is done or in doing than in the outcome (product) or in doing nothing.
Pretends.	Extent—Proportion of time during which there are overt indicators the child is assuming different character roles, pretending to be doing something, pretending something is happening that is not, or pretending an object or person is something other than what it actually is. Skill—The degree of conviction and ease with which the child pretends.
Incorporates objects or other people into play in novel, imaginative, unconventional, creative, or variable ways.	Extent—Proportion of time during which the child (a) uses objects commonly thought of as toys in ways other than those the manufacturer clearly intended, (b) incorporates objects not classically thought of as toys into the play (e.g., bugs, jars, cans, table legs), or (c) uses one toy or object in a number of different ways.
Engages in challenges (motor, cognitive, or social).	Extent—Proportion of time during which the child engages in activities that require him or her to "stretch" a little. Intensity—Degree of challenge accepted by the child.

Continued.

TABLE 4-3	Definitions of ToP Items—cont'd
Item	**Description**
<u>Negotiates</u> with others to have needs or desires met.	Skill—<u>Ease</u> and <u>finesse</u> with which the child verbally or nonverbally asks for what he or she needs.
Plays <u>with</u> <u>others</u>.	Extent—<u>Proportion</u> of <u>time</u> during which the child interacts in any way with other children or adults involved in the same or similar activity.
Plays <u>interactively</u> with others.	Extent—<u>Proportion</u> of <u>time</u> during which the character of the activity would change dramatically if more than one child were not present. Skill—<u>Ease</u> with which the child sustains an interactive (cooperative or competitive) activity.
Assumes <u>leadership</u> role.	Extent—<u>Proportion</u> of <u>time</u> during which the child has been responsible for setting the agenda. Skill—<u>Ease</u> with which the child assumes and executes the leadership role.
<u>Enters</u> a group already engaged in an activity.	Skill—<u>Ease</u> with which the child does something to become part of a group already engaged in an activity; the action is not disruptive to what is going on.
<u>Initiates</u> play with others.	Skill—<u>Ease</u> with which the child approaches others and initiates a new activity or makes a <u>major</u> change to the direction of an ongoing activity.
<u>Teases</u> <u>or</u> <u>jokes</u> with others (verbally or nonverbally).	Extent—<u>Proportion</u> of <u>time</u> during which the child engages in teasing or razzing behavior or incorporates verbally transmitted jokes or funny stories into play with others. Teasing is done "with a glint in the eye rather than out of blackness in the heart." Intensity—<u>Degree</u> to which the teasing or joking approaches but does not cross over "the edge." Skill—<u>Ease</u> and <u>cleverness</u> with which the teasing or joking is accomplished.
<u>Clowns</u>.	Extent—<u>Proportion</u> of <u>time</u> during which the child engages in exaggerated or "galumphing" behavior especially (but not necessarily only) with the intent to gain others' attention.
<u>Shares</u> play things, play equipment.	Extent—<u>Proportion</u> of <u>time</u> during which the child allows others to play with toys, personal belongings, or playmates or on equipment the child is currently using.
<u>Gives</u> clear facial and body <u>cues</u> appropriate to the situation and that say, "This is how you should act toward me."	Extent—<u>Proportion</u> of <u>time</u> during which the child acts in a way to give out clear messages about how others should interact with him or her.
<u>Responds</u> to others' facial and bodily cues.	Extent—<u>Proportion</u> of <u>time</u> during which the child acts in accord with others' play cues. Skill—<u>Ease</u> and <u>smoothness</u> with which a child responds to the cues of others.
<u>Maintains</u> cohesiveness of <u>play</u> <u>frame</u>.	Extent—The <u>proportion</u> of <u>time</u> during which the child maintains the flow and cohesiveness of the play activity.

the conceptual framework from which the ToP has been developed can be used by therapists to systematically examine playfulness in their young clients. Two case examples follow in which the use of this model will be illustrated.

CASE EXAMPLE 1: WILL

Will is a 2½-year-old boy developing typically. He was observed for 15 minutes on the playground of the day-care center in which he spends five mornings each week. Also on the playground at the time were several classmates and two adult day-care workers.

The playground is a large area that contains several pieces of equipment. These include a slide, a climbing apparatus shaped like an inverted **U**, and two large unconventional pieces of play equipment. One is shaped like an insect with an open barrel for a body and six long pole legs that hold it up off the ground. The second is a swaying wooden bridge bounded on both sides by a platform. At the end of one platform is a slide; at the end of the other is a ladder.

Will began his morning recess alone on the climbing apparatus. He climbed the first few bars, which were arranged essentially vertically in relation to one another. When he reached the upper section where the bars are arranged more horizontally in relation to one another, he dropped down between them, hanging by his hands from one bar. In an attempt to prepare himself to move to the next bar, Will began swinging his body. However, this seemed too difficult, and he let go and fell to the ground, landing on his bottom.

Will brushed himself off and ran to join his classmates on the slide where they were being supervised closely by one of the day-care workers. Will took several turns on the slide. The first few he did in the conventional way—seated. Each time he got to the bottom, he waited for David, a classmate, giving clear nonverbal cues that he wanted to race back to the end of the line. Once he slid down before Shanda, another classmate, was off the end of the slide and ran into her. Both giggled, but Will's actions resulted in a reprimand from the day-care worker.

At one point, Will climbed the slide, pausing at the top to view a large truck going by. From his vantage point, he began stamping his feet and yelling repeatedly at his classmates, "Hey guys!"

Finally ready to descend the slide again, he began to position himself prone, head first down the slide. However, this appeared too scary and he immediately began to reposition himself feet first. This position still was not acceptable to the day-care worker who began shouting, "On your bottom, Will!" Will immediately sat up, but turned so his back was facing the bottom of the slide, another position unacceptable to the day-care worker. Will managed to reorient himself supine so that he was going feet first down the slide, but even this was not acceptable to the daycare worker, who made him get off the slide until he was ready to "go on his bottom."

A temper tantrum ensued, and then Will, banned from the slide, spent several minutes playing in the sand underneath it. When he finally resumed his play on the slide, he climbed the ladder, cutting into line in front of two other uncomplaining classmates and unobserved by the day-care worker.

Will jumped off the bottom of the slide and ran over to the swinging bridge where he spent the next few minutes. Twice he sat down at the top of the bridge and began sliding down it—either because of its resemblance to a slide or because he was fearful of the steep angle of descent. At one point he stood up in the middle portion of the bridge and began stomping his feet. This caused two of his classmates who were standing on one of the metal platforms to begin doing the same thing. This stomping lasted several seconds. On one of his descents from the bridge via the short slide, Will chose to stand. He took a couple of steps and either lost his balance or, out of fear, sat down quickly.

Will's final activity on the playground was climbing on the insect. He and one of his classmates began by banging on the "face" of the insect. He then climbed up into the body and began to lean out onto the legs. This resulted in a reprimand from one of the day-care workers who yelled, "You get back!" Will complied, but seconds later was back hanging.

The day-care worker had moved out of sight, and Will and Lisa, a classmate, began a game where one stood on the edge of the insect's body holding onto the legs. "Ready, set, go!" was followed by hanging from the legs as long as possible before jumping to the ground. Once Will landed on his bottom, apparently biting his tongue. Once he accidentally let go with one hand and hung briefly from the bar by the other hand. Once Lisa was behind Will and apparently felt he was taking too long so she kicked him gently. He reprimanded her, "Don't kick me!"

Despite the "difficulties" encountered in this activity, it persisted for approximately 7 minutes, longer than any other activity during the session. It ended only because the children were called to return to the classroom.

Will's Playfulness Profile

Will's scores on the ToP are shown in Table 4-4. By examination of the scores of the items associated with each of the elements (see Figs. 4-11 through 4-14), a playfulness profile has been created for Will. This is shown in Fig. 4-15. Each element is discussed separately in the following subsections.

Intrinsic motivation

The placement of the marker along the continuum representing motivation is far toward the intrinsic end, since Will received high scores on all the items reflecting that element. Despite the warnings of the day-care workers, Will remained actively and intensely engaged in gross motor activities (for which there is no expected outcome) most of the time. Will was obviously exuberant, laughing and shouting, much of the time. However, he was sometimes so focused on the challenge of the activity that he did not demonstrate manifest joy. This is commonly observed in players of all ages. In fact, manifest joy seems to be observed only in certain kinds of activities.

Whereas it is clear that Will was intrinsically motivated, the exact source for the intrinsic motivation is not described by these observations. It seems likely that Will was motivated by mastery of the environment (White, 1959) and by the sheer sensation associated with the activities (Caillois, 1979). He also may have been motivated by his need to make a statement of his identity seen in his repeated engagement in banging, shouting, and other loud activities.

Internal control

The placement of the marker along the continuum representing control is about midway. Will received higher scores on items that reflect self-control than on those that reflect shared control. This is to be expected, given his age. Will appears to feel safe and to be the decision-maker with regard to the activities and their level of challenge most of the time. In fact, when the day-care workers attempted to modify his behavior, he took control either by waiting until they were not looking or by going off to another activity. His temper tantrum reflected his age-related lack of skill with negotiating. Although Will readily shared the climbing equipment and played interactively much of the time, he only rarely took a leadership role. When he did, however (mostly to initiate noise making), he did so quite skillfully. That is, the other children followed his lead very easily.

Suspension of reality

The placement of the marker on the continuum representing suspension of reality is quite far toward the "not free" end. That is, aside from his frequent engagement in mischief and occasional teasing and clowning, this transaction appeared quite bound by objective reality. Pretending was notably absent. As much as anything, Will's performance in this area may have been a reflection of two related factors: his age and the type of activities he selected. The challenge of the equipment and the sheer sensation associated with sliding, jumping, and hanging from the bars may have been sufficient to motivate this 2½ year old. At an older age, he might have been more apt to convert the slide into a car or himself into a superhero. One other aspect of suspension of reality, use of objects in variable or unconventional ways, occurred only some of the time. When Will attempted to use the slide in variable ways, the day-care worker stopped him. Whereas Will did use the insect in varying ways, he really did not use any of the equipment in unconventional ways. These devices are all meant for climbing, sliding, and jumping. Climbing, sliding, and jumping is what he did with them.

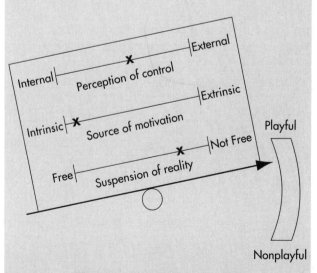

FIG. 4-15 Will's playfulness profile.

TABLE 4-4   Will's Scores on the ToP

TEST OF PLAYFULNESS (ToP)—Adapted

Name: Will	EXTENT	INTENSITY	SKILLFULNESS
Age: 2 1/2 years	3 = Almost always	3 = Highly	3 = Highly skilled
Date: 8/15/94	2 = Much of the time	2 = Moderately	2 = Moderately skilled
Place: daycare playground	1 = Some of the time	1 = Mildly	1 = Slightly skilled
	0 = Rarely or never	0 = Not	0 = Unskilled
	NA = Not Applicable	NA = Not Applicable	NA = Not Applicable

Item	Ext	Int	Skill	Comments
Is actively engaged.	3	3		
Appears self-directed. Decides what to do and how to do it.	3			
Appears to feel safe.	3			
Demonstrates obvious exuberance, manifest joy.	2			
Tries to overcome difficulties, barriers, or obstacles to persist with an activity.		3		
Actively modifies complexity and/or demands of activity.			2	
Engages in mischief or commits a minor infraction of the implicit or explicit rules.	2	2	3	
Repeats actions, activities; stays with same basic theme.	3			
Engages in process aspects of activity.	3			
Pretends.	0		NA	
Incorporates objects or other people into play in novel, imaginative, creative, unconventional, or variable ways.	1			
Engages in challenges (motor, cognitive, or social).	2	2		
Negotiates with others to have needs or desires met.			0	
Plays with others.	3			
Plays interactively with others.	2		3	
Assumes leadership role.	0		NA	
Enters a group already engaged in an activity.			NA	
Initiates play with others.			3	
Teases or jokes with others (verbal or nonverbal).	0	NA	NA	
Clowns.	1			
Shares playthings, play equipment.	3			
Gives facial, verbal, and body cues appropriate to the situation and that say, "This is how you should act toward me."	3			
Responds to others' facial or body cues.	3		3	
Maintains cohesiveness of play frame.	3			

Framing

Will seemed quite good at all the items related to framing. There were no obvious points at which he failed to interact with others in expected ways and it would have been quite easy to know how to interact with him. Further, the play session seemed quite cohesive.

Summary

When viewed summatively, Will's profile describes a relatively playful child. Were he to be observed in an environment more geared toward keeping him safe through means other than controlling his activity (e.g., covering the playground surface with soft landing material), his playfulness might have been even more apparent.

CASE EXAMPLE 2: MEGAN

Megan is a 2½-year-old girl who is experiencing delays across all domains of development. One of Megan's parents greatest concerns is that Megan "does not play well."

Megan was observed at the special education preschool she attends five mornings each week, as she and her classmates engaged in an obstacle course activity. Also involved in the obstacle course were several classmates and four staff members. The obstacle course consisted of three areas: a barrel turned on its side to create a tunnel, a small wooden slide, and a rocker board large enough for four children to sit on simultaneously.

Megan began the obstacle course with the barrel. She crawled into the middle of it, assumed a W sitting posture, and remained there, despite the urgings of a staff member who tried several tactics to entice Megan out of the barrel. Finally, she and the other staff members broke out into song, "Where is Megan, Where is Megan? …" When nothing else worked, the staff member slanted one edge of the barrel slightly, forcing Megan out.

The slide was the next activity in the obstacle course. Megan clearly did not want to go on the slide. She attempted several times to return to the barrel and then just to wander away. A hypervigilant staff member drew Megan back each time by holding her hand or guiding her shoulders. Although Megan did not look happy, she did not protest.

The staff member "facilitated" Megan's ascent up the stairs of the slide by holding her at the hips and shifting her weight. When Megan reached the top of the slide, she sat down with painstaking care and began sliding, her legs widely abducted to control her speed, a look of terror on her face. Despite her caution, Megan nearly fell backward as she slid downward.

The third activity in the obstacle course was the rocker board. As the children sat on the board, a staff member rocked it and sang, "Row, Row, Row Your Boat." Megan approached the board with caution. She waltzed around the edge of it for several seconds asking, "Boat?" One of the two staff members stationed at the rocker board echoed her words. Finally Megan was lifted onto the rocker board where she assumed a W sitting posture. Each time she assumed a W sit, a staff member moved her legs into the long sitting position. However, when Megan attempted to maintain that position, she slowly sunk into the board as it rocked.

Finally free of the board, Megan returned to the barrel. She crawled in the "wrong" end, encountering Ricky, a classmate, halfway. When Ricky exited, Megan moved to the edge of the barrel, poked her head out, and began barking like a dog. Another time, she edged her way out of the barrel and, when "discovered" by a staff member, drew back quickly, a big grin on her face. Unfortunately, the staff member did not pick up on Megan's

peek-a-boo cues. The staff member tried ignoring Megan's obstinate refusal to leave the barrel, but Megan continued to play in the barrel, rocking it slowly and carefully side to side. After a few seconds, the staff member announced that it was time for circle. She again picked up one edge of the barrel, and Megan crawled out reluctantly.

Megan's Playfulness Profile

Megan's scores on the ToP are shown in Table 4-5. Through examination of the scores of the items associated with each of the elements (see Figs. 4-11 through 4-14), a playfulness profile has been created for Megan. This is shown in Fig. 4-16. As with Will, each of the elements of playfulness is discussed separately before summarizing Megan's playfulness profile.

Intrinsic motivation

The mark on the continuum representing motivation is rather far toward the "extrinsic" side. That is, most of Megan's motivation for engaging in the obstacle course seemed to come from outside—primarily from staff members. Although she was doing process-focused activities much of the time, she seemed to have no choice about participating and there was little intensity to her actions. That is, she seemed simply to be "going through the motions." When she wandered off or balked at an activity, a staff member physically manipulated her onto the equipment.

There were a few times when Megan seemed to act out of intrinsic motivation, most notably in the barrel. She seemed then to be seeking interactions typical of much younger children (e.g., peek-a-boo) or low-intensity sensory stimulation (e.g., rocking ever so slightly in the barrel).

Internal control

The marker on the continuum representing control is placed far toward the "external" side. Megan seemed to have little control of her own actions or of the outcomes of the activities. In fact, much of the time she did not even appear to feel safe. Megan did receive a high score on "challenges"; however, it is likely this was artificially inflated since the challenges were imposed externally and seemed far too great for her skills. When she tried to modify the challenges downward (e.g., W sitting), a staff member immediately increased them again. Although Megan did play with other children and thus shared the equipment some of the time, these, too, seemed generally to have been imposed on her.

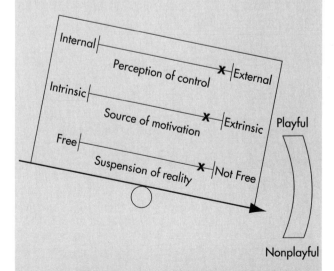

FIG. 4-16 Megan's playfulness profile.

TABLE 4-5   Megan's Scores on the ToP

TEST OF PLAYFULNESS (ToP)—Adapted

Name: Megan Age: 2 1/2 years Date: 7/12/94 Place: preschool classroom	EXTENT 3 = Almost always 2 = Much of the time 1 = Some of the time 0 = Rarely or never NA = Not Applicable	INTENSITY 3 = Highly 2 = Moderately 1 = Mildly 0 = Not NA = Not Applicable	SKILLFULNESS 3 = Highly skilled 2 = Moderately skilled 1 = Slightly skilled 0 = Unskilled NA = Not Applicable

Item	Ext	Int	Skill	Comments
Is actively <u>engaged</u>.	2	0		
Appears <u>self-directed</u>. Decides what to do and how to do it.	0			
Appears to feel <u>safe</u>.	1			
Demonstrates obvious <u>exuberance</u>, manifest joy.	0			
Tries to overcome difficulties, barriers, or obstacles to <u>persist</u> with an activity.		1		
Actively <u>modifies</u> complexity and/or demands of activity.			0	
Engages in <u>mischief</u> or commits a minor infraction of the implicit or explicit rules.	0	NA	NA	
<u>Repeats</u> actions, activities; stays with same basic theme.	2			Staff determined
Engages in <u>process</u> aspects of activity.	2			Staff determined
<u>Pretends</u>.	0		NA	
Incorporates objects or other people into play in novel, imaginative, creative, <u>unconventional</u>, or variable ways.	0			
Engages in <u>challenges</u> (motor, cognitive, or social).	2	3		too great!
<u>Negotiates</u> with others to have needs or desires met.			NA	
<u>Plays</u> <u>with</u> <u>others</u>.	1			
<u>Plays</u> <u>interactively</u> with others.	0		NA	
<u>Assumes</u> <u>leadership</u> role.	0		NA	
<u>Enters</u> a group already engaged in an activity.			0	under duress
<u>Initiates</u> play with others.			0	staff didn't read cues
<u>Teases</u> or <u>jokes</u> with others (verbal or nonverbal).	0	NA	NA	
<u>Clowns</u>.	0			
<u>Shares</u> playthings, play equipment.	1			
<u>Gives</u> facial, verbal, and body <u>cues</u> appropriate to the situation and that say, "This is how you should act toward me."	1			
<u>Responds</u> <u>to</u> others' facial or body <u>cues</u>.	NA			
<u>Maintains</u> cohesiveness of <u>play</u> <u>frame</u>.	NA			set

Suspension of reality

The marker on the continuum representing suspension of reality is placed all the way to the "not free" end. That is, Megan seemed unable to suspend any of the constraints of reality during the obstacle course. She did pretend briefly (i.e., barking like a dog while in the barrel). However, her cues were ignored by the staff. Her feeble attempts at mischief (i.e., remaining in the barrel when she was supposed to move to the next activity) also were largely unsuccessful.

Framing

Although Megan did give out a few relatively subtle cues about how others should interact with her, they went largely unnoticed. Perhaps that was because they tended to reflect the play of children much younger than Megan and thus were "undesirable" behaviors. Megan seemed unaware of any cues given by children around her although there was little encouragement of interaction between the children.

Summary

When viewed summatively, Megan's profile describes a very nonplayful child. Although this profile may reflect Megan's general nature, it also is possible that any tendencies toward playfulness she may have are being "squelched" by an overly controlling human and nonhuman environment.

CONCLUSIONS

In this chapter, it has been argued that play differs in many ways from the other primary occupations. Thus whereas it may be perfectly appropriate to evaluate an individual's abilities in self-care or work by evaluating their performance of self-care or work activities, this approach may not apply well to play. Instead, it may be more important to assess an individual's playfulness than his or her performance of particular play activities. Assessment of playfulness can be done in the context of any activity (play or nonplay). However, the chances of seeing playfulness may be greatest during play.

A model is also provided for the evaluation of playfulness and an assessment is introduced based on that model. Although it is not yet possible to derive meaningful composite scores from the assessment, the model and the assessment items have been used here to illustrate the evaluation of two young children, one developing typically and one experiencing developmental delays.

REVIEW QUESTIONS

1. What is meant by the phrase "operationalizing the elements of playfulness"?
2. Discuss the concept of framing and how it is operationalized in the ToP.
3. What are the four dimensions measured by the Test of Playfulness (ToP)? Define each one, and describe the behaviors and behavioral qualities that each one addresses.
4. How can the ToP be used in clinical practice to generate a playfulness profile for a child? Sketch an example to show a colleague what a playfulness profile may look like.

REFERENCES

Barnett, L. A. (1990). Playfulness: Definition, design, and measurement. *Play & Culture, 3,* 319-336.

Bateson, G. (1971). The message, "this is play." In R. E. Herron & B. Sutton-Smith (Eds.). *Child's play* (pp. 261-269). New York: Wiley & Sons.

Bateson, G. (1972). Toward a theory of play and phantasy. In G. Bateson (Ed.). *Steps to an ecology of the mind* (pp. 14-20). New York: Bantam.

Brooks, L. (1995). *Reliability and validity of the revised Test of Playfulness.* Master's thesis. Colorado State University, Ft. Collins.

Bundy, A. C. (1991). Play theory and sensory integration. In A. G. Fisher, E. A. Murray, & A. C. Bundy (Eds.), *Sensory integration: Theory and practice* (pp. 48-68). Philadelphia: F. A. Davis.

Bundy, A. C. (1992). Play: The most important occupation of children. *Sensory Integration Special Interest Section Newsletter, 15(2),* 1.

Bundy, A. C. (1993). Assessment of play and leisure: Delineation of the problem. *American Journal of Occupational Therapy, 47,* 217-222.

Caillois, R. (1979). *Man, play and games.* New York: Schocken.

Connor, F. P., Williamson, G., & Seipp, J. M. (1978). *Program guide for infants and toddlers with neuromotor and other developmental disabilities.* New York: Teacher's College Press.

Csikszentmihalyi, M. (1975a). *Beyond boredom and anxiety: The experience of play in work and games.* San Francisco: Jossey-Bass.

Csikszentmihalyi, M. (1975b). Play and intrinsic rewards. *Humanistic Psychology, 15(3),* 41-63.

Csikszentmihalyi, M. (1990). *Flow: The psychology of optimal experience.* New York: Harper Perennial.

Fisher, W. P. (1993). Measurement related problems in functional assessment. *American Journal of Occupational Therapy, 47,* 331-338.

Gaik, S., & Rigby, P. (1994). *A pilot study to address the reliability and validity of the Test of Playfulness (ToP)—Research Version 2.2 and to compare the playfulness of children with physical disabilities with age-matched able-bodied peers.* Research report submitted to the Neurodevelopmental Clinical Research Unit. Available from second author, Hugh MacMillan Rehabilitation Centre, 350 Rumsey Rd., Toronto, Ontario, M4G 1R8, Canada.

Harkness, L. (in preparation). *Validity and reliability of the Test of Playfulness with children with disabilities.* Master's thesis. Colorado State University, Ft. Collins.

Hutchinson, G. (1995). *Validity of the Test of Playfulness with toddlers.* Master's thesis. Colorado State University, Ft. Collins.

Kielhofner, G. (Ed.). (1985). *A model of human occupation.* Baltimore: Williams & Wilkins.

Kooij, R. V. (1989). Research on children's play. *Play & Culture, 2,* 20-34.

Kooij, R. V., & Vrijhof, H. J. (1987). Play and development. *Topics in learning Disabilities, 1,* 57-67.

Lawlor, M. C., & Henderson, A. (1989). A descriptive study of the clinical practice patterns of occupational therapists working with infants and young children. *American Journal of Occupational Therapy, 43,* 755-764.

Lieberman, J. N. (1977). *Playfulness: Its relationship to imagination and creativity.* New York: Academic Press.

McNicholas, B. (1995). *Environmental influences on a test of playfulness.* Master's thesis. University of Illinois at Chicago.

Metzger, P. (1993). *Validity and reliability of a test of playfulness.* Unpublished masters thesis. University of Illinois at Chicago.

Morrison, C. D., Bundy, A. C., & Fisher, A. G. (1991). The contribution of motor skills and playfulness to the play performance of preschoolers. *American Journal of Occupational Therapy, 45,* 687-694.

Neumann, E. A. (1971). *The elements of play.* New York: MSS Information.

Rubin, K., Fein, G. G., & Vandenberg, B. (1983). Play. In P. H. Mussen (Ed.). *Handbook of child psychology: Vol. 4, Socialization, personality and social development* (4th ed., pp. 693-774). New York: Wiley.

Stone, F. (1991). *A descriptive study of the use of play in occupational therapy.* Unpublished masters thesis. University of Illinois at Chicago.

Tyler, R. G. (in preparation). Influence of gender and environment on the Test of Playfulness. Master's thesis. Colorado State University, Ft. Collins.

White, R. (1959). Motivation reconsidered: The concept of competence. *Psychological Review, 66,* 297-323.

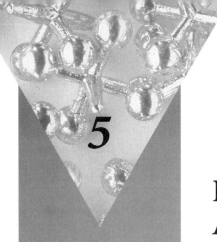

5

FAMILY NARRATIVES AND PLAY ASSESSMENT

Janice Posatery Burke and Roseann C. Schaaf

A life lived is what actually happened. A life experienced consists of the images, feelings, sentiments, desires, thoughts, and meanings known to the person whose life it is…A life as told, a life history, is a narrative, influenced by the cultural conventions of telling, by the audience, and by the social context. (Bruner, 1984, p. 7)

As we move toward the twenty-first century, occupational therapy services continue to evolve and expand. Therapists find themselves surrounded by a myriad of social, cultural, economic, political, and pragmatic issues that affect the children they serve and the service they deliver. How therapists are to integrate these modern-day demands with their professional commitment to the occupational needs of children and their families is one of the major challenges to the field today.

In sorting through the complex issues that have impacts on service delivery during these volatile days of health care reform, therapists must constantly weigh children's needs with service delivery parameters. Among the most pressing delivery forces to be reckoned with are the demands to reconfigure practices to provide effective and efficient service. These must be carefully considered in relation to therapist's professional focus on the occupational roles of children: player, family member, student, and friend. This chapter seeks to identify a strategy for maintaining an occupational therapy focus on the occupational roles of children and families as the primary forces for setting the context for a child's growth and development. With this dual focus an occupational therapy approach to play assessment is considered that uses techniques and methods derived from a narrative perspective.

Play is a primary occupation of childhood and has been recognized and appreciated as such especially within the occupational therapy literature (Florey, 1971, 1981; Reilly, 1974; Takata, 1969, 1974). A consideration of play within the context of the family life story allows the therapist to see the child as part of a family unit, where certain behaviors and activities are more highly valued than others. Intervention that is aimed at the major occupational roles of the child, that of the player, interwoven into a particular family pattern gleaned through the family story (use of narrative techniques) is the approach endorsed in this chapter.

EXTERNAL FORCES SHAPING OCCUPATIONAL THERAPY

The multidimensional quality of occupational therapy practice calls for understanding the whole person, for looking at the everyday adaptive demands put on the individual so as to create opportunities for growth and change. In addition to thinking about children and their environments, occupational therapists are finding themselves considering shrinking health care dollars, greater demands for their time to be used effectively and efficiently (i.e., seeing more patients for shorter lengths of time), administrative directives that ask them to move toward consultative models and managed care models, and pressure from third-party payers. This complicated picture of health care delivery requires a shift in treatment priorities, patterns of practice, and strategies for solving patient needs.

Legislative mandates such as those found in PL 102-119 (The Individuals with Disabilities Education Act Amendments [IDEA], 1991), serve as an example of an external force that is also contributing to a reshaping and restructuring of pediatric occupational therapy. No longer satisfied with a traditional model of treatment, wherein the therapists as the experts provide one-to-one intervention based on goals that have been developed and designed by them, the new public law directs therapists to provide family-centered care. This family-driven intervention includes goals that have been generated through a process of collaboration and mutual problem solving by a team that has the family as a central participant. This new profile of collaboration has asked occupational therapists to think, work, and communicate in ways that support the reconfigured form and structure of the collaborative team (Burke & Schaaf, in preparation). But how do therapists open their thinking to incorporate such a radically different approach to care? How do they ensure that they can positively affect a child's occupations as player? How do therapists successfully move from the role of expert to one of collaborator? How do they successfully embrace family members as equal partners? How do therapists design intervention that addresses the family as a unique social and cultural unit? To begin, therapists will need to broaden their thinking about families, and then add to their repertoire of interactional and communication skills to develop new and innovative approaches to play assessment.

CURRENT DAY PRACTICE PROBLEMS

In pediatric practice today, therapists commonly observe and assess children using many formal and informal instruments to understand deficit states such as limited play interactions, sensory integration dysfunction, gross and fine motor delays, and difficulties in acquiring social, cognitive, and adaptive skills. Following assessment, therapists are then faced with the formidable challenge of transforming their findings into intervention plans. It is not uncommon, however, for therapists to find that their intervention plans are unsuccessful, primary caregivers are overwhelmed with their already full schedules, families are unable to work with their child who reportedly becomes fussy and uncooperative, or families try to implement plans but can't seem to do it "the right way." In turn, therapists may become disheartened with parents who do not follow their home programs, labeling them noncompliant and resistant or as lacking follow through.

Among the reasons that contribute to this lack of connection between the therapist's assessment of a child's problem and the parent's concerns is the therapist's failure to consider the child within the context of the family. This includes recognition of a family's values, goals, and aspirations for their child, for other siblings, and for the family itself along with the realities of that family's life. Without fully exploring these concerns, the therapist has created an intervention plan in a vacuum and has failed to set the problems that truly have meaning for this child and this family, given the context of their lives. Schön (1983) has written about this critical phase of professional problem setting process using the notion of "naming and framing." For Schön, professionals must be careful to "name the things to which [they] will attend" and "frame the context in which [they] will attend to" (p. 40).

It is the contention of the authors of this chapter that several important ingredients are missing from the assessment and intervention plan that has been outlined above. First and foremost, it must be remembered that the primary membership for children is that of family and that each family has its own unique system of communicating and behaving, of setting priorities and goals. When therapists fail to interview parents and other key family members as part of their assessment they have excluded critical information. Second, these authors believe serious consideration must be made of children within their occupational roles (player and family member). Armed with these two additional ingredients, the child as a member of a family and as a player, the therapist is more likely to deliver a relevant and useful assessment. But how are these viewpoints transformed into a useful approach to assessment?

In this chapter storytelling is proposed as a strategy for therapists who wish to address physical, psychosocial, and cognitive needs of a child while placing these needs within the context of the realities of any given family. Storytelling provides the platform for the therapist to ask Who is this family? Who is this child? What is this family asking for? What can I do to help this family and child?

It is these authors' belief that the most effective approach to assessment is for therapists to develop the knowledge and skills that allow them to identify the key issues for any given child and family and design an effective plan to address those issues. This means providing the most relevant and meaningful therapy possible given the parameters of the intervention demands. These authors further contend that a focus by therapists on play offers a particularly insightful mechanism for understanding and interacting with families and children

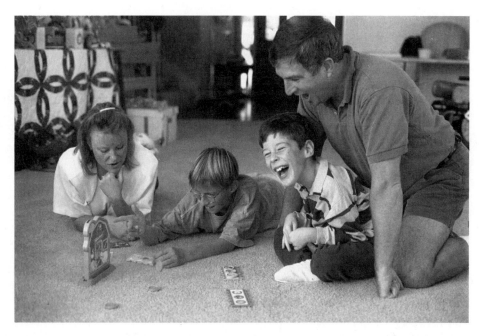

FIG. 5-1   A family-centered, narrative approach entails seeing the child as a family member and player, rather than as a diagnosis. (Courtesy Shay McAtee.)

with respect for, recognition of, and emphasis on the culturally, ethnic, and socially driven values of a family.

CENTERING THE FAMILY IN CARE

The family-centered legislation directs therapists to see the child as part of a family unit. In their interpretation of this mandate, Hanft et al. (1992) called attention to the following key components of family:

- Each family is a unique interactional system that can be described through its members, organization, and behavior.
- Families have routines and traditions that help them maintain their equilibrium or status quo.
- Families have imaginary boundaries that, together with their family rules, let members know how to behave within their system or subsystem.
- Just as individuals proceed through developmental stages, families move through a "life cycle".

Congruent with a focus on the family, occupational therapists are finding great utility in the view of the child as an occupational being with definable roles and skills that permit successful enactment of these roles. Now, instead of seeing a child through her diagnosis, "a 3 year old with Down syndrome and moderate retardation," the child is cast in her occupational roles as "Marie, the youngest child in a family of four, player, and preschooler in an early intervention center."

This broadened view of role behavior within a family unit is complemented by the use of a narrative approach. Narrative calls for understanding a person within the context of his or her life story (Fig. 5-1). It provides a valuable strategy for developing a fuller picture of the kinds of behaviors and activities that are most important for children to learn given

their particular life situations. A child, Marie, for example, is now seen in the context of her family and the occupational roles she holds in it. She is the youngest member of a large extended family. The children in the family are valued for their playfulness and enthusiasm for fun. The family cherishes their time spent together and frequently uses weekends and holidays for outings such as trips to the zoo, picnics at the beach, and walks to the park.

USING NARRATIVE TO UNDERSTAND INDIVIDUAL EXPERIENCE

How Humans Make Meaning

Advocating for a contemporary understanding of the importance of meaning in individual lives and the "processes and transactions involved in the construction of meanings," Bruner (1990, p. 33) calls for a folk psychology. This orientation allows us to focus on the autobiographies each of us constructs and carries in our own minds, stories that form a personal point of meaning but also a cultural cohesion.

Folk psychology consists of culturally shaped notions that individuals use to "organize their views of themselves, of others, and of the world in which they live" (Bruner, 1990, p. 137). Folk psychology is a:

> set of more or less connected, more or less normative descriptions about how human beings "tick," what our own and other minds are like, what one can expect situated action to be like, what are possible modes of life, how one commits oneself to them, and so on. (p. 35)

Folk psychology is organized by individuals using narrative and storytelling (including myths). Using stories, our

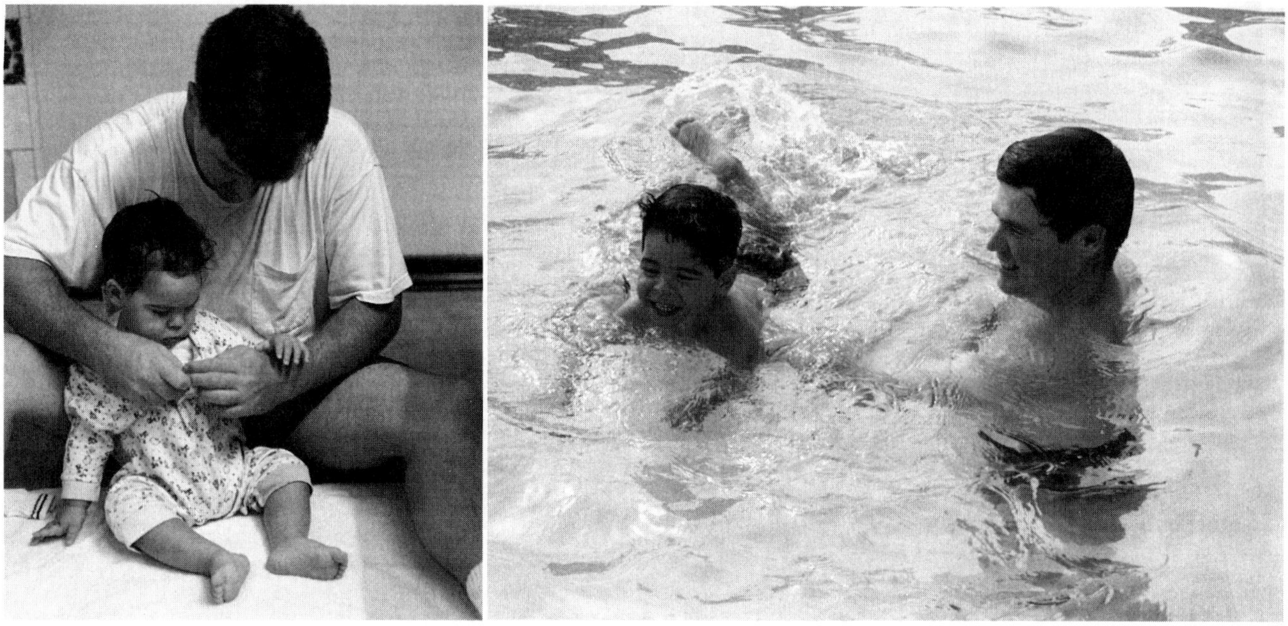

FIG. 5-2 Narratives capture the moments that leave marks on people's lives. These moments may be part of the everyday routine **(A)** or they may be emergent in novel or unstructured situations, as when a child performs a new skill for the first time **(B)**. (Courtesy Shay McAtee.)

lives take on a meaning based on a shared "cultural system of interpretation" (Bruner, 1990, p. 33). The cultural system serves as a model for imposing various patterns on the unfolding story. These patterns are deeply embedded with meanings. As meanings are learned and internalized they become guides and controls for actions. A self grows from "experience in a world of meanings, images and social bonds, in which all persons are inevitably involved" (Rosaldo, 1984, p. 139).

Humans frame their life experiences into storied form to ensure that the event, experience, or feeling is remembered. Valued objects, places, and experiences are preserved in stories that illustrate their importance and meaning to a person, and in this way they help in the development of the self (Rosaldo, 1984, p. 135). In addition, Bruner (1990) suggests that narratives are useful vehicles for "negotiating and renegotiating meanings by the mediation of narrative interpretation" (p. 67). When stories are told to others they are "in some deep sense a joint product of the teller and the told" (p. 124), underscoring the importance of the "transaction" between the parties.

Narratives are particularly meaningful when they capture "moments of crisis. . . [and] alter the fundamental meaning structures in a person's life" (Denzin, 1989, p. 70). Called "epiphanies," these narratives capture the "interactional moments and experiences which leave marks on people's lives" (p. 70). Denzin uses this notion to capture the everyday "ritualized" experiences as well as the "totally emergent and unstructured" (p. 71). In whatever situation, epiphanies allow people to convey meanings and to "relive and reexperience" (p. 71) something that has happened through a narrated story (Fig. 5-2, *A* and *B*.).

The families occupational therapists work with have had significant experiences that have marked their lives and shaped their stories. That therapists can draw out the meaning of these events through stories provides them with an exciting methodology for designing uniquely individual models of care. Parents who are able to tell a therapist about their shock and disappointment of first learning that their newborn child was disabled as well as their surprise and hope when their child later learned to sit up, played peek-a-boo, or showed his or her awareness of music are supplying the richly detailed information that allows the therapist to understand how families construct their lives, the kinds of behaviors that they hold in highest regard, and what they look for and value in their children.

Stories also provide ways to understand a person as an individual with a social and culturally constructed structure (Denzin, 1989). They provide opportunities to see the culturally specific actions, behaviors, and reciprocity of motives that drive individual meanings (Burke, 1993a). Let us turn next to an examination of the role of the therapist in understanding meaning.

Connected Knowing As a Way to Uncover Meaning

Within the feminist stream of literature, authors have looked at the type of knowledge that is valued by different types of people. One such type has been termed "connected knowing." "Connected knowing" refers to a way of understanding a person as a person, "an attempt to achieve a kind of harmony with another person in spite of difference and distance, . . . to enter the other person's frame to discover the

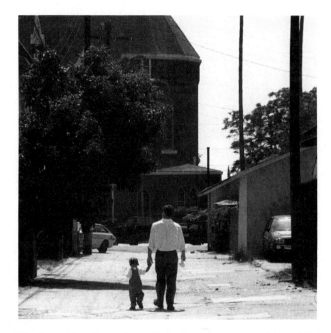

FIG. 5-3   Use of narratives allows therapists to move beyond their stereotypical views of family life. One kind of nontraditional family, for example, consists of father and child. (Courtesy Shay McAtee.)

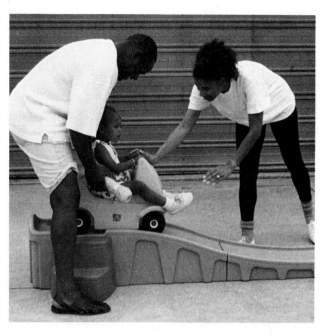

FIG. 5-4   Inquiries about play lead to greater understanding of the family's values and goals by revealing how the family defines fun, how its members spend time together, and what play environments and materials are accessed by them. (Courtesy Shay McAtee.)

premises for the other's point of view" (Belenky et al., 1986, p. 101). This way of knowing is differentiated from an impersonal, autonomous, or separate orientation or what is termed a "separate knowing."

It is the notion of connected knowing that provokes scholars to become intrigued with alternative ways of understanding the world, with individual experience and thought as compared to traditional "hard" or positivist logic. "Connected knowing builds on the subjectivists' conviction that the most trustworthy knowledge comes from personal experience rather than the pronouncements of authorities" (Belenky et al., 1986, p. 113).

In addition to this view of other ways of knowing, connected knowers seek to uncover methods for "gaining access to other people's knowledge" (Belenky et al., 1986, p. 113). As a centerpiece for this process, connected knowers believe "to understand another person's ideas is to try to share the experience that has led the person to form the idea" (Belenky et al., 1986, p. 113). In a connected knower dialogue, talk is found that is "intimate rather than impersonal, relatively informal and unstructured rather than bound by more or less explicit rules" (Belenky et al., 1986, p. 114). Similarly, connected knowers spend more time listening to others and are nonjudgmental. When occupational therapists incorporate these types of ideas, they move away from the professional authority role wherein they impose a quantitative view on the child and family and move toward an orientation that asks, How is this family unit special? What matters most to this family? What occupational therapy information, skills, and techniques may be helpful to this family as they move toward their goals? For one family, mealtime may be a highly valued activity because both mother and father have always considered this to be a nurturing and emotionally enriched

interaction. Another family may take all of their meals separately, valuing the social and emotional quality of such activity very little, but may instead place preference on playful interactions that occur in the evening after bathtime and before bed. Yet another family may value weekly worship services, holidays, and other similar special occasions as a time for the family to gather as a unit.

The use of narratives and life stories provides a way to understand children and families in the context of their social, economic, political, and cultural world and allows therapists to move beyond their stereotypical views of how family life is constructed and enacted, leaving behind value judgments about who should be in a family and what a family should do with its time (Fig. 5-3). For example, a common stereotype is that families have two parents, they spend time together in the evenings and weekends, they go on vacations to the mountains and to the grandparents for Thanksgiving, and they like to go camping in the summer and sledding in the winter. A family story perspective invites a positive, value-free inquiry that asks, Who is this family? What do they like to do? What kind of activity is the most meaningful? What activities are the most important? the most fun?

Play provides a unique window into the life of the child and family (Schaaf & Mulrooney, 1989; D'Eugenio, 1986). Given that people interact in patterns of behavior that are culturally meaningful, the ways a family engages in play can be expected to reflect their culturally driven values and purposes. Inquiries about play offer opportunities to understand the specific ways a family spends time; how it defines fun; the type of interactions, toys, and play materials that are most valued; and the availability and use of play environments (see Fig. 5-4). This culturally oriented glimpse into a family's life also provides a way to understand the environmental forces that shape play.

WITHIN OCCUPATIONAL THERAPY: A VIEW OF PLAY

In a modernized interpretation of occupational therapy, Mary Reilly (1971) urged her contemporaries to move beyond the medical orientation on pathology so as to get at the real problems of their patients—the occupational dysfunction that was experienced when a person became disabled or chronically ill. For Reilly, such a proposal "would include not only the concerns for pathology correction but also for habit restructuring and for the environmental engineering of the opportunities and rewards associated with life adaptation" (p. 245).

Using the organizing principle of role behavior Reilly conceptualized the unique and vital focus for the profession as the occupational behavior of persons with disability and disease. Early in the development of this concept Reilly (1962) suggested that humans have "a vital need for occupation and that [their] central nervous system demands the rich and varied stimuli that solving life problems provides . . . This is the basic need that occupational therapy ought to be serving" (p. 5) to facilitate the healing process in their patients.

Reilly conceptualized occupational roles along a continuum associated with various stages in the evolution of an individual's development, for example the occupational roles of player, student, worker, and retiree. Each role provides opportunities for important learning and practice to ensure success in each of the subsequent roles to be acquired. Reilly wrote, "a child's ability to play, to explore his environment, to exercise his motor skills are the foundation for his later school experiences. The problem-solving processes and the creativity exercised in school work, craft and hobby experiences are the necessary preparations for the later demands of the work world" (p. 6). For Reilly and her associates (Bailey, 1971; Florey, 1971; Matsutsuyu, 1971; Shannon, 1972; Sundstrom, 1972; Takata, 1969), play was conceptualized as a primary occupation of childhood that not only ensured human adaptation but also provided the critical foundation for later childhood, adolescent, and adult successes.

Play As a Marker in Childhood Role Behavior

In numerous exploratory studies and through assessments developed by occupational behaviorists, exemplars of successful player role enactment have been uncovered. These included the importance of human interactions, play with nonhumans, and the physical environments as well as creativity and individual style as demonstrated in preferences and experiences (Burke, 1993b; Florey, 1981; Hurff, 1974; Knox, 1974; Michelman, 1974; Takata, 1974).

As people move about their lives they create experiences that allow them to find meaning and realize their values. Those events and experiences are socially and culturally con-

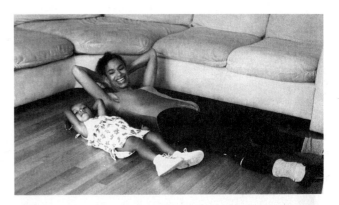

FIG. 5-5 Stories concerning the child's role as player reflect the values, interests, and meanings of the family. A favorite story for the mother in this photograph is how one day her toddler spontaneously and enthusiastically joined in with her exercise routine. This is a particularly meaningful occupation for this mother, who is a performing dancer. (Courtesy Shay McAtee.)

structed and form a pattern of stories reflecting their importance. For young families, stories concerning the child's primary occupational role as player prove to be particularly useful for understanding family culturally derived values, interests, and meanings (Fig. 5-5).

DISABILITY AND FAMILY STORIES

People reflect their everyday experiences, their hopes for the future, and their memories of the past through stories. Storytelling is a basic human way of dealing with reality. All people form stories about their pasts, presents, and futures. Through stories, people chronicle their lives, remembering and reminiscing about the past, marking significant events as they unfold, and spinning the dreams of their futures (Burke, 1993a). Families are immersed in the storytelling process as they plan and ready themselves for a baby's birth. A parent remembers the birth of sisters and brothers, cousins and neighbors and begins to construct a tale about the soon-to-be birth of his or her own child. Using culturally, ethnically, and socially constructed value systems the parent tells him or herself stories about who this child will be, special qualities that the child will have, how life will unfold (Burke, 1993a). Stories such as "My little girl will love her older sister; they will do everything together and be best friends" or "My son will love to play with cars and trucks, and when he is old enough we'll make models together and race them" are typical of how parents begin to picture their futures.

For some people the storyline may already be established when the child is born (Fig. 5-6). Although minor modifications may be in order when the child is not the imagined sex, size, or temperament, these parents for the most part hold to the storyline they have created about their child and family life, and they work hard to see that the story unfolds as expected (Burke, 1993a). At the other end of the continuum, some new parents may have only a vague notion about their

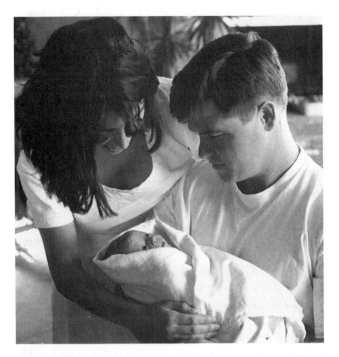

FIG. 5-6 For many parents, a storyline about who their child will be is already established by the time the child is born. (Courtesy Shay McAtee.)

child's story but soon find it is quickly filled in as the baby is born and moves into their life.

The reality of the birth of a disabled, premature, high-risk, or otherwise ill baby wreaks havoc on both ends of the storyline continuum. Parents are typically unprepared for the dramatic changes in plot and storyline that they face and often have few experiences to draw on as they search for clues to how to think about and respond to the situation. In ways that are similar to the dilemmas of adults who recount their own struggles with illness and disability (Frank, 1991; Price, 1994), parents also search for ways to understand what is happening to their family and how their experiences are going to have an impact on their life story. Questions as basic as whether the child will live or die, be able to walk and talk, play with other children, dress her- or himself, and go to school dominate and threaten their life world. In such instances, parents are faced with the task of refabricating and reconstructing a new, tentative, or interim story about their child so as to begin to integrate the experience into their lives (Burke, 1993a).

These situations are often even more complex when parents have very little experience with the issues they are facing, never having known an infant with a similar diagnosis, having few interactions with people who are disabled, and having few past experiences with health care professionals. Frequently, parents expect that their child will be like another they know, the only similarity being the term "disabled or special needs," while not realizing the great variation that is inherent in such a label. In these types of situations parents may be at a loss when it comes to generating storylines and scenarios for family life with a child who has special needs. Parents and caregivers may ask, will I ever play with

my child? Will he or she be able to climb on the jungle gym, ride on the carousel?

STORYTELLING AS A STRATEGY FOR OCCUPATIONAL THERAPISTS

Storytelling gives therapists a method for entering into and assisting a family as it begins to construct a vision for the future. Stories have been documented as an effective clinical strategy for problem solving among therapists, and between therapists and patients. "The narrative nature…manifests itself not only in the work therapists do to understand the effect of a disability in the life story of a particular patient, but also in the therapist's need to structure therapy in a narrative way, as an unfolding story" (Mattingly, 1991, p. 1000).

A narrative approach requires that therapists take the time to examine two points of view, one of the person receiving the care, and the other of the professional delivering it. From the patient's point of view the therapist would ask, "What does this person want?" to gain a greater understanding needs, motives, and individual meanings. Taking the practitioner's perspective the therapist would ask, "What can this person give?" This opening to narrative material may provide the tools for examining and charting the boundaries that encircle treatment (Burke & Frank, 1994).

Techniques that include the use of settings, materials, or props may prove to further facilitate the eliciting of the patient's story. In her work with children and families Shirley Kramer devised an assessment tool called "A 'Snapshot' and 'The Developing Picture' " (Hanft, et al., 1992). Using a piece of paper to represent a page from a scrapbook the therapist asks parents "to close their eyes and capture the very first visualization which comes to them when they think about [their] child." In the second part of the assessment, the parent is asked to "think about the 'snapshot' you just took. How would you like to see [it] change or develop?" (Appendix J) In both situations Kramer uses the scrapbook page as a physical prompt to evoke in a sense a "story" of family life, goals and dreams, and fears and problems as they are experienced now and as they look in the distant future. It is through this family story that therapists may find a prime entry point for assisting the family as it struggles with a particular dilemma the members wish to resolve in order to reach their future dream (My son is sitting in his highchair drinking from a cup, My daughter is riding a trike by herself, He's holding a pencil and writing his name). Because this assessment focuses on a picture that the family selects as meaningful, the therapist is more assured that intervention, consultation, and collaboration are considered valuable to the family. In the instance of working with children and their families two primary stories emerge: the story for the family and child, and the story for the therapist. The family and child story is considered the same unit, especially during the early years, since young children are thought to follow the story as it is constructed by the family.

With this expanded view of the person's story, the therapist begins to infer, examine, and understand motives; works to understand how a person feels; and forms a realistic picture of a person's illness experience as well as the therapist's own experience of treating the person. This ability to move closer to the intimacy of the illness experience and away from the sterility of a pathology focus so prevalent in medicine allows for a "sympathetic accompaniment" (Frank, 1991) with the patient that further legitimizes the illness experience (Kleinman, 1988).

Narrative and storytelling provide occupational therapists with an opportunity to develop a family-centered plan for intervention. Using such an approach the therapist moves away from seeing each treatment interaction as an individual experience where skill acquisition is noted within the occupational therapy (OT) setting. In contrast, the use of narrative allows the therapist to focus on interactions and interventions as a series of events that tie together within the OT environment and beyond. The therapist in this instance moves away from seeing Joey as a participant in OT, showing gains in fine motor skills as evidenced by a more mature pincer grasp when using the therapy putty, or showing gains in attention as demonstrated by an increase in concentration up to 5 or 6 minutes while balancing on the surfboard. Instead, this therapist sees this child as developing play skills to support age-appropriate play behaviors and family roles that require fine motor and attention skills. Given this orientation, the therapist talks regularly with the family to gain its members' perceptions of whether the skills noted in the treatment are generalizing to valued family activities at home. This view provides an opportunity to see interactions with patients as unfolding (Joey is becoming more of a neighborhood player) rather than fixed and to some extent predictable (Joey holds objects using a unrefined three-finger grasp and will improve to a mature grasp within 6 weeks). In this way, storytelling allows health care providers to acknowledge how much they rely on stories to understand the children and families that they treat, how profound the effect of illness and disability is on a family's life and on the way children play, and how illness affects the meaning and purpose of everyday lives.

For people with chronic illness, being ill is just another way of living (Frank, 1991). Although difficult for practitioners with a strictly medical orientation to acknowledge and accept, life with illness requires patients and their families to think about and act on ways to lessen the interruptions or minimize the inconveniences of poor health while still providing opportunities to live active and engaged lives. This requires moving away from placing people in categories of disease to seeing each person as an individual with particular feelings and experiences and with a family who are the "other halves" (Frank, 1991) of the illness experience.

Therapists can create stories in a process of "narratively structured treatment" (Mattingly, 1991, p. 1003) in an effort to center on the individual. By combining expertise in assessment of functional skills and observations of interactions in the human and nonhuman environment with an analysis of play as occupation, and with stories gathered from the family, the therapist begins to create a story about the child. Along with creating a story of the child and family, the narrative approach gives the therapist a strategy "to structure therapy in a narrative way, as an unfolding story" (Mattingly, 1991, p. 1000). For example, given a family story that indicated value placed on family outings, the therapist might develop intervention strategies that assisted the family in meeting their goals, such as providing an adaptive car seating for a child with severe spasticity or suggesting strategies for keeping a child with sensory defensiveness calm during a car ride.

Establishing Startpoints in Assessment

Occupational therapists traditionally have utilized both formalized and nonformalized methods of assessment. An important adjunct to traditional types of data gathering can be found in play observations and dialogues with the child and family in their natural environments. Through nonintrusive observation and documentation of play in a child's natural environment, valuable information regarding the child's ability to enact player and family roles is collected (Burke, 1993b). Information such as the use of play objects, play spaces, play interactions, and play opportunities is easily derived through such play observation and dialogues. By approaching the concept of play as a view to a child's competence, we are able to enter a child's world for the purpose of collecting important information that will contribute "to design[ing] and develop[ing] activities that will be role-specific and address underlying areas of need" (Schaaf and Burke, 1992, p. 1).

Play observation and history taking (dialogues) have proved to be valuable tools for occupational therapy. Takata (1969) recommended taking a play history to gain information regarding the materials, actions, people, and settings that are part of the child's play environment. Findings from the history can be analyzed using a taxonomy of play that classifies play behaviors according to ages and stages of play. (see Chapter 2). D'Eugenio (1986), Schaaf and Mulrooney (1989), and Schaaf and Burke (1992) have elaborated on the concept of play observation as a "window" that allows the therapist to collect information on both a child's competence in occupation and the underlying obstacles to successful occupational role enactment. Schaaf and Mulrooney (1989) specifically developed a framework for assessment of young children that utilized play observation as a means of gaining insight into the child's strengths and needs, as well as a means of assessing the environmental issues that had an impact on the child's ability to play. They recommended incorporating play into both assessment and intervention to enhance overall development and skills. Such occupational therapy–based approaches to play provide a suitable foundation for incorporating family narratives into both assessment and treatment.

Sample Storylines about Play

To examine the use of narrative and storytelling as a strategy for providing meaningful family-centered care, two types of storylines are next discussed as they have an impact on play behavior. These storylines illustrate the intimate relationship between specific neurologically based problems (as manifested in sensory processing and temperament characteristics) and general play behaviors. Each demonstrates the profound effects of dysfunction on the development and enactment of occupation. These storylines are first examined in light of their impact on play behavior and are later used in the presentation of case stories.

Storyline 1. Play and Sensory Processing Issues. The viewpoint of play as a reflection of the child's ability to process and integrate sensory information for adaptive behavior was introduced by Ayres (1972) as part of the sensory integrative process. She set forth the supposition that play was reflective of the child's sensorimotor systems and that difficulty in integrating and processing sensory information would result in difficulty interacting in the environment in activities such as play. A child with normal sensory integration, Ayres felt, would seek play experiences to further growth and development; on the other hand, a child with dysfunction in sensory integration would often avoid or not know how to engage in normal growth-perpetuating play experiences. A child with a dysfunction may seek ways to fulfill the intrinsic need for environmental and sensory input, but these may be maladaptive in nature. These concepts were further explored by Schaaf et al. (1987) in two case studies that examined the relationship of play behavior to sensory integration. These studies found that when children with sensory integrative dysfunction components to their disability were involved in a therapeutic program which addressed their underlying sensory integrative needs, they demonstrated positive changes in play behavior over the course of therapy.

A narrative approach can serve to broaden the occupational therapist's application of sensory integrative theory. Specifically, it assists the therapist in formulating a story about a child that incorporates specific sensory processing information into a broader perspective of the child as a player and family member (Box 5-1).

Storyline 2. Play and Temperament Issues. Building on the notion that play is a reflection of underlying neurobehavioral substrates, the examination of individual temperament as an important influence on play provides a critical approach to the examination of a child's story. Play observation can provide a valuable means for gaining information about factors related to temperament, such as the capacity for self-regulation, engagement, attention, and action (Anzalone, 1994). Authors such as Porges (1993), Brazelton and Lester (1983), Als (1986), Bates (1989), and Carey (1983) have directed attention to the relationship of temperament to later behavioral styles such as those observed

> **Box 5-1**
>
> **COLLECTING SENSORY PROCESSING INFORMATION**
>
> Does the child:
>   tolerate various types of sensory input?
>   crave certain types of stimulation?
>   avoid specific sensory inputs?
>   use self-stimulating behaviors?
>   seem fearful of movement?
>   avoid balance activities?
>   use hands for tactile exploration?
>   show variety in types of activities in terms of sensory input?
> In addition, the therapist will ask:
>   What is the family's definition of this child's problem?
>   What are the family's beliefs about the origins or reasons for the problem?
>   What are the typical interactions that occur within the everyday life of this family?
>   How does this child respond to these interactions?
>   How would the family like things to be different? Which specific interactions are identified as suitable for change?
>   What are the times, preferences, and points in the day that the family finds appropriate to work on specific interactions they have identified?

in play. Using a model developed by Chess and Thomas (1989), these authors conceptualize temperament as an expression of an underlying reactive or self-regulatory process. The child demonstrates either maladaptive, avoidance responses to environmental–sensory input or adaptive, approach responses toward the people and objects in the environment.

The impact of sensory processing and temperament on play is implied using the terminology "goodness of fit," which refers to the match between the child and the environment. A goodness of fit occurs when "capacities, motivation, and temperament are adequate to master the demands, expectations, and opportunities to promote positive development," whereas a poorness of fit occurs when the "child's characteristics are inadequate to master environmental challenges and leads to maladaptive functioning and distorted development" (Chess and Thomas, 1989, p. 380). This concept of fit implies a strong relationship between the child's temperament and his or her ability to interact with the environment in positive, growthperpetuating ways, such as through play. Because play is related to temperament, observations of the child's capacity for self-regulation, engagement, attention, and action provide valuable cues about a child's areas of strength and need.

To understand the impact of temperament on the child's story the therapist can use play observation as well as interview to collect specific information (Box 5-2). This information is integrated with other assessment findings to provide a fuller understanding of the child as player and family member.

Making Observations About Play

Along with providing insight into the child's sensory integrative abilities and temperament, observation of play also provides cues to the child's interests and ability to socialize, attend, use manipulative skills, use large motor skills, and interact with objects and people in the environment. Information in these areas can be gained by considering the child's skills, habits, routines, and interests. Box 5-3 represents a compilation of inquiries about these aspects of the child's play.

Additional areas to consider when collecting information about a child's play include issues related to skill development and the environment (Box 5-4). Further guidelines for appraising the impact of the human and nonhuman environments on a child's play are included in Box 5-5.

The child's story is formulated based on interviews and play observations as well as the use of assessment instruments that collect and analyze traditional performance-based information (Fig. 5-7). Similarly, a family story is formed as a result of interactions with the family. Key factors related to these stories are considered using the matrix depicted in Fig. 5-8. The use of this type of framework provides a method for prioritizing observations made of the child with the concerns of the family. In this way, areas such as strengths and needs of the child as observed in human and nonhuman environments are combined with the priorities and values from the family story to identify plans for occupational therapy input.

The Therapist's Story

Information about the childs' story, as gained through play observation, is considered with the family story to create a therapist's story. In part, the goal of this story is to provide a

---

Box 5-2 **TEMPERAMENT, PLAY, AND BEHAVIOR**

Is there an inherent rhythmicity in this child's play or is the play scattered and disorganized?

Does this child appear comfortable and confident in play environments? How is this enacted?

How does this child make the transition from one activity to the next?

How does this child make the transition through quiet play to active play?

What level of arousal does this child demonstrate during play?

Does this child demonstrate strategies for self-calming or self-organization to regain composure after a period of disorganization?

Does the child stay organized during changes in the levels of environmental stimuli? during periods where multiple stimuli are present?

Does the environment support or inhibit playful interactions?

Box 5-3 **PUTTING IT ALL TOGETHER IN PLAY**

ATTENTION: Is the child able to attend to stimuli in the environment? sustain attention? for what amount of time?

EXPLORATION: Does the child explore objects and people in the environment?

MANIPULATION: How does the child manipulate objects?

INITIATION: Does the child demonstrate intrinsic motivation to initiate play? in what type of situations? with whom?

DEMONSTRATING VARIETY: Does the child play with a variety of toys?

DIVERSITY: Does the child demonstrate diversity in play? Does the child use toys and objects in different ways?

INTERACTION: Does the child include others in play? Who are the others? When does this occur?

CREATIVITY: Does the child create play spaces and objects from the environment?

Box 5-4 **SKILL DEVELOPMENT AND THE ENVIRONMENT**

SKILLS
Does the child have the skills to support play?
Gross motor skills?
Fine motor skills?
Visual skills?
Language and cognitive skills?

ENVIRONMENT
What kinds of people are present and available for play?

What kinds of nonhuman factors are present or available for the child?

What is the relationship between the internal (motivation) and the external (environmental press)? How does this affect this child's play?

Do the child's play spaces facilitate or stifle play?

Do the available toys facilitate or stifle play?

Is the environment safe for play?

Is the environment organized for play?

PLAY ENVIRONMENTS

PLAY ENVIRONMENT: NONHUMAN
Are the basic needs of the family being met in terms of adequate food, clothing, housing, nurturing, and caring?

What are the child's main play environments including the home, day-care or school?

Is there adequate physical space for play?

Are there safety hazards in the play environment?

Is there any organization to the play environment in terms of toys or play spaces?

Are toys accessible to the child?

Are developmentally appropriate toys available to the child?

Is there freedom to explore the environment?

Is the level of stimulation in the environment conducive to play or is there lack of stimulation, or overstimulation, in the environment?

Are there established routines for sleeping and feeding?

PLAY ENVIRONMENT: HUMAN
Do the people in the child's environments (parents, teachers, caregivers) value play? what kind of play?

Are play interactions and synchrony (i.e., responsiveness to child's cues, availability to the child) evident?

Are there opportunities for the child to interact with or play with others?

FIG. 5-7 A matrix of the child's story.

FIG. 5-8 A matrix of the family's story.

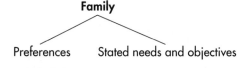

meaningful way to address specific issues that have been specified by the family. Therapists take this information but also look to the future (Mattingly, 1991), asking, Who will this child and family be in 3 years? in 5 years? Consideration of the family, the child, play, and the environment are all folded into storytelling. The information is initially organized by the therapist by simply compiling it as illustrated in Figures 5-8 and 5-9. These figures provide a framework for developing a synthesis of the family and child stories to be used, in turn, as a basis for a meaningful treatment plan focusing on play skills and interactions. In a sense, this framework is the beginning of a storyboard for the family, sketching out a picture of who this child and family is now and who they may become in the future, a story that the family may very well take up and continue to develop after therapy has ended.

The following case examples demonstrate the use of storytelling by two occupational therapists. These stories include the collection of assessment information about a child's play, the family's story, and the therapist's story. The cases illustrate two different ways of constructing child and family narratives.

CASE STORY 1: FINDING MY PLACE

Stephen lives with both parents in a middle-class home. His mom, Phyllis, works as an assistant in a large architectural firm. His father, Paul, is a businessman. Both parents are friendly and talkative. Their original story of family life has been modified somewhat because of their son's complicated medical and developmental picture. For example, Phyllis had planned to return to work full time with a babysitter at home for her child but changed that plan in response to her son's many needs. Both parents are actively involved in their family story, using their parenting roles to help them understand their son and make sense of their future.

Stephen is seen by an occupational therapist in his home as part of his early intervention program. He is considered to have significant sensory processing difficulties as well as developmental disability. Three days a week he attends an early intervention center program. Two other days are filled with visits from his therapists.

During a typical home visit Marge (the occupational therapist) and Phyllis exchange many ideas about why Stephen may be acting as he is, changes each has seen, and ways that interactions may be modified. Their conversation is filled with ideas about using playful

Environment		Child	
Strengths	**Needs**	**Strengths**	**Needs**
Child focused, safe, organized	Opportunities to explore environment	Attends for short periods	Manipulative skills
Lots of toys		Social	Exploration skills
Parents as playmates	Developmentally appropriate toys		Diversity in play behaviors (tactile, vestibular)

FIG. 5-9 The therapist's view of Stephen.

situations, toy objects, songs and jingles that would spark Stephen's attention and curiosity about his world. For example,

Phyllis: I just bought several more of these squeaky toys, he seems to really recognize them.
Marge: I know he really likes them. He plays with them a lot at school.
Phyllis: Let's try the "Find It game" to see what he thinks.
Marge: Good. Do you want to hold him or shall I?

In their interactions Phyllis and Marge engage in a constant give and take of ideas. Equally interesting is how they share responsibility for initiating treatment sequences and playful interactions with Stephen. How did they get to this point? And how similar are their stories for Stephen?

The following stories have emerged over the course of informal conversation and direct inquiry between the parents and therapist. The stories are told by the therapist.

How Phyllis Tells Her Story to Stephen's Therapist

Phyllis sees her 2½ year old son as having the ability to act at a much higher level than his present behavior demonstrates. She sees his difficulties as problems with hearing and seeing, understanding sensory information, and sitting balance. Phyllis and her husband are confident that given time and the right kind of intervention their son will have far more ability then it now appears. They expect that Stephen will talk, go to school, play, and have friends. Although they see Stephen as "always having some problems" their story for him is fairly close to a typical childhood with minor modifications (He will need a speech therapist, perhaps tutors, He may not be great in sports).

Both parents enjoy their interactions with Stephen, which includes feeding, bathing, dressing, and playing with him. Stephen has favorite toys, including rattles that make noise, soft rubbery toys that squeak, and toys with vibration such as the bumble ball. He enjoys being sung to and playing social games such as pat-a-cake and peek-a-boo. He likes being in water and is enrolled in a swimming program at the local community pool.

Thoroughly enjoying the mothering role, Phyllis is very optimistic about Stephen. She feels she knows how to work hard for success and believes that if she is diligent in researching her son's problems, finding the best resources and therapists, and providing a stimulating home environment, she and her husband can help Stephen "overcome" his difficulties. Although Phyllis expects this to take time (up to 3 more years), she is willing to work hard for the end result.

Phyllis says that she never even considered the possibility of having a child with a problem. She had a typical pregnancy, labor, and delivery. There is no history of this type of problem in her family. Her only sister, Sue, is married with three healthy, active children.

Phyllis considers herself to be the type of person who is used to struggle. She always had to work hard for what she earned. Although a good student in school, Phyllis needed to study hard. She was social and active in high school and college but again needed to try hard and to look for second chances and special breaks to get what she really wanted. Her work career has unfolded in a similar pattern of hard work and payoff. She is pleased with her job and, although she puts in many long hours, she feels the fruits of her efforts are well worth it.

How Paul Tells His Story to Stephen's Therapist

Paul was and continues to be overwhelmed by the complexity of issues that surround his son's health. He is repeatedly surprised that in spite of their attention to prescriptive orders from doctors and specialists Stephen's problems persist and he is concerned at what he calls "a lack of progress." Paul views his wife as the emotionally stronger one and counts on her to deal with the medical care and therapy needs for their son. He is eager to support his wife as she increases her involvement in therapy with their son and decreases her work responsibilities. He feels his greatest contribution is in support, encouragement, and just plain manpower whenever possible.

Paul has had minimal exposure to people with disabilities. He grew up across the street from a boy who was mentally retarded. For the most part Paul remembers his neighbor as slow mentally but normal physically. Paul feels frightened for his wife and son and wishes there were something he could do to protect them both from the ongoing pressures of Stephen's problems. He is hoping that eventually all will work out and has his fingers crossed that the next several years will make a difference for his family.

The Therapist's Story

Marge's story for Stephen contains some additional information compared to the family story. Marge has been monitoring her evolving story in an effort to keep from moving too quickly to a view of Stephen's future needs, thus overshadowing the parents' concerns and focus on the present.

In Marge's eyes, Stephen is a child who is "severely involved." She sees him as a boy who may have vision deficits, significant sensory integration dysfunction, and definite cognitive limitations. Marge expects Stephen to require specialized care and schooling as he gets older and that he probably always will depend on adults to initiate and follow through in all aspects of his behavior, including play, learning, and social interactions.

Marge has worked with many children who have levels of ability similar to Stephen's. Similarly, she has also worked with families who are deeply resolved to work hard and solve their child's problems; however, she also respects the unique history and special concerns of each family. In this instance, Marge sees this family as having some very definite overall characteristics, including a high level of expectation, a history of success and perseverance, little experience with physical or cognitive disability, and limited emotional support and resources from families and friends. Although Phyllis and Paul have been very open and candid regarding some of their difficulties with the constant demand of Stephen's care, Marge does not feel she knows whether or not these parents have deeper questions and concerns about his future and whether their sense of the future is realistic.

In considering Stephen's sensory processing characteristics, Marge has considered the questions listed in Box 5-1. Marge feels that Stephen has definite sensory processing deficits. He is hypersensitive to light touch and seeks proprioceptive and vestibular input. Marge has noticed that Stephen enjoys rocking when left alone and she has observed several other self-stimulatory behaviors, including head shaking and seeking visual input by pressing on closed eyes. Questions regarding visual and hearing abilities are still unanswered, although Marge suspects that Stephen has serious limitations in these areas that, when combined with his cognitive and sensory deficits, are going to present challenges to the child and family throughout his life.

As Marge asked herself questions regarding this family's story she began to formulate a picture of their beliefs, hopes, and dreams. To Marge, it seems that Stephen's parents define his problem as a deficit state, something that with the right amount of treatment and care can be fixed or overcome. Stephen's parents enjoy many playful interactions with their son over the course of the day. This family values closeness, being able to talk with, be with, and play with one another. They are affectionate with each other, enjoying kissing and hugging. Stephen is very responsive to his parents; he smiles and laughs to their playful touch and voice. Paul and Phyllis both would like to be able to go on outings with their son. They have long dreamed of typical family trips to amusement parks, zoos, and similar attractions. Both are interested in Stephen's looking like other children and responding appropriately when faced with new yet safe and secure situations, such as petting a dog or holding a kitten, and being friendly when meeting new children and visiting friends and relatives.

Taking these priorities into account Marge collected information about Stephen's play behaviors and social interactions. When Marge considered the questions listed in Box 5-2 (temperament, play, and behavior) she gained insight into how Stephen's play and social interactions were affected by his temperament. Marge noted that Stephen's play was organized as long as an adult structured the interaction and provided the rhythmicity for it. In addition, Stephen had strong preferences for play spaces and play materials and exhibited disorganization in his behavior when new toys or different spaces were used. Teachers reported similar behaviors at school, characterizing Stephen as liking things his way. Similarly, his teachers have noted that Stephen has difficulty changing from one activity to the next (play time to snack time, quiet play to noise group play), even when those activities follow a prescribed order. Unscheduled and atypical situations present considerable difficulty for Stephen and can put him out of sorts for the rest of the day. These would be important details to share with Stephen's parents and to consider when moving toward play and social goals.

In making observations and inquiries into the specific qualities of Stephen's play, Marge has found that Stephen has difficulty attending during his play because of environmental distractions, such as sounds from others; noises outside of the room, such as a car sound or children singing; and touch, including extraneous touch from others who are playing nearby or who walk by and touch from the physical qualities of play materials. Typically, Stephen will spend up to 10 minutes in play with repeated breaks in his attention over that period. Exploration, manipulation, and initiation are all limited by temperament and self-organization characteristics. Stephen's play is guided by his strong and narrow preferences for certain people, settings, and materials. He is most content when he is playing with a familiar adult.

Stephen's limitations in play are influenced by his deficits in gross motor, fine motor, and language and cognitive skills. Many of his skills are typical for a child who is between 18 and 22 months old. Although Stephen has the opportunity to function in several rich and varied environments (home, early intervention center) he maintains a distance from novel objects, novel situations, and unfamiliar people. To some extent his own limited preferences have kept him from experiencing variety in his play repertoire, including play companions, play spaces, and play materials.

Figs. 5-9 and 5-10 summarize the therapist's view of Stephen and his family's story. They provide some footing for the therapist, who must now get down to the business of creating a viable plan for occupational therapy input to this child and family.

As Marge considered her understanding of this child and his family she acted on information that would facilitate the family story. Fortunately she is able to provide intervention in the family home using the child's own toys and other familiar objects and in the early intervention setting. Because of her experiences in both environments she is able to learn about and work toward goals and objectives that are valued by the family.

Based on her play assessments and interviews with both parents, Marge had some particular issues to address in treatment: increasing play behaviors, including those that incorporate the parents' interest in having Stephen differentiate toys by touch (finding the ball when given a choice of a ball or a bottle) and increasing his responsiveness to simple commands (Give me your hands, Look over here); developing strategies for family outings (ideas for places to go and ways to facilitate Stephen's participation) and increasing Stephen's spontaneous interactions with people and novel settings. Emphasis on increasing social play, providing opportunities for modulated responses to new stimuli and situations, and problem solving with parents before outings and family events were all included in the treatment plan. In addition, the therapist was interested in developing a long-term goal with the family designed to facilitate a future picture of Stephen that would take into account the nature of his cognitive, visual, and sensory deficits and the potential long-term impact of these deficits on their personal life worlds. At the conclusion of her assessment, Marge asked, Will Stephen be able to fulfill the occupational roles that his family anticipates for him? How will the family modify their occupations in response to Stephen's trajectory of development? How can she best facilitate the family story and a goodness of fit in the evolving roles?

Summary

Priorities for Stephen's occupational therapy intervention were defined through several key avenues of input. The therapist developed an ongoing relationship with the family that allowed her to understand their family story as it related to their primary concerns for their child's needs. These needs were intimately tied to the family's social and cultural view of who they were themselves and what they would like their lives to be like. The therapist used those considerations to guide her assessment of Stephen in his primary occupational role of player. She also used narrative strategies to create a picture of Stephen as a player and family member, which lead her to ask how Stephen will fulfill his roles of player and of family member. Informed by the family story, the therapist designed treatment strategies that were based on the family's definition of their child as well as on her professional knowledge of how play could be used as a focus for occupation based intervention.

Family	
Preferences	**Stated needs and objectives**
Clean, neat, orderly play	Strategies for family outings including maintaining organized behavior, continued development of social and interaction skills, attention to sensory integration deficits and hand skills
Adult directed and controlled experiences	
Maintain homeostasis and provide experiences that are known to be preferred by Stephen	

FIG. 5-10 The family's story: Stephen, Phyllis, and Paul.

CASE STORY 2: RESCUE ME

The story of Monica demonstrates how the birth of a child with special needs reshapes the family storyline and its impacts on the family's routines and values. It also demonstrates how the telling of the story uncovers opportunities for further assessment and intervention, and how play observation can provide a window into the child's and family's strengths and needs. Finally, this story demonstrates the effects of reshaping the play environment to enhance the competence of the child and the family as they enact their daily routines and create a long-term vision for their life.

Monica is a child with pervasive developmental disorder. She is a bright, beautiful, and energetic youngster who fails to interact with her environment in meaningful and purposeful ways. Although she has a strong drive to act, her actions are dominated by a variety of self-stimulatory behaviors ranging from hanging upside down on furniture, to placing inappropriate objects into her mouth, and to making gestures with and talking to her hands. She gives the impression of being locked in her body because of an intense and insatiable need for sensory stimulation, while at the same time begging for someone to rescue her from her driving urges so that she may play in the world of objects and people.

The Family Story
The story begins with Monica and her family. Monica is the second child of a middle-class, Caucasian family who reside in a suburban neighborhood. Her medical and early developmental history were unremarkable with the exception of her sleep patterns, which were irregular, at best. Mrs. C, Monica's mother, reports that as an infant, Monica would bang her feet into the wall forcefully in an attempt to get to sleep. This intense banging caused Monica actually to break through her crib one evening. Monica's irregular sleep patterns and frequent waking episodes during the night disrupted the family's sleep routines and placed them under enormous stress. The older child would awake frequently because of the disruption that Monica made during the night. Mrs. C felt increasingly tired and irritable because of lack of sleep and Mr. C's work began to suffer.

The family was concerned about Monica's sleep behavior; however, the family pediatrician assured them that there was no cause for worry and advised Mrs. C to calm down, saying that the baby and the rest of the family would in turn be able to calm down. This advice did not comfort the family. By the time Monica was 18 months old, the family had become increasingly overwhelmed by her increasingly difficult behaviors. They began to notice her delays in acquiring both language and social interaction skills.

By actively networking through the community, Mrs. C was able to access community support systems and was able to contact a citywide program to obtain a comprehensive evaluation for Monica. Based on this evaluation at 20 months of age, Monica was diagnosed with pervasive developmental disorder with borderline developmental delay and severe language delay. Although the diagnosis was troubling, it also provided a degree of relief for Mrs. C because she no longer felt Monica's behavior was a result of something she was doing wrong. She also remembers feeling positive that now she had a direction for addressing Monica's needs and enrolled her in a local preschool program for children with special needs.

Monica's problem behaviors and constant needs continued to dominate this family story. Although the preschool program offered some assistance with Monica's care, the family continued to feel stressed about her behavior at home. Left unsupervised, Monica was a danger to herself as well as to her older brother. She quickly learned to unlatch the front door and run out to the street. She would scream, hit, pinch, or bite when her brother tried to prevent her from leaving the house or engaging in other dangerous play. Although the family fenced in the yard to provide a safe play area for Monica, she quickly mastered climbing the fence. Mrs. C was

no longer able to work outside the home, which created a significant financial stress for the family.

Daily family routines were also significantly altered by Monica's behavior. Family meal time was one of many battle grounds for Monica. She refused all but a limited variety of foods while continuing to have difficulties remaining seated at the table. She disliked having clothing on her body; thus dressing became a wrestling match that often ended in a tantrum. Teeth brushing was impossible unless Mrs. C physically restrained Monica.

Despite the chaos created by Monica the family remained committed to helping her in any way possible. Because of a close extended family, the grandparents offered considerable assistance with both children and provided periods of respite for the parents. Mrs. C continued to pursue any services that she felt would be helpful for Monica, including behavioral and speech therapy in the home and occupational therapy at a local clinic.

The family has always been able to look past Monica's disability and see her as a bright, beautiful, energetic youngster, with special needs. They continued to maintain a strong hope that once her behavior was under control and her language emerged Monica would be able to function independently. Using the snapshot exercise described earlier in this chapter, Monica's parents talked about their future vision for her. They hoped to see Monica grow up to be self-sufficient, use language with a true communicative intent, be able to socialize with others, and have a life that did not include special education.

Listening to the family story gave the therapist the opportunity to engage in connected knowing and to enter the family's frame to "discover the premises for the other's point of view" (Belenky et al., 1986, p. 101). The therapist was able to gain insight into how Monica's special needs shaped the family storyline. It was obvious that the family valued children and were willing to make the children the focus of their lives. The physical and emotional home environment echoed this value. Although they were overwhelmed with the situation that Monica's needs created, they continued to seek answers and solutions for them. Aware of the needs of their other child as well, the family sought balance and stability in their lives, as well as ways to enhance Monica's behavior and functioning. As noted earlier in this chapter, family's establish patterns of behavior that are culturally meaningful, and the ways a family engages in play reflect their culturally driven values and purposes. Although Monica had significantly disrupted this family's patterns they continued to engage in an active process of redefining their patterns, seeking a fit between values and behaviors.

The following section describes how play observation guided subsequent adaptations of the play environment to assist the family in meeting their valued goals for Monica and to reestablish a degree of stability and balance in the family.

The Therapist's Story
The therapist enters the story with a deep understanding and reverence for the beliefs that Reilly (1962) set forth regarding human occupation. Monica was not able to realize this endeavor of human occupation. Her behavior was driven by her intense need for sensory input. Because the stimuli were not grounded in meaning, they simply perpetuated a vicious cycle of aggressive, sensory-seeking behavior. She was unable to utilize sensory input for adaptive, purposeful interactions with her environment. As a result, play, as we define it, did not exist for Monica.

Observation of Monica's unstructured time provided a valuable vehicle for observing and interpreting her play behaviors and needs. In addressing the questions related to sensory processing as presented in Box 5-1, it became evident that Monica craved sensory input and used self-stimulating behaviors to gain it. She used her hands (and any other part of her body for that matter) not for exploration but merely for stimulation. She required an extremely high and constant level of input. She was in perpetual motion. When deprived of this level of activity, Monica became aggressive and agitated and frequently would hold tantrums and scream for long periods.

Examples of Monica's spontaneous behavior included running around the room and banging into a large upholstered chair, hanging upside down on the couch, walking across the top of the couch to the window ledge and jumping onto a large pillow on the floor, and finally running over to her mother and pulling up her shirt for a back rub. Monica also sought oral stimulation using an object such as a plastic dinosaur or her fingers to provide the desired input. She enjoyed playing outside on a swing set and enjoyed running around the fenced yard using blades of grass to visually self-stimulate as she ran in circles. Monica utilized all types of sensory input for self-stimulation, including visual, tactile, vestibular, and proprioceptive. In contrast, Monica demonstrated a severe aversion to imposed stimulation such as her mother combing her hair, or the therapist attempting to engage her in sand play.

A typical day for Monica began after a night of interrupted sleep followed by difficulty waking in the morning. Breakfast was unpredictable, since Monica's tolerance for foods varied greatly on any given day. If presented with a food that was not tolerable, Monica would have a tantrum and run away. Dressing and grooming were also difficult since she disliked putting clothes on and had severe aversive reactions to having her hair combed and her teeth brushed.

Monica rode the bus to school and returned each day at 3:15 pm. The afternoon and evening hours were characterized by the behaviors previously described. Monica enjoyed watching videotaped movies. Bedtime often spanned several hours. Monica was difficult to calm down at the end of the day, and once asleep she would wake at unpredictable times and remain awake and active for several hours. She would often go to her parents' bed and keep them awake for several hours during the night.

Monica's behavior was characteristically driven by her sensory processing dysfunction and her temperament, which included an extraordinarily high level of activity with little or no rhythmicity in her interactions. In reference to Box 5-2 and Box 5-3, which address issues of temperament and level of play, Monica's behavior was interpreted as in a constant state of overarousal. She is unable to maintain periods of focused attention for purposeful behavior, is guided by her own internal rhythms, and is driven by a need for a high level of stimulation. Monica is unable to engage in even the lowest level of play since she cannot sustain her attention to materials or actions with the exception of self-stimulating objects and behaviors. Exploration, manipulation, variety, diversity, interaction, and creativity in play, as described in Box 5-3, are not possible at this point given Monica's preoccupation with sensory stimulation.

The next level of assessment gained through play observation is designed to clarify information regarding skill development (Box 5-4). Monica demonstrated highly developed motor skills, especially in the area of gross motor development. She was able to climb, balance, motor plan, and execute quite sophisticated motor activities such as pumping a swing, pedaling a bike, and climbing a metal fence. She demonstrated no fear of movement and her coordination was excellent. Fine motor and visual motor skills, although not formally assessed, appeared age appropriate and certainly ade-

Environment		Child	
Strengths	**Needs**	**Strengths**	**Needs**
Variety of play spaces	Safety of play areas	Cute appearance	Improved sensory processing abilities; dominated by self-stimulation
Abundance of toys	Point out toys that are developmentally appropriate; decrease potential for over-stimulation (remove toys that are likely to elicit self-stimulation or overstimulation); opportunities for proprioceptive-based play	Motor skills	Graded, adaptive responses to sensory input (in constant motion; often a danger to self)
Variety of people to "play" with	Create situations for safe interactions; discuss calming strategies with parents, grandparents, siblings	Manipulative skills	Use of hands for adaptive behaviors (does not use hands for exploration)
		Strong needs	Transition into directed activities rather than tantrums and screaming
Chaotic because of M's behavior	Structure environment for play	Loving child	Regulation of sleep–wake cycles
			Increase repertoire of foods she will tolerate
Clear routines	Adaptations to sleeping environment to encourage state regulation; establish cues for routines, such as a song before meal time	Independent mobility	In constant motion
		Potential for language	Improve organizational behavior through play

FIG. 5-11 The therapist's view of Monica.

Family

Preferences and strengths	Stated needs and objectives
Feel overwhelmed by M's vast needs	Work with family to identify priorities
Want child to appear normal	Strategies to regulate M's sleep Strategies to decrease self-stimulating behaviors
Want to engage in family outings	Work with family to identify and initiate play and leisure activities that M can tolerate
Concerned about nutritional intake and oral hygiene	Address oral hypersensitivities
Have established long-range vision	Work with family to implement vision by accessing needed services for M and adapting home environment
Would like M to engage in independent play	Adapt play environment for safety

FIG. 5-12 Monica's family's story.

TABLE 5-1   Intervention Strategies for Monica

Goals	Intervention Strategy
Short-Term	
Decrease extreme activity level	Use of weighted vest in the home
	Use of weighted blankets at night combined with large pillows to create a proprioceptive nest
Establish regular sleep patterns by providing sensory input to maintain sleep state	Consider use of a vibrating surface for sleeping and comfort object (doll, blanket, pacifier, or a chewy toy) to restore sleeping state when awakened during the night
Decrease tactile hypersensitivity	Initiate rapid, firm pressure brushing routines (Wilbarger & Wilbarger, 1991)
	Use of oral desensitization and stimulation techniques
	Use of Nuk brush for teeth brushing
Increase proprioceptive input	Use of trampoline in the home
	Wearing weighted vests on walks
	Pulling a wagon on walks
	Respond to requests or signals for deep pressure with massage
Long-Term	
Increase exploration of environment through play	Introduction of developmentally appropriate play objects
Develop play skills	Encourage exploration, manipulation, initiation, diversification, interaction
	Create play situations.
Independence in self-care and routines of daily living	Provide opportunities to develop dressing skills and grooming skills such as washing hands before snack

quate for developmentally appropriate, functional behaviors such as feeding, dressing, and using crayons. Cognitively, Monica's abilities were more puzzling. Although she was limited by a severe language delay, she appeared to be able to solve complex problems to have her needs met. Spontaneous language, although meaningless, demonstrated a wide range of skills. For example, Monica was able to verbalize intricate strings of words such as, "Stop it yellow, I'm coming over to get you." She was able to memorize long phrases and paragraphs from the videotaped movies she watched. Her potential for language seemed excellent, but like her other behaviors, her language was inaccessible to the people around her.

An important area for assessment and intervention with Monica and her family was the environment. The environment is seen as providing the context within which behavior occurs, as well as supporting children's play (through exploration) and motor skill development (through movement and exercise). Consideration of the environment includes human and nonhuman characteristics that have an impact on the child's play. Use of Box 5-5 to structure the observation of Monica's environment revealed many positive characteristics of the play environment. There is adequate space and time for play, there are varied play objects and opportunities for different

types of play (quiet play, active play, social play). Attention has been paid to safety as well as to developmental appropriateness of play objects. In terms of the human environment, there is access to a variety of people (siblings, parents, grandparents, peers) to facilitate purposeful interactions. At this time Monica is unable to access these environmental supports. Her sensory processing dysfunction drives her intrinsic motivation toward activities that are self-stimulating rather than interaction oriented.

Summary

This unfolding of the story provides insight into Monica and her family that can be organized as shown in Figures 5-11 and 5-12. This organization provides direction for intervention, which addresses the sensory processing dysfunction that underlies Monica's extreme activity level, her inability to establish patterns of sleep, her self-stimulating behaviors, and her inability to sustain focused attention for purposeful behavior. Based on these findings, an approach combining traditional sensory integrative intervention with environmental adaptations in the home was initiated. Examples of intervention strategies are listed in Table 5-1.

CONCLUSION

Much information about a child can be gained as a therapist creates stories through assessment and observation of play, as well as informal dialogues and interviews with a family. Organization of this information into a usable format for analysis and synthesis provides the therapist with a structure for developing intervention priorities that flow from the integration of the therapist's view of the child with the interests and values of the family as expressed through the family's story. Assessment that is narrative in nature; focused on family-driven values, interests, and concerns; and oriented to the occupation of the child as a player yields useful and highly relevant data to guide successful occupational therapy interventions.

REVIEW QUESTIONS

1. The authors describe some of the current practice problems in pediatrics. Discuss these, considering implications for intervention and assessment.
2. Define "folk psychology." How is this linked to narrative?
3. Describe how therapists can use storytelling to assist families as they prepare to care for a disabled child.
4. Discuss the storylines (1) play and sensory processing issues, and (2) play and temperament issues. How can the therapist integrate these storylines into a broader perspective of the child?
5. What is a "family story"? What is a "therapist's story"? How does the therapist integrate these in an assessment, in order to plan intervention?

REFERENCES

Als, H. (1986). *A synactive model of neonatal behavioral organization: Framework for the assessment of neurobehavioral development in the premature infant and for support of infants and parents in the neonatal intensive care environment.* New York: Haworth Press.

Anzalone, M.E. (1994, July). Mother-infant play: Developmental level and exploratory style. Paper presented at the Annual Conference of the American Occupational Therapy Association and the Canadian Association of Occupational Therapists, Boston, Massachusetts.

Ayres, A. J. (1972). *Sensory Integration and learning disorders.* Los Angeles: Western Psychological Services.

Bailey, D. (1971). Vocational theories and work habits related to childhood development. *American Journal of Occupational Therapy, 25,* 298-302.

Bates, J. E. (1989). Concepts and measures of temperament. In G.A. Kohnstamm, J. E. Bates & M. K. Rothbart (Eds.). *Temperament in childhood* (pp. 3-26). Chichester, England: John Wiley and Sons.

Belenky, M. F.; Clinchy, B.; Goldberger, N. & J. Tarule (1986). *Women's Ways of Knowing. The Development of Self, Voice, and Mind.* New York: Basic Books.

Brazelton, T. B., & Lester, B. M. (1983). *New Approaches to developmental screening of infants.* New York: Elsevier.

Bruner, E. (1984). The opening up of anthropology. In Bruner, E. M., (Ed.). *Text, play, and story: The construction and reconstruction of self and society.* Washington, D.C.: The American Ethnological Society.

Bruner, J. (1990). *Acts of meaning*. Cambridge, MA: Harvard University Press.

Burke, J. P. (1993a). Illness Narratives. Unpublished paper. University of Pennsylvania.

Burke, J. P. (1993b). Play: The life role of the infant and young child. In Case-Smith, J. (Ed.). *Pediatric Occupational Therapy and Early Intervention*. Andover, MA: Andover Publishers.

Burke, J. P., & Frank, A. (1994, July). Narrative rehabilitation: The untaught half of occupational therapy. Paper presented at the Annual Conference of the American Occupational Therapy Association and the Canadian Association of Occupational Therapists, Boston, Massachusetts.

Burke, J. P., & Schaaf, R. C. (in preparation). Clinical reasoning strategies in family centered care.

Carey, W. B. (1983). Intervention strategies using temperament data. In Brazelton, T. B., & Lester, B. M. (Eds.). *New Approaches to developmental screening of infants* (pp. 245-257). New York: Elsevier Science Publishing Co.

Chess, S., & Thomas, A. (1989). Issues in the clinical application of temperament. In Kohnstamm, G. A., J. E. Bates & M. K. Rothbart (Eds.). *Temperament in childhood* (pp. 377-386). Chichester England: John Wiley and Sons.

Denzin, N. (1989). *Interpretive Biography*. Newbury Park, CA: Sage Publications.

D'Eugenio, D. (1986). Infant play: A reflection of cognitive and motor development. In Pehoski, C. (Ed.). *Play, a Skill for Life*. Rockville, MD: American Occupational Therapy Association.

Florey, L. L. (1971.). An approach to play and play development. *American Journal of Occupational Therapy, 25,* 275-280.

Florey, L. L. (1981). Studies of play: Implications for growth, development, and for clinical practice. *American Journal of Occupational Therapy, 35,* 519-524.

Frank, A. (1991). *At the Will of the Body*. Boston: Houghton Mifflin.

Frank, A. (1992). What kind of phoenix? Illness and self-knowledge. *Second Opinion 18,* 31-41.

Hanft, B., Burke, J. P., Cahill, M., Swenson-Miller, K., Humphry, R. (1992). *Working with families: A curriculum guide for pediatric occupational therapists*. Chapel Hill, NC: Frank Porter Graham Child Development Center.

Hurff, J. (1974). A play skills inventory. In Reilly, M. (Ed.). *Play as exploratory learning: Studies in curiosity behavior*. Beverly Hills, CA: Sage Publications.

The Individuals with Disabilities Education Act Amendments of 1991 (IDEA). Oct 7, 1991, PL 102-119, 105 Stat. 587.

Kleinman, A. (1988). *The illness narratives*. New York: Basic Books.

Knox, S. (1974). A play scale. In Reilly, M. (Ed.). *Play as exploratory learning: Studies in curiosity behavior*. Beverly Hills, CA: Sage Publications.

Matsutsuyu, J. (1971). Occupational behavior: A perspective on work and play. *American Journal of Occupational Therapy, 25,* 291-294.

Mattingly, C. (1991). The narrative nature of clinical reasoning. *The American Journal of Occupational Therapy, 45,* 998-1006.

Michelman, S. (1974). Play and the deficit child. In Reilly, M. (Ed.). *Play as exploratory learning: Studies in curiosity behavior*. Beverly Hills, CA: Sage Publications.

Porges, S. W. (1993). The infant's sixth sense: Awareness and regulation of bodily processes. *Zero To Three, 14,* 12-16.

Price, R. (1994). *A whole new life*. New York: Atheneum.

Reilly, M. (1962). Occupational therapy can be one of the great ideas of 20th century medicine. *American Journal of Occupational Therapy, 16,* 1-9.

Reilly, M. (1971). The modernization of occupational therapy. *American Journal of Occupational Therapy, 25,* 243-246.

Reilly, M. (1974). Defining a cobweb. In Reilly, M. (Ed.). *Play as exploratory learning: Studies in curiosity behavior*. Beverly Hills, CA: Sage Publications.

Rosaldo, M. (1984). Toward an Anthropology of Self and Feeling. In Shweder, R. A., & LedVine, R. A. (Eds.). *Culture theory: Essays on mind self, and emotion*. Cambridge: Cambridge University Press.

Schaaf, R. C., & Burke, J. P. (1992). Clinical reflections on play and sensory integration. *Sensory Integration Special Interest Section Newsletter, 15,* 1-2.

Schaaf R. C., & Mulrooney, L. (1989). Occupational therapy in early intervention: A family-centered approach. *American Journal of Occupational Therapy, 43,* 745-754.

Schaaf, R. C., Merrill, S. C. & N. Kinsella (1987). Sensory integration and play behavior: A case study of the effectiveness of occupational therapy using sensory integrative techniques. *Occupational Therapy in Health Care, 4,* 61-75.

Schon, D. (1983). *The Reflective Practioner*. New York: Basic Books.

Shannon, P. (1972). Work-play theory and the occupational therapy process. *American Journal of Occupational Therapy, 26,* 169-172.

Sundstrom, C. (1972). The physiological aspects of work and play. *American Journal of Occupational Therapy, 26,* 173-175.

Takata, N. (1969). The play history. *American Journal of Occupational Therapy, 23,* 314-318.

Takata, N. (1974). Play as a prescription. In Reilly, M. (Ed.). *Play as exploratory learning: Studies in curiosity behavior*. Beverly Hills, CA: Sage Publications.

Wilbarger, P., & Wilbarger, J. (1991). *Sensory defensiveness in children aged 2–12*. Santa Barbara: Avanti Educational Programs.

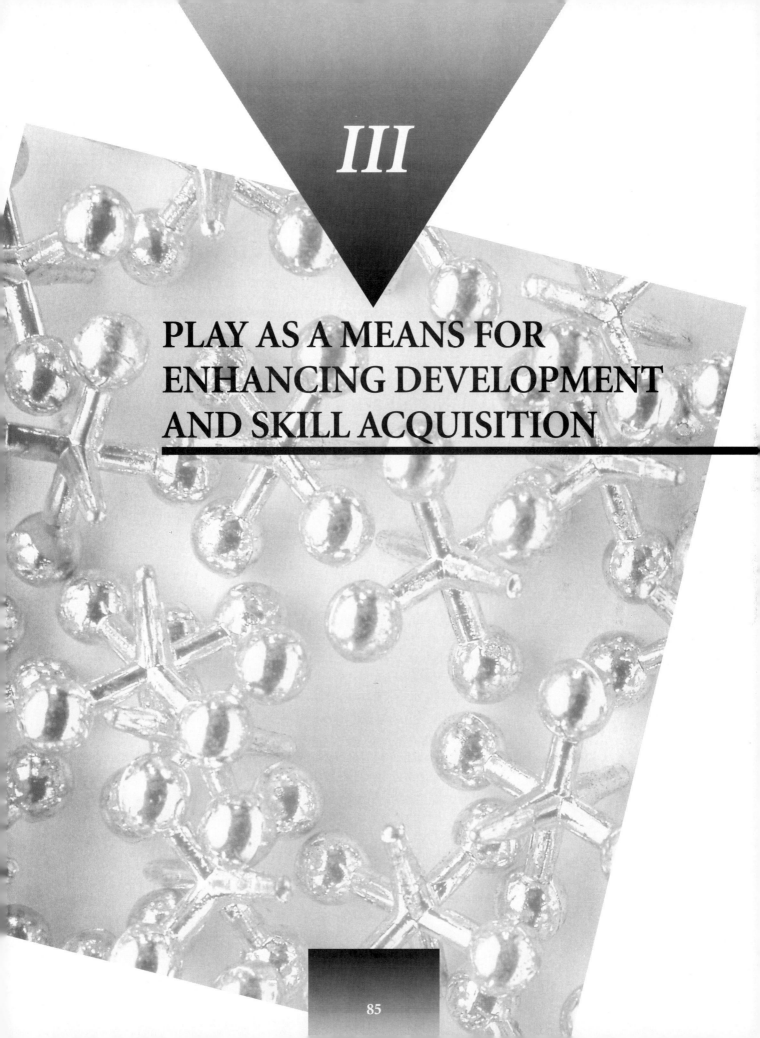

III

PLAY AS A MEANS FOR ENHANCING DEVELOPMENT AND SKILL ACQUISITION

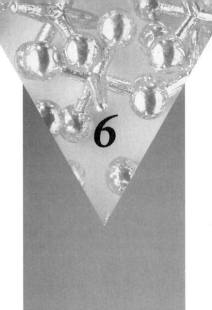

6

THE POWER OF OBJECT PLAY FOR INFANTS AND TODDLERS AT RISK FOR DEVELOPMENTAL DELAYS

Doris Pierce

TAPPING THE THERAPEUTIC POWER OF OBJECT PLAY

Object play is the predominant waking activity of the young child. Few are the pediatric occupational therapy sessions that do not rely on object play for their therapeutic outcomes. How, then, can object play be most effectively applied by occupational therapists to facilitate development in young children at risk for delays? This chapter offers a discussion of the sources of power in object play applications, the types of goals addressed in play-based interventions, and the use of object play in the treatment of young children.

An Occupational Science Approach to Object Play

The promise that occupational science has made to occupational therapy is that, through its contributions to the field's understanding of occupation, therapists will bring the applications of occupation to bear in increasingly potent ways (Clark et al., 1991). Occupational science has not yet produced much research to enhance the field's understanding of human activity. However, for this author, combining occupational science training with daily practice has provided a fertile ground for considering how these promised applications may work in pediatric practice.

A hallmark of human evolutionary adaptation is the reliance on alterations of the physical environment (Chapple & Coon, 1942; Moore, 1992). Human occupations involve a striking variety of material culture: crops, shelters, domesticated animals, vehicles, tools and machinery, aesthetic and ritual objects, clothing, information records, foods, medicines, and toys. Complex manipulations of physical objects in space and time are an essential aspect of the human occupational nature. Henderson (1992) argues that occupational therapy has neglected examination of human spatial skills in near and far space. Her argument can be extended even further to propose that humans require spatial skills not only for managing bodily movements in space but also for managing complex relationships between themselves and a variety of physical objects. It is in object play that the early foundation is laid for these adult interactions with the physical world.

Occupational Therapy for Infants and Toddlers at Risk for Developmental Delays

Pediatric occupational therapists often treat infants and toddlers at risk for developmental delays. These infants can present with unclear diagnoses and a medical history that may or may not include prematurity, birth complications, irregularities of muscle tone, questions surrounding hearing and vision, and respiratory and feeding problems. In addition to the therapeutic needs of the child, the therapist is often dealing with a family in turmoil. The unclear prognoses for these young children demand strong assessment and acute observation for setting treatment goals. The play deficits of children with physical, developmental, intellectual, environmental, or psychological problems are also documented in the literature (Dee, 1974; Gralewicz, 1973; Howard, 1986; Kalverboer, 1977; Mack et al., 1982; Mogford, 1977; Vandenburg & Kielhofner, 1982; Wehman, 1977; Wehman & Abramson, 1976).

DESIGNING FOR POWER IN THERAPEUTIC OCCUPATIONS

How are the most effective object play interventions created? What are the sources of power in a successful therapeutic application of occupation? Occupational therapists are quite good at the breakdown of activity into components or at analyzing the weaknesses and strengths of a patient's performance. This facility is not surprising considering its similarity to many forms of reductionist thinking in the medical milieu. However, creative design of occupations that will draw a patient toward goals with the greatest efficacy is something that is not well understood. This is a critical ability that is assumed to be acquired through practice. Creating new treatment ideas is often dismissed as simple pragmatics or "recipe book." Like very young children in object play, we are good at taking apart but not yet so good at putting together.

Occupational therapists currently create intervention activities by combining in-depth knowledge of a subskill area with a superficial grasp of the occupation to be used as an intervention. This is not the fault of the therapist but reflects the paucity of literature on the dynamics of everyday occupations. Generation of effective therapeutic occupations depends on the ability of the therapist consistently to design activities that are intact, appealing, and custom fitted to the goals of the patient.

Therapist Design Skill

The design skill of the therapist is essential to therapeutic outcomes. Of course, the therapist also requires skills of empathy, assessment, goal setting, and management of the occurring treatment session. However, creating activities that are effective in reaching goals is the most demanding and least well understood of the therapist's skills. Occupational therapists working with children do original problem solving for every treatment. The repeated effort to tailor several maximally intriguing activities for every treatment session can be extremely demanding, especially for the new therapist.

All treatment settings contain barriers to creative design. The effectiveness of play-based interventions can be limited by time pressures, limited play object choices, lack of understanding of normal play patterns, and a clinical culture that favors component level interventions over intact occupational applications. Some of these barriers are more easily corrected than others. The importance of identifying barriers to creative design is twofold. First, recognizing barriers to excellence in treatment design positions the therapist to change those barriers if the opportunity arises. Second, the therapist's realization that limited efficacy of treatment may not be entirely his or her fault reduces frustration and burnout.

Generating effective object play interventions is a design process. In the applied field of architecture, the creative skills of practitioners is carefully nurtured. The phases of the design process are described as recognition of a problem to be solved, analysis, definition, generating solution options, selection, implementation, and evaluation of the implementation's success (Koberg, 1981). If therapists were to broaden their conceptualization of their own professional development to include these critical design skills, they could be easily acquired. Methods of attending to therapist design skill might include readings on design, topical journaling regarding treatment design experiences, an efficacy evaluation routine, or a therapist discussion group that met periodically.

Sources of Power in Therapeutic Occupations

Occupational Intactness. The *intactness* of an occupation is the degree to which the activity used as an intervention is whole. That is, it occurs in the natural condition in which it is to be found in daily life, rather than as it is used as an intervention. The natural conditions of an occupation include the patient's senses of choice, space, time, and social situation usually associated with that occupation. The importance of self-direction to therapeutic gains is especially supported in pediatrics by the work of Ayres (1985). The usual spatial context of an occupation is rich with cues, opportunities, and affordances that can have positive effects on outcomes. The usual social context of an occupation similarly supports performance, as well as conferring a more positive identity than is conferred on a child by a medical setting. The wholeness of the temporal context of the occupation includes the tempo, length, sequence, time of day, and frequency of the activity.

The intactness of an occupational application is a difficult thing to maintain in most occupational therapy practice settings. The sensory integration approach, for example, depends on a spatial condition that is very specifically controlled by the therapist and unlike most usual activity settings of a child. This is not to say that these treatment context choices are not justified. Still, it is important to recognize that these contextual choices, although they may bring effectiveness in some ways, also dilute effectiveness in others. If the therapist remains attuned to these contextual factors, some amelioration may offer itself, such as the opportunity to offer the treatment in another setting or to normalize aspects of the clinical setting.

Occupational Appeal. The *appeal* of the therapeutic occupation is the attractiveness of the activity to the patient. To create occupational applications with high appeal, the therapist depends on empathy for how his or her patient sees the world. Another factor in the appeal of an activity is developmental fit, or the degree to which the activity fits the current abilities and social identity of the individual. A strong understanding of normal object play is especially useful for creating play-based interventions that offer good developmental fit to children at risk for delays. The motivational value of the offered activity depends on novelty, complexity, sensory properties, and the object's exhibition of independent responses and responsiveness to the child. (See "Motivational Properties in Therapeutic Object Play" in this chapter.) Choosing play objects that are irresistible but not overwhelming requires both acute therapeutic judgment and access to a well-stocked toy storage room.

Occupational Goal Fit. The goal fit of the designed activity assures that the application is clearly targeted on treatment goals. It is possible to design an intact and appealing occupation that does not result in any therapeutic gains. This can be a result of poor fit between identified goals and the selected intervention and reflects a failure in design skill. The occupational therapist is required to perform a constant mental balancing act, blending occupations that will be engaging for the patient with those that will produce gains in goal areas. Therapists can feel, by their own levels of satisfaction at the end of the session, whether the correct balance has been struck.

TYPES OF GOALS IN PLAY-BASED INTERVENTIONS

In the developmental interventions of pediatric occupational therapists today, psychology is the extradisciplinary literature base and play is the action reality. This fragmentary relationship between therapists' daily use of play and their training in development influences practice in two negative ways. Therapists are pushed toward reductionistic goal setting at the level of subskills. They are pushed away from intervention at levels of whole occupations by the inadequacy of the play literature.

Play and Development: Creating Play Interventions from a Subskill Literature

Play and development are related and intertwining concepts (Hutt & Hutt, 1970; Kalverboer, 1977; Kielhofner & Barris,

1984; Piaget, 1952, 1962, 1976; Rosenblatt, 1977). "Play" is a cultural and relatively amorphous term referring to the activities of children. It has been widely credited as a source of learning and a critical sphere for normal development (Florey, 1981; Piaget, 1962; Reilly, 1974; Robinson, 1977). On the other hand, "development" is a term that refers to the subskills that support play actions (such as perception, movement, and cognition). Both concepts refer to the capacities of children but at different levels of wholism. The greatest challenge of using a play-based approach to occupational therapy for children at risk for delays is that the therapist must create therapeutic applications primarily from a literature that does not describe children's play. This requires an intuitive leap from the underlying developmental subskills of play to the creation of play applications.

Goal Types in Play-Based Interventions

There are four ways in which occupational therapists currently use object play. These are described only briefly here, from the simplest to the most sophisticated and wholistic level of play-based intervention. The more thorough discussions in the following chapter sections are thereafter presented in the reverse order, from most wholistic to least, so as to begin with a basic discussion of normal object play development.

The simplest use of object play in treatment is as a therapy lure or as a reward for performance of the activity that generates the therapeutic change. Whether this is truly a type of treatment goal is debatable, since the play does not directly generate changes but serves only to keep the child engaged. Perhaps it serves the goal of the therapist by keeping the session going. This is the lowest skill level in the use of object play in treatment. The play is not an intact occupational application, since the object interactions do not occur in the same time as the therapeutic activity. Still, therapy lures can be useful in motivating a child to engage in other activities. (See "Motivational Properties in Therapeutic Object Play" in this chapter.)

The most common use of object play is to facilitate acquisition of the developmental components underlying play. In keeping with the fragmented developmental literature on which they depend, pediatric occupational therapists tend to focus on the isolated skills that underlie successful engagement in childhood occupations: primarily sensory, motor, and cognitive goals. (See "Using Object Play to Address Common Developmental Component Goals" in this chapter.)

Less often, therapists think in terms of facilitating the child's ability to negotiate the spatial, temporal, and social dimensions of the environment. Those who set goals that are addressed by object play in this sophisticated way are usually more experienced therapists who have immersed themselves in an understanding of play. (See "Using Object Play to Develop Environmental Negotiation Skills" in this chapter.)

Most rare of all is the pediatric occupational therapist who construes treatment goals in terms of desired patterns of occupations. These therapists address the individual child's skills and the dimensions of that child's environment as they combine to enable a more desirable occupational pattern for the child. An occupational pattern is the way in which an individual's abilities and repertoires are manifested within the context of daily life as a series of activities. Examination of an individual's occupational pattern can reveal competence, developmental delay, strengths in some types of occupations and weaknesses in others, a poor fit between individual and context, or other insights. Therapists must always keep in mind that it is this occupational pattern, beyond the clinical setting, that they are targeting for change. Therapists who are setting goals and designing play-based interventions at the level of occupational patterns are rare master therapists who are able to treat within the complexity of whole, naturally occurring occupations without completely reducing them to a component skill perspective (Box 6-1). (See "Using Object Play to Alter Occupational Patterns" in this chapter.)

USING OBJECT PLAY TO ALTER OCCUPATIONAL PATTERNS

The most sophisticated level at which occupational therapists set goals and attempt intervention is in the alteration of real occupational patterns. This section offers theoretical and empirical perspectives on normal play development to support therapists' interventions at this master level of practice within the daily activities of their young patients. Establishment of developmentally appropriate

---

Box 6-1   **INTRODUCING ROBERTO**

I met Roberto during his initial assessment at 5 months corrected age. He was a small male infant, born 6 weeks prematurely and displaying the features of Nager acrofacial dysostosis syndrome: deafness, micrognathia, preauricular tags, atresia of external ear canals, hand and arm malformations, and cleft palate. The thumb of his right hand showed no active movement. The musculoskeletal structures of his left shoulder, arm, and hand were irregularly formed: missing and incompletely developed portions of the rotator cuff, shortened humerus, synostosis and shortening of the radius and ulna, and a missing left thumb.

Beyond Roberto's upper extremity movement limitations, he also exhibited overall weakness, no functional grasp, and a strong tendency toward a right asymmetric tonic neck reflex position. He was not holding up his head, reaching, or sitting without full support. He was considered to be at risk for cognitive delays (Fig. 6-1). Because of his micrognathia, cleft palate, and tracheostomy, he was completely dependent on gastrostomy feedings. He was also chronically ill because of his bronchopulmonary dysplasia and required frequent suctioning.

In-home occupational therapy was initiated twice weekly shortly after Roberto's evaluation. Over the course of treatment, Roberto moved from very hesitant engagement to enthusiastic and creative play with objects. After a year of treatment, he also underwent hand reconstructions. He was discharged when he moved away, at 2 years of age, with only minimal developmental delays.

In each of the remaining boxes in this chapter, examples are provided from Roberto's treatment sessions to illustrate how the concepts discussed in the chapter can be translated into practice.

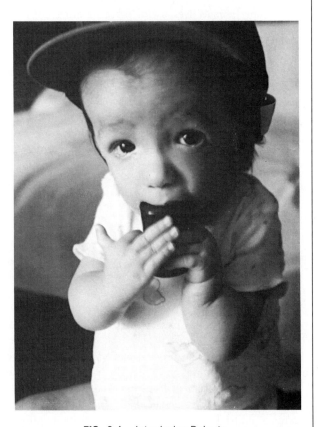

FIG. 6-1 Introducing Roberto.

self-care and play are the occupational pattern areas most often addressed in occupational therapy with very young children.

At all goal levels, an understanding of play development is also necessary for the generation of effective treatment ideas. Unfortunately, research on the normal development of play is somewhat limited. Therapists bridge the gap between the generality of theory and daily requirements for fresh treatment ideas by building a personal repertoire of play choices through trial and error, interactions with normal children, and observations of other therapists. The following review provides a much richer base from which to consider the integrity of play patterns in children at risk and to generate ideas for intervention than can the sum of any individual therapist's experiences.

Drawing from Extradisciplinary Perspectives on Normal Play Development

Setting goals at the level of changes in occupational patterns first requires an examination of existing patterns. The therapist can use family interview, observations, or more formal play assessments. From this initial picture and discussions with the family, the therapist can then begin to plan for treatment. Several areas of the play literature supply perspectives useful for generating both goals for altering occupational patterns and ideas for play-based interventions.

Piaget's Play Theory. Piaget (1952, 1962) emphasizes the development of cognition from play experience. According to Piaget (1962), practice games predominate before the age of 2 years. Within practice games, Piaget delineates three categories. Mere practice games are reproductions of actions for the sake of exercising power over the environment. Later, they are replaced by fortuitous combinations, which are playful repetitions of discovered object combinations. Last in practice games is the class called "intentional combinations," in which the child deliberately designs action sequences that are repeated for the sake of play. The change from practice games to symbolic games at approximately 2 years of age is distinguished by the use of imaginary objects and settings (Piaget, 1962).

Occupational therapists working with very young children draw on Piagetian play theory primarily in their efforts to move the child from a passive lack of engagement with play objects to simple productions of effects on objects. Therapists with an interest in play theory may even attempt to facilitate advancement from one Piagetian play stage to the next. However, Piagetian theory is primarily used in terms of understanding the subskill of cognition within the childhood occupation of play. It is imprecise in describing the actual repertoire of play actions, the sequencing of those actions, or the influence of environmental characteristics on the child's play.

Pretend Play. Pretend activities begin to emerge during the second year, increase for 3 or 4 years, and then taper off (Fein, 1981). Although pretend increases over the early years, it is still a relatively infrequent play form, reaching a maximum of 37% of play acts in kindergarten children (Rubin et al., 1976). Pretend play is at first, at around 12 months, referenced only to the self (Piaget, 1962). Later, pretend is directed toward an other, such as a doll (Fein, 1981).

Pretend play is not a primary concern for occupational therapists working with infants and toddlers since the youth and developmental delays of these children often place them at a less sophisticated play level than that of pretend. It is important that therapists recognize that children of less than 2 years of age are generally playing in very concrete terms. Although pretend play acts, such as talking on a play phone, may hold the child's interest momentarily or stimulate some imitation, they are unlikely to produce the enthusiastic play engagement of a more developmentally appropriate activity. Recognition of the developmental complexity of pretend play will steer the therapist working with a very young child toward concrete object play strategies more likely to generate therapeutic gains.

Studies of Infant Play with Objects. As a group, the studies of infant object play confirm the existence of a variety of partial patterns in the development of infant–object interactions. Actions serving to explore the physical properties of objects (mouthing, handling, and others) increase in complexity, moving away from just mouthing and toward inclusion of vision, touch, and sound. Action fit becomes more specifically tailored to the object (Palmer, 1989; Rochat, 1989; Ruff, 1984). Rochat (1989) studied the actions of 6- to 12-month-old infants who were offered hand-sized objects while being held in their mothers' laps. The infants performed the following broad range of actions: three types of fingering, mouthing, switching objects between hands, dropping, other releases, waving, banging on the table, banging between hands, slapping on table, dangling, pulling on a part of the object, scooting, pressing on the table, squeezing, and touching to face.

Developmental progressions in object play can also be seen in increasingly precise grasp, increasing appropriateness of object use, object separations and combinations, and the phases of pretense–symbolic object play. Fenson et al. (1976) showed changes in predominating play acts from close visual and tactual examination with mouthing at 7 months, to simple physical relating of objects at 9 months, to increasing diversity, symbolic activity, and sequential play by 20 months. Belsky and Most (1981), observing free play with standard objects in infants from 7 to 21 months old found that there were developmental progressions in the emergence of manipulation, use of objects in ways identified as their usual functions, object combinations, and increasingly complex pretend play.

Largo and Howard's (1979) laboratory study of children from 9 to 30 months old interacting with a standard set of toys demonstrated that exploration through mouthing, manipulation, and vision dominated at 1 year. Container play was most prevalent at 15 months. Functionally appropriate object play emerged at the beginning of the second year. Grouping behavior, the physical ordering of objects with like characteristics, began at 18 to 24 months of age. Representational doll play, such as pretend infant caregiving, predominates at 18 to 30 months.

Occupational therapists working with young children at risk for developmental delays must distill guidelines for treatment from this limited body of research as best they can. Developmental trends in this group of studies can serve as ends, or goal targets, for play development as well means in the design of developmentally appropriate therapeutic activities. It is clear from this review that changes gradually appear in the simple exploration of objects, from simple mouthing to very specific fit of action to object. Simple physical relating of objects begins at 9 months and then develops into the increasingly complex object relations of container play and other combinations. Use of objects in functional, or culturally expected, ways emerges at 12 months of age. The emergence of pretend and symbolic play is evident at approximately 18 months, at first directed toward the self and with real objects and then moving into being directed toward others and completely imaginary objects. If the therapist can find the place on these play progressions that fit the at-risk child with whom he or she is working, the power of the treatment will be greatly enhanced.

Reilly's Rules: A Legacy of Disciplinary Play Research

Reilly's Rules of Motion, Objects, and People. Mary Reilly (1962, 1974) was one of the first occupational therapists to write on children's play. She hypothesized that children learned rules of people, objects, and movement during play. Reilly defined rules as symbols derived from and guiding interaction with the environment. Reilly's student, Robinson (1977), further elaborated on how rules were acquired in the arena of play.

Intrigued by Reilly's concepts and the central role that object play held in pediatric occupational therapy, this author completed a preliminary theoretical description in the late 1980s of rules of objects (Pierce, 1991). That study produced a descriptive taxonomy of three types of object rules learned in object play in children up to 2 years of age. Object property rules are the child's internal representation of the object's static and dynamic properties, such as shape or direct responses to action. Object action rules are the child's action repertoire, such as simple direct actions on objects and such strategies as repositioning an object to continue an interaction with it. Rules of object affect are the factors the child actively manages in selecting objects and keeping the emotional experience of play at an enjoyable level, such as novelty, sensory potency, and responsivity.

As this chapter is being written, its author is immersed in the next study in this occupational therapy exploration of infant play with objects. The current study is to produce a more comprehensive theoretical description of the normal developmental progressions in the temporal and spatial dimensions of natural infant interactions with physical objects in the home. It is hoped that the current study offers occupational therapy a much clearer picture of normal patterns of infant–object play so as to generate strategies for intervention from the strategies of normally developing infant players. If therapists begin to base their play interventions in an understanding of the usual development of whole, naturally contexted object play, they may more effectively generalize to changes in the everyday pattern of occupations.

This developing line of disciplinary research describes many dimensions along which the occupational therapist can work with the young child at risk for delays. It differentiates aspects of object play that have been only superficially described previously: how the young child builds through play experience an understanding of the action potentials associated with objects, the developmental changes in object combinations from simple approximation to complex tool use, the strategies that maintain play sequences, and how the child balances factors to keep play enjoyable (Pierce, 1991). Soon, new occupational science research is likely also to describe how young children develop action sequencing and space use in object play.

Occupational Pattern Goals for Young Children at Risk for Delays

For a young child at risk for delays, the acquisition of normal patterns of play is both an important goal and a powerful means through which to reach other goals. The foregoing review of primary areas of research on object play offers both new and experienced therapists perspectives from which to draw in generating goals and interventions.

Goals for Establishing Developmentally Appropriate Play Patterns. Goals that are intended to facilitate developmentally appropriate play in the child's daily life can range from the broad to the specific. Of course, what a desirable goal is depends on the judgment of the family. It may be helpful to describe to family members what usual patterns of play are at the age of their child and to inquire as to the importance of these patterns to them. Usually, this is a goal area that is shared in its valuing by both family and therapist. Goals for establishing developmentally appropriate play can address the frequency or amount of the child's play time, the types or developmental complexity of the child's play content, and the availability of play objects that facilitate the type of play toward which the family and therapist wish the child to move.

Establishing developmentally appropriate play is accomplished through therapist-facilitated play progressions. The child's play competencies must be accepted as they are initially found. If the child is not playing, then the goal will be for the child to engage briefly by showing interest in objects. The therapist gradually facilitates the child along aspects of developmental play complexity. These aspects are described in the foregoing review of primary theoretical and empirical perspectives on play. The object play research suggests several continua along which to advance: increasing specificity of exploration of a single object, learning object functions, changes in physically relating objects, and, at later ages, different types of pretense. The occupational therapy research line started by Mary Reilly and now ongoing suggests other areas to consider: building a broad repertoire of object uses, moving through a variety of increasingly complex object combinations, using strategies to maintain play with an object, and increasing independence in play initiation and discontinuation (Box 6-2).

Object Play and Establishing Patterns of Self-Care. Object play can also be used to establish more normal occupational patterns in self-care for children at risk for developmental delays. Generally, object play is used to facilitate childhood self-care by blurring the markers that identify an activity as either play or self-care. Objects associated with the desired self-care arena can be included in playtimes. This familiarizes the child with them and provides a gradual approach to what may be an anxiety-provoking experience. An example of this is food play, in which the child is encouraged, but not required, to taste a food as it is manipulated for the sake of play alone. If the child is willing to engage in the self-care activity only briefly, it may be tried in alternation with a play activity. Finally, if the child is an unenthusiastic participant in the self-care activity, the activity can be made more enjoyable by infusing it with a playful spirit. This can be done through inclusion of play objects in the activity (for ex-

---

Box 6-2 ESTABLISHING PLAY PATTERNS FOR ROBERTO

At the time of evaluation, Roberto was not playing. The first step was to coax him into simple, brief explorations of objects. This required a volume of novel, responsive, and mostly hand-sized toys. Later, use of larger objects in simple motor play was incorporated, such as pulling up, supported standing play (Fig. 6-2), reaching for and pursuing objects short distances, and, last, climbing. Developmental changes in physically relating objects were facilitated: from simple single-object exploration, to interactions with multisite toys such as busyboxes, to object pounding and other single-object movements within reach, to simple approximations of objects, to disassociating objects in provided combinations, to intentional combinations of objects, and, last, to appropriate use of one object on another in a simple tool pattern.

The objects used in Roberto's play progression are too numerous to describe. Often I left objects for a period, if they were especially successful or timely for the goal progression. It goes without saying that a therapist using play-based interventions requires a large toy storage area. The family was also very creative in identifying and inventing challenging play objects for Roberto, since I always explained to them why Roberto was being encouraged into certain types of play.

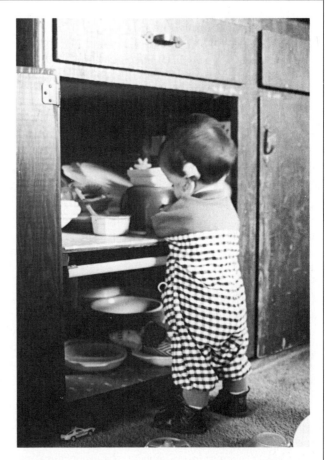

FIG. 6-2 A normal play pattern: unloading a cupboard in a supported stand.

ample, tub toys or a musical potty chair) and placing an emphasis on just having fun with the activity (Box 6-3).

USING OBJECT PLAY TO DEVELOP ENVIRONMENTAL NEGOTIATION SKILLS

Occupational therapists working with children are most accustomed to thinking of goal setting in terms of a series of intraindividual skills, such as movement, perception, and cognition. However, since occupations are interactions between child and environment, both internal developmental skills and skills for negotiating the environment are required of children. Object play is a natural medium for the acquisition of skills for negotiating the spatial, temporal, and social dimensions of the environment.

Negotiating Infant Space

The negotiation of space is a central skill in the development of the child. Most theories of infant perception and cognition attribute development to active engagement with the environment. Yet, research directly examining the develop-

ment of infants' daily movements through and manipulations of their usual surroundings is rare (Haith, 1990). For infants, the experience of object play is the training ground for understanding the relation of their bodies to their physical world, the arrangement of familiar terrains, and the potential combinations of objects in their world.

Specificity theory (Wachs & Gruen, 1982) describes the potential for the environment to offer particular types of objects at just the right place and time to have a positive impact on development. Providing the appropriate object experience, whether directly or indirectly, just as the child is ready to advance to more sophisticated levels is also the art of therapy. To use object play to address the skills of young children in negotiating the spatial environment, therapists require a basic understanding of the normal development of infant spatial abilities, as well as an understanding of how normal object play develops in spatial context.

Theories of the Development of Spatial Skills.
Piaget: from egocentric to fully coordinated reference systems. Piaget (1952, 1962) describes developmental knowledge gained from the child's actions on the environment as moving from simple sensorimotor representations

---

> ### Box 6-3 ESTABLISHING SELF-CARE PATTERNS FOR ROBERTO
>
>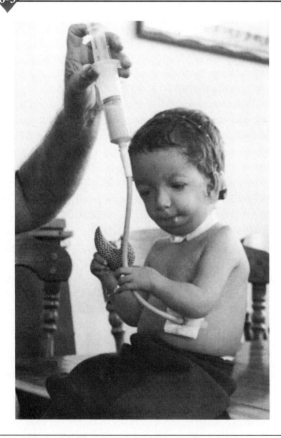
>
> Because of Roberto's age and fragility, toileting and dressing were not a focus of treatment in his case. Feeding was a primary concern. Roberto's micrognathia, cleft palate, tracheostomy, and severe bronchopulmonary dysplasia prevented him from having normal feeding experiences. He was fed by gastrostomy. During the course of treatment, the approach to feeding went through several phases: chewing on safe food and nonfood objects, taking small bites of puree with his gastrostomy feedings, sipping liquids, and eating some small bites of soft solids. Roberto was very interested in experimenting with spoon use, helping with the gastrostomy feedings (Fig. 6-3) and tasting a variety of flavors. Play was used by including feeding objects in treatment sessions, playing with food, encouraging play at home with feeding tools and foods, and working with a variety of toys to desensitize Roberto to textures. This treatment approach was not aggressive in establishing independent self-feeding, because of concerns regarding the impact of feeding on his respiratory status. However, it was aggressive in including Roberto as fully as possible in the occupation of feeding.
>
> **FIG. 6-3** Roberto assisting with his gastrostomy feeding.

of action to more abstract complex representations. Piaget theorizes that the child's spatial representations move from an egocentric reference system in the sensorimotor phase, relating object locations to his or her own body, to an allocentric system in the preoperational phase, representing space in terms of a layout of the environment that is abstracted from the location of the individual. Later, in the period of concrete operations, the child acquires representations of a few fixed regions of the environment. Adults hold a fully coordinated system of reference (Heft & Wohlwill, 1987).

More specifically, Piaget (1952, 1962) proposes that spatial understanding in infancy develops as follows. Up to 4 months of age, infants experience action in space as undifferentiated between themselves and the world around them (Acredolo, 1985). From 4 to 10 months, all observed changes in the surroundings of the infant are egocentrically attributed to the self as the causative agent. At this point, spatial understanding is concerned with how the object is related to the child, rather than how it may be related to other objects or persons. Piaget (1952) proposes that the infant begins physically relating objects to each other around the tenth month and proceeds from there to an increasingly internal representation of objects and their properties in relation to each other by 18 months of age. At 18 months of age the child is still performing most manipulations in the real world, rather than in the abstract (Piaget, 1952).

A part of this increasingly internal infant representation of the world is the acquisition of object permanence, the realization that an object continues to exist even though out of sight. Of all of Piaget's theoretical contributions to an understanding of spatial cognition in infancy, object permanence studies have received the most research attention. Results of studies on this popular topic have been soundly criticized for the difficulty of drawing a meaningful synthesis from the wealth of object permanence studies, all using a variety of settings and test objects, different manipulations of the hidden object and/or the infant, and a great range of accompanying laboratory setting landmarks (Acredolo, 1985). In actuality, acquisition of object permanence is probably an isolated milestone along a developmental progression of spatial negotiation skills.

Gibson's ecological approach to perception. James Gibson (1986), at the peak of a distinguished career in traditional visual perception research, proposed a revolutionary ecological approach to perception. His theory relies on the notion that it is not simply the passive acceptance of visual stimuli and its processing in the brain which results in our conceptions of the environment and its objects. Instead, Gibson proposes it is through the active discovery of the objective properties of the physical environment that people come to understand their surroundings. This claim has been supported by research (Acredolo, 1985; Benson & Uzgiris, 1985; Lockman, 1984; Sophian, 1986; Wellman, 1985).

Gibson's (1986) ecological psychology hypothesizes that the meaningful environment is perceived in terms of me-dium, substance, surface, and affordance. *Medium* could be a liquid, solid, or gas. Each medium offers special characteristics in terms of breathing, locomotion, transmission of light and sound, chemical diffusion, and gravity. *Substances* are portions of the environment that are relatively solid and therefore do not easily transmit light, sound, or smell. The interface of one medium with another forms a *surface,* such as the ground surface at the meeting of solid earth and gaseous air. These surfaces are the areas of the environment at which most perception and action occur. *Affordances* are the opportunities the surfaces provide to the animal or human. For instance, a large and level piece of ground affords humans support. It can be stood upon upright, walked or run upon, danced upon. It cannot, however, be dipped into or poured, or swum through, as can an air–water surface. Objects are solid configurations that are detachable from the environment. These are the primary concepts of Gibson's (1986) theory of perception, in brief version.

Environmental and ecological psychology. Environmental psychology is "a multidisciplinary approach to understanding person–environment interactions" (Cohen, 1987, p. 2). The discipline engages primarily in field research, studying the influence of the environment on individuals in context. One area of research in environmental psychology describes the internal representations, or cognitive maps, of the spatial dimensions of familiar large-scale settings (Evans, 1980; Kaplan & Kaplan, 1981; Lynch, 1960; Neisser, 1976). Most of these cognitive mapping studies have used methods inappropriate to infant research, such as analysis of adult directional narratives and sketch maps.

One exceptional environmental psychology study is Hart's (1979) examination of the free time negotiations of the physical environment by a group of elementary school aged children in a small town. Hart (1979) developmentally described the children's space use throughout their neighborhoods, their knowledge of places, the values and feelings they associated with those places, and the activities they performed in different places.

The term "ecological psychology" most often refers to Barker and Wright's (1955) approach in their landmark study of the spatial and social aspects of childhood in a small midwestern town. They described the role of the behavior setting in shaping the observed actions of the children. It is this somewhat greater emphasis on the dynamics of the environment in the person–environment interaction that distinguishes ecological psychology from environmental psychology (Wohlwill & Heft, 1987). Unfortunately, ecological psychologists usually limit their examination of the environment to social factors (Hart, 1979; Wachs, 1990).

An occupational therapy perspective. Henderson (1992) argues that visual–spatial ability in children is poorly understood in occupational therapy. Further, she states that most evaluations of spatial abilities in children are confined to examination of figural spatial tasks in cognitive space, neglecting evaluation of the role of spatial abilities in the negotiation of the real spaces of daily environments. Henderson

(1992) offers a useful typology of spatial abilities and disabilities in the following. Real space includes peripersonal space (within the range of grasp), near space (space through which a person moves), and far space (seen in the distance). Cognitive space includes "mental images of places and things in places" (Henderson, 1992, p. 4). Grasping this differentiation of types of spatial abilities offers therapists an excellent beginning for understanding infant skills for negotiating space.

Object Play Environments. Theorists and researchers have long touted the effects of the physical environment on development (Hebb, 1949). The consistent feedback available from the physical environment, in contrast to the more variable responses of the social environment, is important for the development of sensorimotor schemata (Piaget, 1952), for learning about the affordances of the environment (Gibson, 1986), and for development of a concept of the self (Neisser, 1991). In studies of the relationship between infant development and the home environment, stronger predictive correlations were found between physical setting measures and developmental scores in later childhood than could be obtained between infant assessments and later developmental scores (Wohlwill & Heft, 1987). Several studies have shown the negative effects on development of restrictions in floor freedom with playpens and other infant care equipment (Ainsworth & Bell, 1974; Elardo et al., 1975; Tulkin & Covitz, 1975; Wachs, 1976, 1979).

Factors in the home environment that appear to have the greatest impact on development include both the characteristics of environmental objects and the ability to access the physical environment. Positive relationships have been found between infant development and in-home object complexity, variety, and responsivity (Bradley & Caldwell, 1984; Clarke-Stewart, 1973; Elardo et al., 1975; Jennings et al., 1979; Wachs, 1976, 1978, 1979; Wachs et al., 1971; Yarrow et al., 1982, 1983). These findings highlight the importance of the occupational therapist's object play interventions. She or he is altering the impact of the physical environment on the child's development, whether introducing the child directly to developmentally challenging objects, helping family members to understand how the home setting influences development, or initiating changes in the child's access to spatial experiences in the home.

The greatest influence on spatial design of occupational therapy clinics serving young children at risk for delays is likely to be the administrative culture that supports that practice rather than the needs of the child for spatial experience. The goodness of fit of settings and young children's needs for spatial development probably range along the continuum of how naturalistic the settings are. That is, from worst fit to best, hospital inpatient, outpatient clinic, sensory integration style private practice, preschool, and in-home practice. The fact that sensory and movement skills are of great interest to occupational therapists does shape the clinic to the needs of the child for spatial experiences to some ex-

tent. However, the field's understanding of the development of spatial skills is presently quite limited (Henderson, 1992). Therefore, the spatial challenges offered by clinical settings, such as horizontal range, vertical levels, and active relations between objects, are not being fully exploited by the practicing therapist.

Using Object Play To Enhance Spatial Negotiation. It is time for occupational therapy to broaden its work with young children at risk for developmental delays beyond mastering the simple challenges of moving their own bodies smoothly through space. The spatial skills required for living in today's technological culture far exceed balance and coordination. Performance of everyday actions requires spatial skills for precise manipulations of peripersonal object combinations, for understandings of large and detailed spatial layouts, and for movement of objects through environmental space. It is time for therapists to extend their grasp of infant spatial skills beyond the blend of visual processing and sensory integration concepts on which they currently depend for these interventions. The ways in which infants acquire these skills in object play suggest a wealth of therapeutic interventions facilitating spatial negotiation skills.

The preceding review of primary theories of spatial skill development provides a good base from which the therapist interested in working on spatial negotiation skills can begin. Using Henderson's (1992) typology, most intervention with young children can be described as occurring in peripersonal and near space. The following discussions of simple movement through object space, object transport, and object manipulations in peripersonal space emanate from this author's current research observations. They suggest some of the spatial dimensions of usual object play that may serve the therapist as either targeted play development goals or as suggestions for the design of creative object play interventions.

Simple movement through object space. In conquering surrounding space, the infant's earliest explorations are visual. Active negotiations of space during play begin with the child's simple movements across level surfaces, perhaps in an attempt to move toward a toy or off of a blanket spread on the floor. These simple negotiations across surfaces bring lessons about traction, differences between level and inclined surfaces, and how to circumvent or clamber over low obstacles. For this phase, sofa cushions, small hills, wedges, ramps, recumbent individuals, single steps, and other low objects are useful.

A more three-dimensional sense of how the infant's body is spatially related to the environment emerges as the child begins to pull up, clamber, and climb up on objects. They then start going around, behind, and under furniture, doors, walls, and anything else of interest. An appliance box with holes cut out can be incredibly motivating in this phase of spatial development. Infants may discover favorite child-sized spaces in the home, such as behind a couch or in a blanket fort built by an older sibling. At some point, most children become intrigued with trying to move through space with vision obscured by a blanket or a bucket over the head. In the second year, infants usually become interested in removing, and later donning, their own and others' clothing.

As the child becomes more adept at locomotion, the distance traveled independently around the home increases. At first, all play is within arm's reach, then mostly within a single room, usually close to a family member. By 9 months, the child ranges easily over the whole house if allowed, usually following or leading a companion. By 18 months of age, a child quite comfortably goes to other rooms of the house without being accompanied. The sum of all of this simple movement experience is spatial skill, as well as the development of cognitive maps of the home landscape.

Object transport. Once the child becomes mobile, he or she transports objects about the environment. Mothers will testify that this seems like a centrifugal process, as objects spread inevitably outward from their starting point but only rarely back. With development, the child's object transports become increasingly intentional and aimed to a specific destination.

The earliest object transport is crawling with an interesting small toy in hand. At times, objects are carried in the mouth. Later, the infant more intentionally carries, pushes, pulls, and rides objects through space. Seeking objects out of sight and occasional placing of objects in a space associated with them emerges around the end of the first year. Propelling objects begins with dropping, then unloading objects off of surfaces and out of cupboards. Later, infants throw, and then kick, objects. Last, the infant player uses one object on another to propel it through space, such as hitting a ball with a bat, and uses containers (purse, wagon, bucket with handle) to transport groups of objects.

Object manipulations in peripersonal space. Some objects afford fine manipulation within the immediate reach of the child. Earliest are exploratory interactions that often include mouthing and handling of surfaces at hand, small hand toys, foods, drinks, and straps and strings. Many of these simple toys are interesting in their high responsivity, producing sounds or movements in reaction to the child's actions. Pounding small objects on available surfaces is probably the earliest object combination. Later, approximating two objects in hand, the classic pounding together of blocks is seen. Also in this period, infants may spend time interacting with busyboxes, multisite toys that offer simple responses to simple actions.

Developmental progressions in object combinations emerges following simple pounding and object release. Occupational therapists would do well to note that, in combinational play, the developmental phase of learning to put together is always preceded by and depends on the taking apart phase. Thus, there will be unnesting and then nesting, disassembling puzzles long before assembling, and knocking down or struggling to take apart block structures before interest in construction. Most complex is tool use, or using one object to affect another: using drawing and eating utensils, for example (Box 6-4).

Negotiating Infant Time

In occupational therapy, the most poorly understood skills for successfully negotiating the environment are those used to organize actions within time. Time is the invisible, and often forgotten, dimension of the context of our actions. Temporal negotiation skills in infancy include the establishment of a biotemporal base rhythm, differentiation between simultaneity and succession, recognition of the temporal sequences in environmental events, and action timing and sequencing. Occupational therapists often intuitively challenge these skills in treatment through the use of object play. However, temporal negotiation skills are rarely acknowledged as goals. Infants' and toddlers' acquisition of skills for sequencing interactions with the physical environment is foundational to almost all childhood and adult occupations.

Infant Biotemporal Rhythms. Most research on the infant experience of time is concerned with physiological processes, or biotemporality. The oscillation durations of biological rhythms include short (heartbeat, respiration), circadian (day length), monthly, circannual, and lifespan.

Little is known regarding differences between adult and childhood biotemporal rhythms or their entrainment to environmental zeitgebers, or time givers. In the human infant, circadian regularity is thought to precede the capability of entraining to environmental cues. In utero, the infant is subject to the circadian rhythms of the mother. The sleep–wake pattern is rhythmic and repetitive at birth. However, the child does not immediately entrain to environmental zeitgebers. Infants alternate between periods of wakefulness and napping around the clock. The periods of sleeping and waking lengthen over the first few months. This free-running rhythm may appear in the early months to reach synchrony with the rest of the family, with the baby sleeping at night. In actuality, it is often merely a congruent free-running oscillation that matches for a few nights to that of the entrained family's sleep–wake cycle. Then the oscillations continue into completely incongruent patterns to the despair of the baby's parents. By about the twentieth week of life, the human infant begins to achieve true synchrony through entrainment to light and social cues (Moore-Ede et al., 1982).

Later in infancy and toddlerhood, a rhythm of daytime sleep and activity is established within the activity patterns of the family. By 9 months of age, this pattern is clearly settled into between one and three predictable nap periods each day. As the child matures, the awake periods lengthen and the nap periods decrease in number. Typically, the midday nap is retained until about 4 years of age. This midday slump in energy level is also typical of adults and is retained in many cultures as a usual rest time for all ages (Moore-Ede et al., 1982).

Temporal Cognition in Childhood. Research on temporal cognition in childhood has focused on children of sufficient

▼ **Box 6-4** **WORKING ON SPATIAL DEVELOPMENT WITH ROBERTO**

Roberto's weakness and need for frequent suctioning limited the development of his spatial skills. The family kept him close to the suction machine instead of allowing his exploration of home spaces. However, with my encouragement and attractive spatial play objects, Roberto began to venture out and explore, although his skills were delayed. His resistance to crawling, because of his shoulder weakness, also impeded his early experiences of space use. We incorporated a lot of upright spatial exploration. Roberto was encouraged to spend time in cruising and supported standing play and in unloading a small kitchen cupboard full of hand-sized toys and Tupperware.

In the area of peripersonal manipulations, Roberto spent time unloading small toys out of bags, boxes, and crates, and later placing pegs and stickers and other objects on, in, and through other objects. We pushed balls around the house, climbed up and down the stairs, and clambered over disassembled couches. We also spent time outside when the weather permitted, despite Roberto's fears of the texture of the grass. The family became receptive to the therapist's encouragement to take Roberto as many places as they could, using the portable suction machine.

In Roberto's case, the goals that primarily addressed spatial negotiation skills included an increased variety and number of everyday spatial object play, broader and more frequent independent ranging in home space, initiating horizontal and then three-dimensional movements in space, and a developmental progression through object combinations and tool use (Figure 6-4, *A, B,* and *C*).

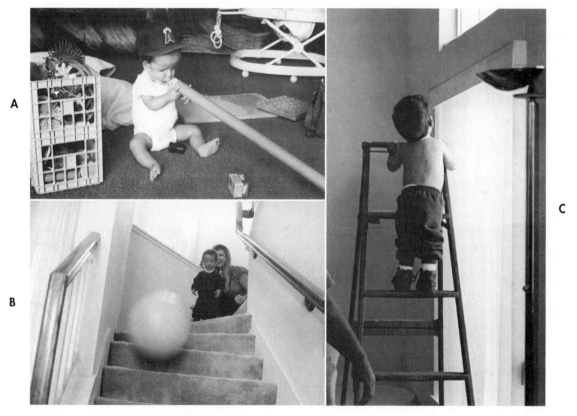

FIG. 6-4 Exploring home space: **A,** Roberto watching a bearing roll down a tube. **B,** Roberto rolling a ball down the stairs. **C,** Roberto up a ladder.

age to articulate their perceptions of the world around them. The perception of time in the most immediate sense includes differentiation between simultaneity and succession, perception of order and interval, and estimation of duration. Memory processes are inseparably tied to these percep-

tual abilities (Fraisse, 1963). Piaget (1971) envisioned the child's growing capacities as internal representations emerging from their actions on the world, changing from simple reflexive action to anticipation of future events and a practical series of actions to reach an envisioned end. Piaget

(1971) and Fraisse (1963) detailed the older child's abilities to manage abstract estimations of time, recalling the order of events, estimating duration, and understanding order and duration separately. Once the child is able to reverse constructions, a more complex set of logical operations can be used to access time. All of these abilities contribute to a developmental expansion of temporal horizons. Temporal horizons are the lengths of time to which the child can project events into the past or into the future from the present.

The research on temporal skills of older children provides a framework for describing the antecedent understandings of time that may be held by infants and toddlers. A newborn seems to live in the moment, with little awareness of the sequences in which its experience is embedded. In the early months, infants begin to differentiate between simultaneous and successive events. They demonstrate recognition of the sequences observed around them by their responses, such as turning to see an approaching person appear around a corner, or attempting to escape the approach of a suction bulb. At 6 months of age, the infant clearly demonstrates intentional action sequences, such as wriggling toward a desired object or pounding an object repeatedly on a surface. They hold in mind a desired object for a short period after it disappears but then can be distracted by another interesting object. Later, the infant shows frustration when anticipated outcomes fail to materialize and persists in searching for desired objects out of sight.

At later ages, the infant progresses to increasingly complex sequences of action. By 1 year of age, the infant is using fairly sophisticated sequences of instrumental planning, such as transporting an object to use as a step to reach a counter or handing pieces of laundry out of the dryer for mother to fold. Ayres (1985) discussed some aspects of action sequencing and timing in her work on praxis, primarily in relation to movement skills. Piaget (1952) also discussed the infant's evolving complexity of action in the progression in the first 2 years from primary to tertiary circular reactions. However, this literature does not begin to describe the sophistication of the 2 year old's understanding of household routines and the potential series of object combinations available in play.

Research on infant understandings of temporality is extremely limited at this time. However, infants do demonstrate a maturing understanding of the temporal context of their own actions and the actions of those around them. Occupational therapists working with children at risk for developmental delays need to consider skills for negotiation of time when setting goals for facilitating development through object play.

Using Object Play To Facilitate Temporal Negotiation Skills.

Although occupational therapists are not accustomed to thinking in this way, object play is easily used to facilitate improved temporal skills in young children. The place to start is at the base of temporal skill development: biotemporal rhythms.

Establishing regular biotemporal rhythms. The establishment of regular biotemporal rhythms provides the base from which to build temporal skills. This is especially critical for children recently discharged from the hospital, where they may not have been exposed to the normal light and activity cues that usually entrain the infant biological clock.

To begin, record a log of a minimum of 1 week of the child's sleep–wake rhythm. This will sensitize the parents to the biotemporal rhythm and provide the therapist with information. If there is no recognizable pattern, the immediate goal becomes to facilitate one's solidifying. If there is a pattern in need of change, select with the infant's caregivers the pattern toward which they wish to aim.

Changes must be made in very small increments, and in the direction of lengthening awake periods and moving them later rather than shortening them or moving them earlier. The primary tools that can be used to influence the sleep–wake pattern are exposure to light, hunger–satiation, activity context, and object play. Exposure to the light at the beginning of the child's day and during active play times and limitation of light exposure at sleep times assists entrainment of temporal patterns. A predictable schedule of feedings also helps, especially the avoidance of hunger during desired sleep periods. A sleep routine can be created by the family, including favorite toys or blankets, feedings, music, rocking, or sequencing ties to other activities, such as bathing or dinner. The activity context of the family's actions surrounding the child also influence the child's sleep–wake pattern. For example, if the family is doing energetic actions around the child, he or she is more likely to remain awake, and vice versa. Last, keeping motivating play objects until the end of the desired awake period can be used to extend the rhythm toward the goal pattern.

Facilitating temporal awareness. Infants first acquire awareness of temporal sequences by recognizing temporal patterns in the activities surrounding them. For this reason, it is important that infants at risk for delays be included as much as possible in these patterns. During everyday household activities, infants can be included through being placed at a good vantage point for observation, by being allowed to handle and play with the objects involved, and by participating in other simple ways. The temporal pattern of the activity can be accentuated by making eye contact or doing a simple repetitive play action with the child at repeating points in the activity. For instance, every time that mom reaches for another diaper to fold, she may momentarily drape it over the baby's face and then pull it away, creating a repeating game.

The infant's anticipation of events can be facilitated through cuing. The therapist or the caregiver can call the infant's attention to impending events, such as a toy that is about to produce sound, or a bottle that is going into the microwave. Selection of toys that lend themselves to demonstrating strong repeating patterns also assists in acquisition of temporal awareness. An example of a strong repeater is a Jack-in-the-box. Involving the infant in a pattern of turn taking also facilitates this skill.

Facilitation of normal patterns of play sequences in therapy is difficult because of the lack of literature describing these developmental patterns. It is not difficult to create activities for the simple pattern of a single action and response, but the patterns beyond that are not well understood. At 6 to 9 months old, the infant plays with a series of small hand-held toys, grasping, mouthing, banging, passing them from one hand to the other, and dropping them. Often, the same objects are returned to over and over, as long as they remain within reach. For this phase, the sequence requires a large number of small objects with which to repeat similar actions. As infants mature, they appear to play longer with an object, performing a related series of actions on it. By 18 months, they are performing longer instrumental combinations of objects. Research describing these lengths and sequences in play is needed to support therapeutic facilitation of temporal skills in infants and toddlers (Box 6-5).

Box 6-5   **FACILITATING TEMPORAL NEGOTIATION WITH ROBERTO**

Roberto's early months of life in a neonatal intensive care unit and his chronic respiratory problems resulted in a completely unpredictable sleep–wake schedule. The establishment of a regular biotemporal rhythm was an immediate goal when therapy began. This process included keeping periodic logs, discussing with the family desired temporal patterns and strategies to reach them, gradually building up a sleep routine, and introducing changes in Roberto's sleep space. Transition from a completely nonpredictable to a settled sleep–wake pattern took approximately 6 months. After that, there were gradual maturational changes in the pattern.

Temporal cognition goals for Roberto included extending his temporal horizons in the anticipation of environmental sequences, learning turn taking, and independently sequencing play actions of increasing lengths (Figs. 6-5, *A* and *B*).

For this, a wide variety of play activities was used, especially games that had strong ending points, such as the collapse of a block structure or production of music. When working with object play of sequences longer than Roberto could maintain on his own, I used chaining, encouraging Roberto to assume a larger and larger portion of the sequence until he performed it all on his own. I often brought these sequence-chaining play objects to treatment several times before Roberto conquered them. At times, I would bring back favorite objects from earlier months to check on how he was remembering the previously learned uses of those objects. I deliberately gave many cues about upcoming portions of the session by putting out the series of activities within view, saying that I was leaving after a certain play object, and using our own unique arrival and leave-taking rituals (Fig. 6-5, *B*).

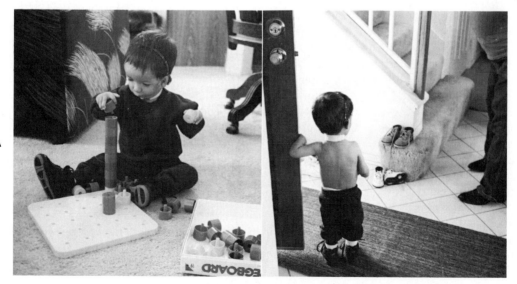

FIG. 6-5   **A,** Roberto in sequencing play. **B,** Roberto participating in a leave taking.

Negotiating the Infant Social Environment

The third dimension of the environment that the young child must learn to negotiate is the social dimension. Object play can be used to facilitate the child's social skills, to draw the family into involvement in treatment, and to establish interactive play in the home.

Sociocultural Impacts on Development. The social dimension of the child's play environment has strong impacts on the infant's development. Research indicates that cultural and socioeconomic status differences shape the daily experience of infants, especially through the pattern of the mother–infant relationship (Bornstein et al., 1990a, 1990b, 1991; Rubin et al. 1976). Infants of specific groups of mothers, such as teenagers or depressed women, are at high risk for compromised development (Coll et al., 1986; Lyons-Ruth et al., 1986). Infants' referencing to maternal facial expressions has been shown to influence their actions with toys (Cohn & Elmore, 1988; Gunnar & Stone, 1984; Hornik et al., 1987; Klinnert, 1984; Walden & Ogan, 1988). A factor analytic study of a home physical environment inventory's predictive validity for intelligence showed the highest dependence on measures of the learning materials provided and the mother's facilitation of her child's development (Stevens & Bakeman, 1985). This research on the impact of the social dimension on infant development supports the importance of the therapist's attention to the infant's social environment and social skills.

Facilitating Infant Social Skills Through Object Play. The social skills of infants and young children generally include the ability to establish bonds with family members, to communicate with others, and to enjoy developmentally appropriate shared activities. All of these are learned through interactions with family members during play or caregiving activities. The most important action the therapist can take in the facilitation of the infant's social skills is to impress on the family the importance of interactive play to the child's development. Families of children at risk for developmental delays are often dealing with critical health issues, in which concerns for the child's health may override the desire to interact in usual, playful ways with the child. Loss of opportunities for play because of a demanding care schedule can also have a negative impact on the child's social and play skills, the family members' enjoyment of their child, and the strength of the emotional bonds between the child and family members. Beyond reiterating to caregivers the importance of social play in the home, the therapist can facilitate social skills in the following ways.

In direct treatment, the therapist can use object play as the basis for his or her interactions with the child. This is best done by providing activities in which an adult's involvement is necessary to continue. This requires the child to communicate with, alternate action with, and anticipate the actions of the therapist. The therapist must focus on understanding and responding to the child's smallest attempts at communication. She or he must also have great patience, repeatedly awaiting the child's action in the shared play sequences. By 15 months, a typically developing child is able to request objects, bring adults to desired objects out of reach, and bring objects to an adult for play. During treatment sessions, the therapist can draw caregivers into interactive play with the child to the extent that they appear to be comfortable. Some explanation of the specific gains that can be expected from offered activities may encourage them to join in, despite how nonserious the activity may seem.

Social object play is easily facilitated in the home. In home programs, every effort should be made to frame all aspects of requested participation in terms of play. Optional ideas for play interactions should be provided frequently and updated regularly. Play at home between treatment sessions should always be inquired about by asking open-ended questions such as "What has been the favorite play object this week?" and finding positive things to say about the value of that play. The therapist may also loan particularly successful or appropriate toys, leaving them with the family between visits. This can be more expensive in terms of supplies but is well justified in its enhancement of therapeutic effect. Suggestions of challenging play objects can be provided at holidays or birthdays if it seems appropriate within the family. If the caregivers and therapist are fortunate enough to share the aims of treatment clearly among them, the family may begin to discover and invent play objects that meet the needs of the child, proudly showing their creations to the therapist (Box 6-6).

USING OBJECT PLAY TO ADDRESS COMMON DEVELOPMENTAL COMPONENT GOALS

Object play is most commonly used by pediatric occupational therapists to address goals targeting development of sensory processing, movement, or cognition. Occupational therapists are comfortable at this level of intervention for several reasons. Our training emphasizes a breakdown analysis of component skills and then setting goals in weak areas of performance. The empirical and theoretical bases for clinical interventions at this goal level are found in focused blocks of literature. Further, designing goals that are delimited to a single area of development is easier, and progress is more readily measured. Many excellent resources exist within occupational therapy for addressing this level. Working at the level of developmental component goals is already familiar ground for most therapists. The contribution of this chapter to those competencies is to support the use of object play to reach those goals more effectively.

Using Object Play to Address Goals of Sensation and Perception

Infant development of sensory and perceptual processes are often of concern to occupational therapists. The infant's

Box 6-6   **USING OBJECT PLAY TO FACILITATE ROBERTO'S SOCIAL NEGOTIATION**

In Roberto's case, the family was very involved in his treatment. His mother was young, his father was out of the country, and there were concerns that his mother would not be able to provide his care while continuing as the sole support of herself and her parents. Institutionalization was a possibility. Roberto was the only young child in the home. He was cared for during the day by his grandparents, both active despite some disabilities.

My first concern was to make the mother more comfortable with her child. She appeared afraid to play with Roberto because of his fragility. At first, we focused on small, quiet, playful interactions that she could share with Roberto. Some of these included holding his gaze on her face or on slowly moving objects that interested him, gentle touching games, and gentle movements to music.

At times, the family was so intent on observing Roberto's interactions with me that it felt like a performance. I was able to draw the family into play at some times and not at others, depending on other household activities. I also found that, when Roberto was feeling uninterested in treatment activities, especially when he was ill, pulling a family member into play would support his motivation nicely. I was pleased that the family was always trying to understand how Roberto could improve his skills. I often left toys for a week or more, and the family would proudly report his exploits with them.

In home programs and in discussions with the family, I tried to provide as many different play ideas as possible. I jotted them down on notes that I stuck on the refrigerator at regular intervals. I encouraged the family to problem solve with me over times when Roberto was not progressing in some area. Roberto's grandfather was especially creative in finding and inventing objects to encourage Roberto's progress (Fig. 6-6).

As is not unusual with children at risk, there was a point at which questions of discipline and limit setting were confronted. After several brief discussions prompted by eruptions of problematic behavior, Roberto's mother established a successful approach to discipline. Roberto's social skills were excellent by his second birthday, despite his limited language.

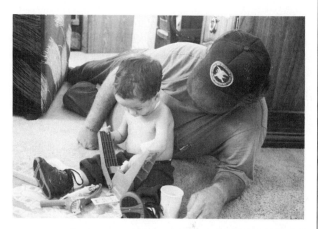

FIG. 6-6   Roberto and his grandfather playing with play dough.

---

processing of visual, tactile, auditory, vestibular, kinesthetic, proprioceptive, and gustatory information are abilities essential to interactions with the physical environment (Ayres, 1985; Neisser, 1976). Generally, therapists writing goals in the area of sensation and perception attempt to make changes in sensation tolerance, perceptual accuracy, and interpretation of perception in the production of an active response.

Thanks to the work of A. Jean Ayres (1972, 1985) and others, occupational therapists are the premier professionals for remediation of perceptual problems in childhood. Amelioration of problems of processing tactile and movement information through interactions with the physical environment is especially strong in the field. Some therapy supply companies are focused almost entirely on offering therapists objects for remediation of sensory processing problems. Some clinical settings are completely designed around offering these challenges. Since therapists are already so resourceful in this area, only brief mention of several types of sensory processing is made here as a spur to thinking about the range of play objects to which therapists have access in their practice for addressing goals of sensory processing.

Tactile Perception. Consistent success in creating object play opportunities to address tactile processing skills depends on a wealth of activity ideas that offer a wide variety of textures. Therapists should inventory their toy cupboards to see whether they have several materials that easily offer complexes of these textures: dry, wet, smooth, rough, moldable, solid, stretchy, particulate, and variations of density and softness of pile fibers. Types of object play used to interact with these textures include simple texture exploration, seeking and matching by touch games, art production, food preparation, and pretend. Textures can also be added to objects used frequently to address other goals, such as balls, swings, and large containers. In some clinics, the "messiness" of some of these potential activities prevents them from being frequently used. This is an unfortunate triumph of housekeeping concerns over the needs of the child. Also, therapists must never forget that providing a tool with which to manipulate a material can provide a graded approach to full contact with an intimidating texture. Rotating different objects for combining with a frequently used textured material also increases the novelty and potential repertoire of actions with which it can be used.

Vestibular Processing and Balance. Processing of movement sensation is most easily addressed through object play involving suspended equipment, such as the variety of swings and platforms typically used in a clinic specializing in the sensory integration approach. Simply staying positioned on these during movement can be the primary activity, or they can be used as the surface on which another type of object play occurs. Object play demanding vestibular processing can also use nonsuspended unstable surfaces, such as a therapy ball or roll, scooter board, incline, skates, riding toys, or surfaces that have give (trampoline, waterbed, piles of cushions). The therapist must control the level of demand the activity places on the tolerance for and interpretation of vestibular input by the child. Safety is always a concern with the use of unstable surfaces. Object play facilitating vestibular processing without using unstable surfaces includes games in which the young child must use extremities to reach, catch, hit, or kick objects without losing balance. Therapists should have quick access to a wide variety of objects that challenge vestibular processing.

Proprioceptive and Kinesthetic Perception. Processing information about limb position is most often challenged in object play incorporating movement, such as those activities just described for vestibular processing. Often, therapists use different weighting strategies to enhance proprioception, such as attaching weights to extremities or around the child's trunk, or using weighted play objects, such as balls, building blocks, or sandbags. Object play involving heavy work, such as lifting, carrying, pulling, or pushing also provides input to the proprioceptive system. Games requiring accurate placement of extremities to make contact with an object, such as catching or hitting something, also require accurate proprioceptive processing. Play in darkness or in which vision is occluded is especially useful for work on proprioception: walking under a blanket, for example. Very fine kinesthetic demand can be provided in games or art projects requiring carefully graded control, such as in placement of a small object through an aperture or drawing within a limited area.

Visual Perception and Coordination. Effective gaze is the base for visual perception. Infants must master gaze localization, fixation, pursuits, and shifts (Erhardt, 1986). Using object play to work on goals of visual perception with very young children usually involves visual seeking of some type of target, whether that be the therapist's face, a place to throw or place another object in a simple game, or an attempt to locate a desired object. Remember that the child must have achieved object permanence to play any seeking games in which the target is largely obscured. Visual perception can also be challenged in combinational play, in which the accurate placement of an object is required. Visual perception of objects in motion is often used when gaze coordination is an issue. Finer visual perception in older children is tapped in many tabletop paper and pencil activities, such as mazes, hidden pictures, writing, and drawing.

Auditory Perception. Object play challenging auditory processing includes games of seeking by sound, simple direction following, sing-alongs, playing simple instruments, childhood chants that cue action (such as Ring Around the Rosey), and objects that give pleasurable auditory responses. For many infants, the problem of auditory defensiveness requires the therapist to monitor closely, and possibly limit, the degree of auditory input in the infant's environment.

Arousal. Therapists addressing goals of sensory processing often also set goals addressing arousal levels in children who appear chronically underaroused or overaroused. Object play to address goals of arousal draw on the same activities just described within the areas of sensory processing. However, in working on arousal, the therapist is more interested in the effects on alertness and its stability than in the accuracy of perception.

Using Object Play to Address Development of Motor Skill

The single most frequently written goal in pediatric occupational therapy is probably a motor goal. Movement goals are very highly valued by families. Since the literature in this area is comparatively well developed both within and outside of the field, a detailed review is not provided within the limited space of this chapter. As with all of the developmental goals, it is assumed that the therapist will seek out research and educational opportunities to stay abreast of this rapidly changing area. For the purpose of discussing how object play can be used to facilitate movement goals, the topic is split into two distinct types of interventions: stability and locomotion, and object contact and manipulation.

Stability and Locomotion. With very young children, movement goals focusing on stability and locomotion can be framed in two ways. One is to target qualities of performance, such as strength, endurance, or coordination. The other approach is to move the child along a familiar developmental progression: head control, turning over, prone propping, sitting, supported stand, pulling up, combat crawl, crawling, cruising, standing, clambering, walking, climbing, and running.

Goals of stability, in which the therapeutic interaction requires the child to remain relatively stationary, require sufficiently engaging object play to incite the child's endurance. Therapists need to offer a variety of play activities at the child's developmental level of object play that challenge the targeted stability skill.

Goals of locomotion use play objects that are interacted with as surfaces or media, as special spaces, as transportable objects, or as therapy lures. "Surfaces" or "media," refer to objects whose appeal is in the experience of moving over or through them. For instance, in working on crawling in very shallow water (medium), or on walking on a trampoline (surface), the play object is not a small, hand-held, manipulable toy, but the thing across (or through) which locomotion occurs.

Special spaces are large stationary objects that offer the child opportunities to go in and out, go under, or go on top of the object. Examples are pools, sandboxes, blanket forts, appliance boxes, and corners behind furniture.

Transportable objects are those that the child can enjoy pushing, pulling, riding, or carrying across a surface. Pushing and riding toys are common on the market and easy to find. Push toys are especially useful for supported walking. However, the therapist needs to have a developmental progression in the motor complexity as well as in the size of the toy. This is problematic for children who are working on locomotion goals at a chronological age at which they are significantly larger than the children for which the toy industry has designed these toys. The therapist must be sensitive to these issues, using object adaptations and a persistent shopping strategy to assemble the appropriately challenging pushing and riding toys. String pull toys are not as easily found as they once were. However, other objects can also be pulled, such as a light wagon, a blanket with a stuffed animal rider, or a long kite tail of silk. Push or pull toys that are also containers offer additional play possibilities.

Carry objects can be anything the child is interested in transporting in arms. Sometimes, this can be made into a game of carrying a series of objects to a container, or incorporated into the getting out or picking up phases of the treatment session. Containers with handles, such as purses or buckets with bails, are especially useful for encouraging object transport.

When viewing movement development goals from the perspective of sensory integrative theory it is important to consider the degree to which offered object play challenges self-directed praxis (Ayres, 1985). The intent to facilitate development of ideation, motor planning, and execution in the very young child may lead the therapist to involve the child to a greater extent in selection and creation of activity choices. This requires the therapist to provide a greater number of custom-tailored activity choices appropriate to the needs and goals of that infant. With a sufficient number before them, their self-directed actions are still likely to serve as a good fit with therapeutic goals. The therapist must work from the child's current level of ability, offering actions of high appeal to draw out just slightly more sophisticated performances each time. Ayres (1985) also emphasized the importance of action sequencing and timing in her work on praxis. Often, a spontaneous game of sequence repetition

and sequence expansion can be generated from the child's initially simpler actions. Therapists must always remember that working on praxis requires object play that is novel, not routine.

Object Contact and Manipulation. As in locomotor goals, goals for hand skills can specify attainment of qualities of performance, such as strength or degree of dexterity, or the goals can follow a developmental sequence. The development of object contact and manipulation skills have not been as linearly described as have gross motor skills. Working from the literature on grasp development can yield goals specifying emergence of specific grasps, phases of eye–hand coordination, midline crossing and bimanual coordination, in-hand manipulation skills, and functional manipulations of objects.

Infant development of reach and grasp passes through these phases: early reflexive grasp that is extinguished by 24 weeks (Gesell, 1940), reaching beginning as early as 8 weeks, object contact at 20 weeks, and successful gross grasp of a cube at 24 weeks (Gesell, 1940; White et al., 1964). As infants gradually gain control over the many degrees of freedom in upper extremity movement, reaching becomes more continuous and precise (Elliot & Connolly, 1973; Gesell, 1940). By 18 months of age, reaching is highly automatic.

Development of eye–hand coordination has been widely described (Bushnell, 1985: Erhardt, 1982: McDonnell, 1979: White et al., 1964: Williams, 1973). Along with the earlier acquisition of visual fixation and tracking skills, prehension is initially accomplished with gaze at the hand, later with gaze primarily for grasp adjustments, and finally with vision fixed only on the object of interest. Increasing differentiation in bimanual coordination is often attributed to the normal development of brain lateralization (Bresson et al., 1977; Fagard & Jacquet, 1989). Exner (1992) has described the wide variety of in-hand object manipulations used by children, although how these emerge in infancy is not yet known. There is also evidence of the infant's adjustment of hand orientation to object characteristics as early as 18 weeks of age, and becoming increasingly sophisticated over time (Lockman et al., 1984; Newell et al., 1989).

Connolly and Dalgleish (1989), in an innovative videotape study of the acquisition of spoon feeding, found the following pattern across development: increasing consistency in type of grasp and in use of the preferred hand, increasing involvement of the contralateral hand in the eating task, changes in patterns of movement, action smoothing, increased visual monitoring of the spoon, and decreased time required to bring the spoon to the mouth.

The specificity and multiplicity of goals in this area precludes a detailed discussion here of the possible object play interventions to reach those goals. The interface of the human hand and the physical environment is such a central crux of human occupation that object play addressing goals of object contact and manipulation can be generated from nearly any activity that is of interest to the child. The therapist simply begins with the developmental object play level of the child, compares that with the object contact or manipulation goal, and then uses his or her creativity to design activities challenging that skill.

Using Object Play to Address Cognition

Because Piagetian theory is the premier window on both infant cognitive development and play development, the relationship of play and cognition is deeply woven for therapists. The following discussion of using object play to facilitate cognition is based on the Piagetian stages found in the sensorimotor period (0 to 2 years). Although it is not possible to discuss Piagetian theory fully within this chapter, his work is recommended to all pediatric therapists who find themselves frequently addressing cognitive development.

The first stage (0 to 1 month) of the sensorimotor period is elementary sensorimotor adaptations. This stage is characterized by simple reflexes, uncoordinated movements, and the first discrimination and recognition of human and nonhuman objects. Selection of play objects for goals at this level of cognition strives simply to focus attention on an interesting object, produce reactions that demonstrate recognition, and provide experiences of reflexive grasp. Objects to attract visual gaze should offer visual contrast or high responsivity. For grasp, the objects must be of hand size.

The second stage (1 to 4 months) involves acquired adaptations. The first primary circular reactions, the child's retention of chance results in play, are seen in this stage. Object play facilitating cognition at this stage uses visual observation of stationary and moving objects, early sound play turn taking, reflexive object holding and moving within the visual field, and mouthing of objects in hand or not in hand. This is a stage at which a large variety of rattles, balls, and other small graspable objects are most useful.

Stage three (4 to 8 months) of the sensorimotor period, intentional sensorimotor adaptations, is dominated by the repetition of discovered patterns. The child begins distinguishing means and ends. Parts of an action are linked in time, but a series of actions are not. At this stage, objects that produce a clear direct response to the child's actions are useful, such as busyboxes, infant keyboards, and percussion toys. The child spends lengths of time simply grasping, handing from one hand to the other, and releasing objects, often until all objects within reach are beyond reach. If the infant is crawling, he or she pursues objects within close visual range. Discovering objects that are partially obscured leads to establishment of object permanence.

The fourth stage (8 to 12 months) involves further formation of concepts regarding the properties of objects. Time, causality, and space relationships begin to form as the child travels through the setting. The child begins to circumvent barriers to reach a desired object, further demonstrating emerging object permanence. Intermediary objects are used to reach goals, as in climbing on something else to get up on the couch, or pulling on a blanket to get a toy that is on it. The child more clearly anticipates outcomes from indicators in the environment. Play strategies from one toy are tried out on another toy. At this age, objects begin to be used in simple combinations, such as banging a spoon on a tray and dumping things out of containers.

The fifth stage (12 to 18 months) is the stage of experimentation. Much time may be spent in what appears to be repetition but is actually subtly varied action. Large numbers of objects are typically engaged over time, yielding what can seem to the parent to be an explosion of toys, pots and pans, clothing, and other objects scattered through the house. Putting in, taking out, transporting, and early matching of parts (pans and lids often) is constant. Children's understanding of how objects can be combined becomes so much more sophisticated by the end of this stage that they begin simple tool use, such as drawing with chalk, stirring with a spoon, or other functional uses of one object on another.

The sixth stage (18 to 24 months) of the sensorimotor period is characterized by the use of mental combinations to invent new means of acting on objects. Many of the "problems" of reaching an end are now encountered and accommodated to internally through mental combinations. This results primarily in a difference in speed of invention in comparison to the previous stage, as well as an abbreviation of object manipulations leading to invention.

Object combinations become even more complex as the child begins simple constructions, continues to develop tool use, and enters fully into imitation of others as a mode of exploring objects.

The sensorimotor period is followed by the preoperational period, which lasts from 2 to 7 years of age. The preoperational period is characterized by the egocentrism of the child, demonstrated in attitudes of animism, realism, and magical thinking. Games of make-believe predominate from 2 to 4 years, giving way to interactive games with increasingly complex shared rules (Box 6-7).

MOTIVATIONAL PROPERTIES IN THERAPEUTIC OBJECT PLAY

The simplest use of object play in therapeutic applications is as a therapy lure, used to motivate the child to engage in another more or less unrelated therapeutic activity. For example, an attractive toy is presented out of reach of a child who is being encouraged to crawl. Play with the toy is brief, however, since it does not encompass a goal on which the child needs to work. The therapy lure is the least sophisticated therapeutic use of object play.

An understanding of the motivational properties of play objects can be used to increase the appeal of play-based activities for goals targeting developmental components, environmental negotiation skills, and occupational patterns. The competence of the therapist in fostering the child's motivation to play is critical to successful intervention with children with disabilities, who are often considered unmotivated. The most draining treatment sessions for this author are those in which the child is lethargic and uninterested.

◤ **Box 6-7** ◢   **FACILITATING DEVELOPMENTAL COMPONENT GOALS WITH ROBERTO**

In the area of sensation and perception, Roberto's goals were primarily focused on reducing his tactile defensiveness. For this, play objects of a variety of textures were used, beginning with less potent textures and working toward more challenging textures over the treatment period (Fig. 6-7). Food textures were explored in play and in brief feeding sessions just before gastrostomy feedings. Additionally, treatment activities initially supported visual development. Auditory experience was also included in many activities since the degree of Roberto's deafness was not clear. The sensory goals were addressed through simple variety in play objects that offered a good developmental fit for Roberto.

Roberto's needs in the area of movement primarily involved upper extremity skills because of the malformations of his hands and left arm and shoulder. Both before and after his hand reconstructions, I selected activities that would challenge the emergence of his ability to grasp and manipulate objects. For this reason, we often spent much of the session seated on the floor playing with small manipulable objects. Treatment also supported the emergence of movement and locomotion skills (Fig. 6-8, A

and B). Although consistently delayed, they were acquired in a relatively normal sequence. The exception to this was crawling, which was difficult because of Roberto's left shoulder malformation. He resisted all but the most interesting activities if they required efforts to crawl. We continued to work with activities that yielded shoulder strengthening, even after he was walking well. Roberto did eventually learn to crawl.

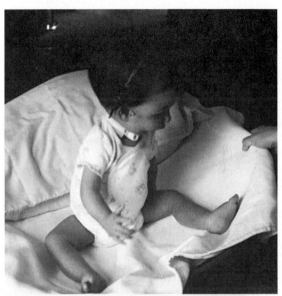

A

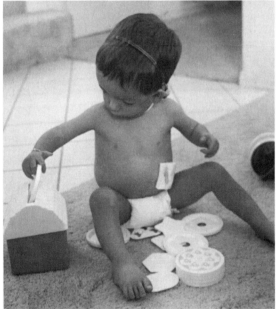

B

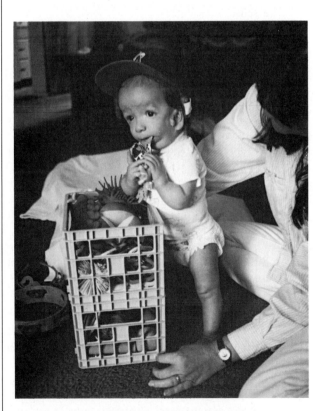

FIG. 6-7   Early work on tactile defensiveness.

FIG. 6-8   **A,** Early work on motor goals: postural stability on a saucer. **B,** Later work on motor goals: grasp and dexterity.

Continued.

FACILITATING DEVELOPMENTAL COMPONENT GOALS WITH ROBERTO—Cont'd

Roberto's cognitive development was at risk because of his deafness, chronic illness, physical limitations, and restrictions to environmental exploration. Cognition was easily supported in this case, simply by assisting Roberto to progress through the developmental levels in normal object play (Fig. 6-9). The object interactions used were too numerous to describe here. However, they roughly included the early use of multiple hand-sized objects for exploration, then objects that provided strong direct responses to the infant's actions or challenged object permanence, later the simplest object combinations, and then container and construction play and more complex tool use.

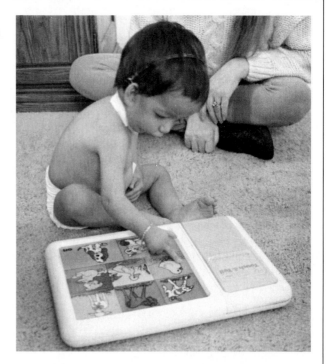

FIG. 6-9   Cognitive goals: picture identification.

Theories of Play Motivation

The motivations proposed for play are as various as the theories of play. In psychoanalysis and gestalt psychology, play is seen as an attempt to reduce inner tension (Erikson, 1950; Slobin, 1964; Wehman & Abramson, 1976). Behavioral psychology views play as response to environmental stimulation and reinforcement (Slobin, 1964). Piaget cites the equilibrium of ego assimilation and accommodation as a general motivator of behavior, functional pleasure as a motivation of play, and mastery as the desired result of learned schemas (Piaget, 1962).

Popular definitions of play usually associate play with fun and pleasure. Actually, research shows that interest is the predominant emotion in children's interactions with toys, with little variation. Joy is observed, but less often than would be expected from cultural representations of play (Phillips & Sellitto, 1990).

Optimal Arousal. Theories of optimal arousal view play as a strategy to maintain a pleasurable emotional state. Arousal is a measure of alertness (Berlyne, 1965). Collative variables, defined as comparison situations resulting in arousal, include novelty, complexity, and incongruity or surprisingness (Berlyne, 1965, 1971; Fowler, 1965; Herron & Sutton-Smith, 1971; Hutt, 1966; Look, 1977; Weisler & McCall, 1976). States

of suboptimal and supraoptimal arousal are aversive. By engaging pacers or optimally arousing stimuli situations, the system is advanced upward along the scale of complexity as the pacers are explored and new concepts incorporated (Ellis, 1973). Resolution of pacers is experienced as pleasurable. Hence the fun of play (Berlyne, 1971; Ellis, 1973).

Novelty-loving species learn to deal flexibly with a changing environment rather than use patterned behaviors. Ellis (1973) postulates that problem-solving skills are acquired through play, motivated by a drive to maintain an optimal arousal level. The potency of novelty in increasing attention span, activity level, exploration, and level of play in preschool children have all been documented (Berlyne, 1971; Butler, 1977; Cantor, 1963; Daehler & O'Connor, 1980; Eson et al., 1977; Faulkender, 1980; Henderson, 1978, 1981; Henderson & Moore, 1980; Hutt, 1966; Lewis, 1978; Scholtz & Ellis, 1975; Sussman, 1979).

Flow Theory. Another useful perspective on the emotional qualities of the play experience is provided by Csikszentmihalyi's (1975) concept of "flow." The flow state is enjoyable and fully involving, a good match of perceived skills and action challenges. It is marked by five conditions: "a merging of action and awareness," "a centering of attention on a limited stimulus field," "a loss of self-conciousness," "control over actions and the environment," and "unambiguous feedback from the environment" (Csikszentmihalyi, 1975, pp. 38-46). This flow state is easily observed in normal infant object play.

Competence and Mastery. The urge for competency was proposed by Robert White in 1959 and adopted by occupational therapy as superior to then-current motivational theories of intraego tension reduction, instinct, and reinforcement (White, 1971). Leon Yarrow and colleagues have produced a body of research linking mastery motivation to cognitive development (Morgan & Harmon, 1984). Mastery motivation and the related concepts of intrinsic motivation and effectance motivation are rooted in the belief that humans naturally possess a motive to control the environment, master skills, and be effective. Standard sets of mastery motivation tasks follow a developmental hierarchy assessing object exploration, persistence tasks (effect production, combinatorial, means–ends, and multipart tasks), preference for challenging tasks (3 years and older), and self-initiated mastery (4 years and older). The strong relationships of infant mastery motivation to later cognitive skills supports the importance of developmental progressions in infant play interactions with objects (Hrncir et al., 1985; McQuiston & Yarrow, 1982; Morgan & Harmon, 1984; Yarrow et al., 1982, 1983).

Selecting Therapy Lures and Enhancing Play Motivation

The characteristics that endow an object with motivational power are subjectively perceived. That is, the past environmental experiences of the child determine the relative play value of any object. A toy or household object can motivate a child to engage it through its novelty, independent responses, responsivity, complexity, or sensory properties.

Novelty. Essentially, novelty is newness. Novelty is most powerfully compelling at the developmental age of about 5 to 9 months. At this peak phase for novelty, almost any new object that can be picked up and explored provides a challenge. Following that period, novelty continues to hold some motivational power, but the object must offer other characteristics that bring it up to the level of developmental challenge that best fits the child.

Independent Responses. Independent responses are qualities of action that the object exhibits independent of any action on it by the child. For example, a windup toy can display independent responses. The object's movements or sounds call the child's attention. Therapists and parents often unconsciously use independent responses to attract children to activities, for instance, by rolling a ball or giving a swing a little push, for instance. One set of objects that provides a great deal of attractive independent responses is animals.

Responsivity. Responsivity is the ease with which the child's action produces some reaction in the object. The response could be a sound, a light, a shape change, or a movement. The classic example of high responsivity is the rattle. The busybox, a multisite responsivity toy, is a modern technological expansion of the same concept. Again, a child of higher developmental level will not be motivated by rattles or busyboxes. The therapist must offer activities of the appropriate developmental challenge. However, any object that responds with a quick and easily observed reaction to the child's action is likely to be more motivating than an object that is unresponsive, is difficult to trigger, or offers a muted response.

Complexity. "Complexity" refers to the challenge to understanding that the object offers to the child. Even for a simple lure, the developmental fit of the play object to the child's current level of play development influences how motivating it is.

Sensory Properties. Sensory properties are the relatively constant and inactive aspects of objects, such as smell, taste, temperature, and texture. The sensory properties of an object can be very motivating for children. However, the degree to which specific properties motivate specific children varies widely. For example, some children climb barriers to play with Gak, whereas others will climb barriers to avoid it. A wide variety of inexpensive objects of high sensory potency can be found in the grocery store (Box 6-8).

ARTISTS ARE ONLY AS GOOD AS THEIR MATERIALS

Object play is the predominant waking activity of the young child. For this reason, object play offers powerful therapeutic effects to pediatric occupational therapists. It is time that occupational therapy began to balance excellent training in breaking down activities with insight into the skills of designing highly effective, intact, appealing, and goal-targeted occupational applications. This chapter has described four levels of sophistication in the therapeutic use of object play: altering occupational patterns, facilitating environmental negotiation, addressing common developmental goals, and using therapy lures.

Artists are only as good as their materials. To provide the most therapeutically powerful object play to children at risk for developmental delays, pediatric occupational therapists have to take their tools seriously. For this to happen, therapists will have to fight against the field's historical tendency to make the most of inexpensive and easily found materials. Today's health care system demands the highest accountability for productive interventions. Therapists need to survey their storage areas and ask themselves whether they have sufficient play objects to provide multiple novel interventions at the complexity of normal play development required by the populations with which they work. Therapists need to address the following questions: Is there some time in the cal-

Box
6-8

MAINTAINING PLAY MOTIVATION WITH ROBERTO

The effort to keep Roberto maximally engaged in the goal-targeted play activities that I brought to his home required constant attention. I selected activities carefully and remarked on their effectiveness in my notes. Often I would record recommendations for the next session while they were fresh in my mind and then review these when next I loaded my car for the day's treatment schedule. I kept Roberto's objects in large canvas sacks that provided plenty of choices, constantly adding and removing things from the selection (Fig. 6-10).

Novelty was maintained by designing many activities to address the same goal areas and rotating their appearance in treatment. This was especially important when Roberto was younger. Many similar toys would be interacted with for short periods. We would continue to use the same activity as long as it was compelling. Later, more challenging and complex offerings were required. I tried to keep all objects in the high-responsivity range throughout treatment. Sensory properties had to be used carefully because of Roberto's tactile defensiveness. The exploration of food tastes and textures was ongoing.

Although this sounds like a lot of design work, it was actually not. Once I had developed a large set of play objects along the normal developmental play progression, it was easy to select several for each session that addressed play development as well as other goals. In working with Roberto, I also began to notice the strong tie between how motivated he was during treatment and how I felt as I left. The effort to provide Roberto with intriguing activities not only enhanced the efficacy of his treatment but made treatment much more enjoyable for me. I have the habit now, when feeling discouraged by a case in which the child is difficult to engage, of mentally focusing on that child while shopping for treatment activity supplies at a favorite toy store or other resource.

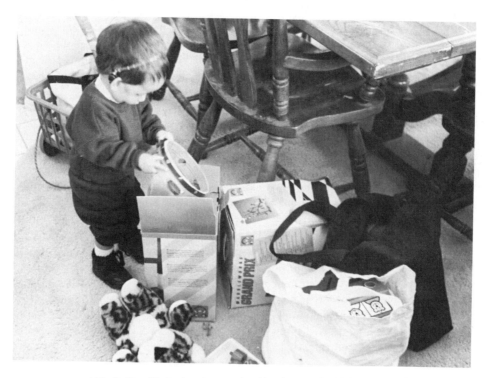

FIG. 6-10 Motivational properties: Keeping novelty high requires choices.

endar each week for treatment design, or must things be grabbed quickly off the shelf? Are multiple resources kept in mind for obtaining new objects? Is the budget sufficient to replenish expendable supplies and regularly import fresh play objects?

Although the therapists' tools may look like fun, they meet very serious goals for their patients. The cost of play objects and a little design time is low in comparison to the benefits that powerful therapeutic applications of object play can yield.

REVIEW QUESTIONS

1. Consider what the author means by "sources of power in therapeutic occupations." What elements of intervention may or may not contribute to this power?
2. Generating effective object play interventions is described as a "design process." Consider ways the therapist can develop her or his design skills.
3. Describe ways the therapist can enhance the occupational appeal of a treatment activity.
4. Describe ways in which occupational therapists currently use object play. Consider the strengths and limitations of these modes of use.
5. Identify ways occupational therapists can use object play to alter occupational patterns. Consider the perspectives on normal play development as you formulate your response.
6. Discuss environmental negotiation skills. Consider spatial, temporal, and social negotiation skills in your answer. Suggest specific therapeutic strategies that can be used to address each of these areas.
7. How do occupational therapists use object play to address sensory, perceptual, motor, and cognitive goals? Describe specific therapeutic strategies in your answer.
8. Consider the theories of play motivation. Review these theories with consideration for how occupational therapists can design effective play experiences.

REFERENCES

Acredolo, L. P. (1985). Coordinating perspectives on infant spatial orientation. In R. Cohen (Ed.). *The development of spatial cognition* (pp. 115-140). Hillsdale, NJ: Lawrence Erlbaum Associates.

Ainsworth, M. D. S., & Bell, S. M. (1974). Mother-infant interaction and the development of competence. In K. J. Connolly & J. S. Bruner (Eds.). *The growth of competence* (pp. 97-118). New York: Academic Press.

Ayres, A. J. (1972). *Sensory integration and learning disorders.* Los Angeles: Western Psychological Services.

Ayres, A. J. (1985). *Developmental dyspraxia and adult onset apraxia.* Torrance, CA: Sensory Integration International.

Barker, R. G., & Wright, H. F. (1955). *Midwest and its children: The psychological ecology of an American town.* New York: Harper & Row.

Belsky, J. & Most, R. (1981). From exploration to play: A cross-sectional study of infant free-play behavior. *Developmental Psychology, 17,* 630-639.

Benson, J. B., & Uzgiris, I. C. (1985). Effect of self-initiated locomotion on infant search activity. *Developmental Psychology, 21,* 923-931.

Berlyne, D. E. (1965). *Structure and direction in thinking.* New York: John Wiley and Sons.

Berlyne, E. E. (1971). *Aesthetics and psychobiology.* New York: Meredith.

Bettelheim, B. (1987). The importance of play. *The Atlantic Monthly,* March, 35-46.

Bornstein, M. H., Azuma, H., Tamis-LeMonda, C., & Ogino, M. (1990a). Mother and infant activity and interaction in Japan and in the United States: I. A comparative macroanalysis of naturalistic exchanges focused on the organization of infant attention. *International Journal of Behavioral Development, 13,* 267-287.

Bornstein, M. H., Toda, S., Azuma, H., Tamis-LeMonda, C., & Ogino, M. (1990b). Mother and infant activity and interaction in Japan and in the United States: II. A comparative macroanalysis of naturalistic exchanges. *International Journal of Behavioral Development, 13,* 289-308.

Bornstein, M. H., Tamis-LeMonda, C., Pecheux, M., & Rahn, C. W. (1991). Mother and infant activity and interaction in France and in the United States: II. A comparative study. *International Journal of Behavioral Development, 14,* 21-43.

Bradley, R. H., & Caldwell, B. M. (1984). The relation of infants' home environments to achieve test performance in first grade: A follow-up study. *Child Development, 55,* 803-809.

Bresson, F., Maury, L., Pieraut-Le Bonniec, G., & De Schonen, S. (1977). Organization and lateralization of reaching in infants: An instance of asymmetric functions in hand collaboration. *Neuropsychologia, 15,* 311-320.

Bushnell, E. W. (1985). The decline of visually-guided reaching during infancy. *Infant Behavior and Development, 11,* 419-430.

Butler, K. B. (1977). *The effects of novelty on the young child's exploration of objects.* PhD Thesis, University of Houston. Order no. 7800536.

Chapple, E. D., & Coon, C. S. (1942). *Principles of anthropology.* New York: Henry Holt.

Clark, F. A., Parham, D., Carlson, M., Frank, G., Jackson, J., Pierce, D., Wolfe, R. J., Zemke, R. (1991). Occupational science: Academic innovation in the service of occupational therapy's future. *American Journal of Occupational Therapy, 45,* 300-310.

Clarke-Stewart, K. A. (1973). Interactions between mothers and their young children: Characteristics and consequences. *Monographs of the Society for Research in Child Development, 38* (6-7, Serial No. 153).

Cohen D. (1987). *The development of play.* New York: New York University Press.

Cohn, J. F., & Elmore, M. (1988). Effect of contingent changes in mothers' affective expression on the organization of behavior in 3-month-old infants. *Infant Behavior and Development, 11,* 493-505.

Coll, C. G., Vohr, B. R., Hoffman, J., & Oh, W., (1986). Maternal and environmental factors affecting developmental outcome of infants of adolescent mothers. *Developmental and Behavioral Pediatrics, 7,* 230-236.

Connolly, K., & Dalgleish, M. (1989). The emergence of a tool-using skill in infancy. *Developmental Psychology, 25,* 894-912.

Csikszentmihalyi, M. (1975). *Beyond boredom and anxiety.* San Francisco: Jossey-Bass.

Daehler, M. W., & O'Connor, M. P. (1980). Recognition memory for objects in very young children: The effect of shape and label similarity on preference for novel stimuli. *Journal of Experimental Psychology, 29,* 306-321.

Dee, V. (1974). *An investigation into the play behaviors of mentally retarded and normal children.* Unpublished master's thesis, University of Southern California, Los Angeles.

Elardo, R., Bradley, R. H., & Caldwell, B. M. (1975). A longitudinal study of relation of infants' home environment to language development at age three. *Child Development, 46,* 71-76.

Elliot, J., & Connolly, K. (1973). Hierarchical structure in skill development. In Connolly, K. & Bruner, J. (Eds.). *The growth of competence* (pp. 11-48). New York: Academic Press.

Ellis, M. J. (1973). *Why people play.* Englewood Cliffs, NJ: Prentice-Hall.

Erhardt, R. P. (Producer and Director). (1986). *Normal visual development: Birth to 6 months* [videotape]. (Available from Erhardt Developmental Products, 2109 Third Street North, Fargo, ND 58102).

Erhardt, R. P. (1982). *Developmental hand dysfunction: Theory, assessment, treatment*. Tucson, AZ: Therapy Skill Builders.

Erikson, E. H. (1950). *Childhood and society*. New York: W. W. Norton.

Eson, M. E., Cometa, M. S., Allen, D. A., & Hanel, P. A. (1977). Preference for novelty-familiarity and activity-passivity in a free choice situation. *Journal of Genetic Psychology, 131*, 3-11.

Evans, G. (1980). Environmental cognition. *Psychological Bulletin, 88*, 259-287.

Exner, C. (1992). In-hand manipulation skills. In Case-Smith, J. & Pehoski, C. (Eds.). *Development of hand skills in children*. Rockville, MD: American Occupational Therapy Association.

Fagard, J., & Jacquet, A. (1989). Onset of bimanual coordination and symmetry versus asymmetry of movement. *Infant Behavior and Development, 12*, 229-235.

Faulkender, P. J. (1980). Categorical habituation with sex-typed toy stimuli in older and younger preschoolers. *Child Development, 51*, 515-519.

Fein, G. (1981). Pretend play in childhood: An integrative review. *Child Development, 52*, 1045-1118.

Fenson, L., Kagan, J., Kearsley, R. B., et al. (1976). The developmental progression of manipulative play in the first two years. *Child Development, 47*, 232-236.

Florey, L. (1981). Studies of play: Implications for growth, development, and for clinical practice. *American Journal of Occupational Therapy, 35*, 519-524.

Fowler, H. (1965). *Curiosity and exploratory behavior*. New York: Macmillan.

Fraisse, P. (1963). *The psychology of time*. Translated by Jennifer Leith from French, 1976. New York: Harper and Row.

Gesell, A. (1940). *The first five years of life: A guide to the study of the preschool child*. New York: Harper & Brothers.

Gibson, J. J. (1986). *The ecological approach to visual perception*. Hillsdale, NJ: Lawrence Erlbaum Associates.

Gralewicz, A. (1973). Play deprivation in multihandicapped children. *American Journal of Occupational Therapy, 27*, 70-72.

Gunnar, M. R., & Stone, C. (1984). The effects of positive maternal affect on infant responses to pleasant, ambiguous, and fear-provoking toys. *Child Development, 55*, 1231-1236.

Haith, M. M. (1990). Progress in the understanding of sensory and perceptual processes in early infancy. *Merrill-Palmer Quarterly, 36*, 11-27.

Hart, R. A. (1979). *Children's experience of place*. New York: Irvington.

Hebb, D. O. (1949). *The organization of behavior*. New York: Wiley.

Heft, H., & Wohlwill, J. F. (1987). Environmental cognition in children. In Stokols, D. & Altman, I. (Eds.). *Handbook of environmental psychology* (pp. 175-203). NY: Wiley.

Henderson, A. (1992). A functional typology of spatial abilities and disabilities. In McAtee, S. (Ed.). *Symposium '92 Proceedings: Current topics in sensory integration* (pp. 1-19). Torrance, CA: Sensory Integration International.

Henderson, B. B. (1978). *Exploratory behavior of preschool children in relation to individual differences in curiosity, maternal behavior and novelty of object*. Thesis, University of Minnesota. Order No. 7800536.

Henderson, B. B. (1981). Exploration by preschool children: Peer interaction and individual differences. *Merrill-Palmer Quarterly, 27*, 241-255.

Henderson, B. B., & Moore, S. G. (1980). Children's responses to objects differing in novelty in relation to level of curiosity and adult behavior. *Child Development, 51*, 457-465.

Herron, R. E., & Sutton-Smith, B. (1971). *Child's play*. New York: John Wiley.

Hornik, R., Risenhoover, N., & Gunnar, M. (1987). The effects of maternal positive, neutral, and negative affective communications on infant responses to new toys. *Child Development, 58*, 937-944.

Howard, A. C. (1986). Developmental play ages of physically abused and non-abused children. *American Journal of Occupational Therapy, 40*, 691-695.

Hrncir, E. J., Speller, G. M., & West, M. (1985). What are we testing? *Developmental Psychology, 21*, 226-232.

Hutt, C. (1966). Exploration and play in children. *Symposium of the Zoological Society of London, 18*, 61-81.

Hutt, S. J., & Hutt, C. (1970). *Direct observation and measurement of behavior*. Springfield, IL: Charles C Thomas.

Jennings, K. D., Harmon, R. J., Morgan, G. A., Gaiter, J. L., & Yarrow, L. J. (1979). Exploratory play as an index of mastery motivation: Relationships to persistence, cognitive functioning, and environmental measures. *Developmental Psychology, 15*, 386-394.

Kalverboer, A. F. (1977). Measurement of play: Clinical applications. In Tizard, B. & Harvey, D. (Eds.). *Biology of Play. Clinics in Developmental Medicine*, No. 62. Philadelphia: J. B. Lippincott.

Kaplan, S., & Kaplan, R. (1981). *Cognition and environment: Functioning in an uncertain world*. New York: Praeger.

Kielhofner, G., & Barris, R. (1984). Collecting data on play: A critique of available methods. *Occupational Therapy Journal of Research, 4*, 150-180.

Klinnert, M. D. (1984). The regulation of infant behavior by maternal facial expression. *Infant Behavior and Development, 7*, 447-465.

Koberg, D. (1981). *The revised all new universal traveler*. Los Altos, CA: William Kaufmann.

Largo, R. H., & Howard, J. A. (1979). Developmental progression of play behavior of children between nine and thirty months. I; spontaneous play and imitation. *Developmental Medicine and Child Neurology, 21*, 299-310.

Lewis, M. (1978). Attention and verbal labeling behavior in preschool children: A study in the measurement of internal representations. *Journal of Genetic Psychology, 133*, 191-202.

Lockman, J. J. (1984). The development of detour ability during infancy. *Child Development, 55*, 482-491.

Lockman, J. J., Ashmead, D. H., & Bushnell, E. W. (1984). The development of anticipatory hand orientation during infancy. *Journal of Experimental Child Psychology, 37*, 176-186.

Look, K. S. (1977). *An occupational therapy view of play and skill in primates and humans*. Unpublished master's thesis, University of Southern California, Los Angeles.

Lynch, K. (1960). *The image of the city*. Cambridge, MA: MIT Press.

Lyons-Ruth, K., Zoll, D., Connell, D., & Grunebaum, H. U. (1986). The depressed mother and her one-year-old infant: Environment, interaction, attachment, and infant development. *New Directions for Child Development, 34*, 61-82.

Mack, W., Lindquist, J. E., & Parham, L. D. (1982). A synthesis of occupational behavior and sensory integration concepts in theory and practice, part 1. Theoretical foundations. *American Journal of Occupational Therapy, 36*, 365-374.

McDonnell, P. M. (1979). Patterns of eye-hand coordination in the first year of life. *Canadian Journal of Psychology, 33*, 253-270.

McQuiston, S., & Yarrow, L. J. (1982). Assessment of mastery motivation in the first year of life. Presented at the annual meeting of the American Psychological Association, Washington, DC, August, 1982.

Mogford, K. (1977). The play of handicapped children. In Tizzard, B, & Harvey, D. (Eds.). *Biology of play. Clinics in Developmental Medicine* No. 62. Philadelphia: J. B. Lippincott.

Moore, A. (1992). *Cultural anthropology: The field study of human beings*. San Diego, CA: Collegiate Press.

Moore-Ede, M. C., Sulzman, F. M., & Fuller, C. A. (1982). *The clocks that time us*. Cambridge, MA: Harvard University Press.

Morgan, G. A., & Harmon, R. J. (1984). Developmental transformations in mastery motivation: Measurement and validation. In Emde, R. N. & Harmon, R. J. (Eds.). *Continuities and discontinuities in develment* (pp. 263-292). NY: Plenum Press.

Neisser, U. (1976). *Cognition and reality*. New York: W. H. Freeman and Company.

Neisser, U. (1991). Two perceptually given aspects of the self and their development. *Developmental Review, 11*, 197-209.

Newell, K. M., Scully, D. M., McDonald, P. V., & Baillargeon, R. (1989). Task constraints and infant grip configurations. *Developmental Psychobiology, 22*, 817-831.

Palmer, C. F. (1989). The discriminating nature of infants' exploratory actions. *Developmental Psychology, 25*, 885-893.

Phillips, R. D., & Sellitto, V. A. (1990). Preliminary evidence on emotions expressed by children during solitary play. *Play and Culture, 3*, 79-90.

Piaget, J. (1952). *The origins of intelligence in children*. New York: International Universities Press.

Piaget, J. (1962). *Play, dreams, and imitation in childhood.* New York: W. W. Norton.

Piaget, J. (1971). *The child's conception of time.* New York: Ballantine.

Piaget, J. (1976). Symbolic play. In Bruner, J. S., Jolly, A., & Sylva, K. (Eds.). *Play—its role in development and evolution.* New York: Basic Books.

Pierce, D. E. (1991). Early object rule acquisition. *American Journal of Occupational Therapy, 45,* 438-449.

Reilly, M. (1962). Occupational therapy can be one of the great ideas of twentieth century medicine. *American Journal of Occupational Therapy, 16,* 1-9.

Reilly, M. (1974). *Play as exploratory learning.* Beverly Hills, CA: Sage Publications.

Robinson, A. (1977). Play, the arena for acquisition of rules of competent behavior. *American Journal of Occupational Therapy, 31,* 248-253.

Rochat, P. (1989). Object manipulation and exploration in 2- to 5-month old infants. *Developmental Psychology, 25,* 871-884.

Rosenblatt, D. (1977). Developmental trends in infant play. In Tizard, B. & Harvey, B. (Eds.). *Biology of play. Clinics in Developmental Medicine* No. 62. Philadelphia: J. B. Lippincott.

Rubin, K. H., Maioni, T. L., & Hornung, M. (1976). Free play behaviors in middle- and lower-class preschoolers: Parten and Piaget Revisited. *Child Development, 47,* 414-419.

Ruff, H. (1984). Infants' manipulative exploration of objects: Effects of age and object characteristics. *Developmental Psychology, 20,* 9-20.

Scholtz, G. J. & Ellis, M. J. (1975). Repeated exposures to objects and peers in a play setting. *Journal of Experimental Child Psychology, 4,* 59-79.

Slobin, D. I. (1964). The fruits of the first season: A discussion of the role of play in childhood. *Journal of Humanistic Psychology, 4,* 59-79.

Smith, M. B. (1974), Competence and adaptation. *American Journal of Occupational Therapy, 28,* 11-15.

Sophian, C. (1986). Developments in infants' search for invisibly displaced objects. *Infant Behavior and Development, 9,* 15-25.

Stevens, J. H., & Bakeman, R. (1985). A factor analytic study of the HOME Scale for infants. *Developmental Psychology, 21,* 1196-1203.

Sussman, R. P. (1979). *Effects of novelty and training on the curiosity and exploration of young children in day care centers.* Unpublished thesis, University of Chicago.

Tulkin, S., & Covitz, F. (1975, April). *Mother-infant interaction and intellectual functioning at age 6.* Paper presented at the meeting of the Society for Research in Child Development, Denver, CO.

Vandenburg, B., & Kielhofner, G. (1982). Play in evolution, culture, and adaptation: Implications for therapy. *American Journal of Occupational Therapy, 36,* 20-28.

Wachs, T. D. (1976). Utilization of a Piagetian approach in the investigation of early experience effects: A research strategy and some illustrative data. *Merrill-Palmer Quarterly, 22,* 11-30.

Wachs, T. D. (1978). The relationship of infants' physical environment to their Binet performance at 2 i/2 years. *International Journal of Behavioral Development, 1,* 51-65.

Wachs, T. D. (1979). Proximal experience and early cognitive-intellectual development: The physical environment. *Merrill-Palmer Quarterly, 25,* 3-41.

Wachs, T. D. (1990). Must the physical environment be mediated by the social environment in order to influence development? A further test. *Journal of Applied Developmental Psychology, 11,* 163-178.

Wachs, T. D., & Gruen, G. E. (1982). *Early experience and human development.* New York: Plenum.

Wachs, T. D., Uzgiris, I. C., & Hunt, J. McV. (1971). Cognitive development in infants of different age levels and from different environmental backgrounds: An exploratory investigation. *Merrill-Palmer Quarterly, 17,* 283-317.

Walden, T. A., & Ogan, T. A. (1988). The development of social referencing. *Child Development, 59,* 1230-1240.

Wehman, P. (1977). *Helping the mentally retarded acquire play skills.* Springfield, IL: Charles C Thomas.

Wehman, P., & Abramson, M. (1976). Three theoretical approaches to play. *American Journal of Occupational Therapy, 30,* 551-559.

Weisler, A., & McCall, R. B. (1976). Exploration and play. Resume and redirection. *American Psychologist, 31,* 492-508.

Wellman, H. M. (1985). *Children's searching: The development of search skill and spatial representation.* Hillsdale, NJ: Lawrence Erlbaum Associates.

White, B. L., Castle, P., & Held, R. (1964). Observations on the development of visually-directed reaching. *Child Development, 35,* 349-364.

White, R. W. (1971). The urge toward competence. *American Journal of Occupational Therapy, 25,* 271-274.

Williams, H. G. (1973). *Perceptual and motor development.* Englewood Cliffs, NJ: Prentice-Hall.

Wohlwill, J. F., & Heft, H. (1987). The physical environment and the development of the child. In Stokols, D., & Altman, I. (Eds.). *Handbook of environmental psychology* (pp. 281-328), NY: Wiley.

Yarrow, L. J., Morgan, G. A., Jennings, K. D., Harmon, R. J., & Gaiter, J. L. (1982). Infants' persistence at tasks: Relationships to cognitive functioning and early experience. *Annual Progress in Child Psychiatry and Development 1,* 217-229.

Yarrow, L. J., McQuiston, S., MacTurk, R. H., McCarthy, M. E., Klein, R. P., & Vietze, P. M. (1983). Assessment of mastery motivation during the first year of life: Contemporaneous and cross-age relationships. *Developmental Psychology, 19,* 159-171.

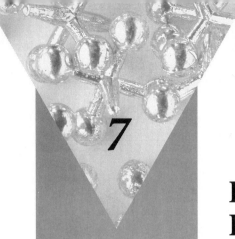

7

PLAY AND THE SENSORY INTEGRATIVE APPROACH

Zoe Mailloux and Janice Posatery Burke

Sensory integration unfolds in a predictable pattern as part of central nervous system development in the human child. The development of sensory integrative skills and behaviors is observed in all aspects of children's lives, including their abilities to maintain a calm and alert state; to develop new skills such as picking up, holding onto, and examining a fuzzy stuffed animal (see Fig. 7-1); and to learn about interacting and relating to others. Similarly, play skills develop in concert with a child's physical, cognitive, and motor abilities that support their emergence. For occupational therapists, interest in and attention to both sensory integration and play provides a complex and intriguing framework for structuring intervention for children who exhibit deficits and related problems in these domains.

The sophisticated relationship of sensory integration to play is dependent on the development of a number of neurobehavioral capacities, including the drive for receiving, perceiving, and integrating sensory information with motor responses. The opportunity to practice and refine sensory integrative behaviors provides the scaffolding for the more complex thinking and doing that emerge in the everyday play of a child. In turn, these play behaviors fuel further sensory integrative development. The interrelatedness of these systems are discussed in this chapter, which is designed to illustrate the role of sensory integrative behaviors in normal play development, discuss how sensory integrative deficits affect play, and describe how play provides a useful construct for addressing sensory integrative deficits.

SENSORY INTEGRATIVE CONTRIBUTIONS TO PLAY DEVELOPMENT

Infancy: The Sensory Beginnings of Play

In typical development, early sensorimotor play is strongly influenced by the drive for sensory and motor experiences. During this stage of play development, basic sensory functions dominate behavior, with infants spending a great deal of time in exploratory play, seeking and experiencing tactile, vestibular, proprioceptive, visual, and auditory input. Infants are captivated by these sensations, and they spend their time searching for new and interesting as well as known and comforting sensory experiences.

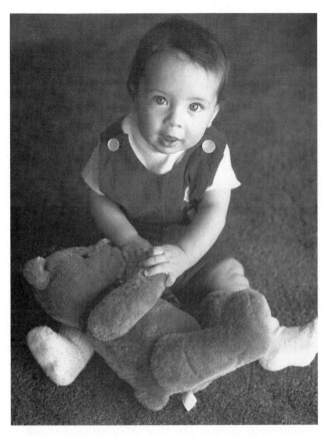

FIG. 7-1 Simple acts such as picking up and holding a fuzzy stuffed animal depend on the integrity of sensory integrative functions. (Courtesy Shay McAtee.)

Along with a natural drive for a variety of sensory experiences, infants begin to experiment with moving their bodies in novel ways (see Fig. 7-2). As infants develop voluntary, controlled movement, they begin to form ideas about what to do and ways to plan that action. This drive is evident in every purposeful action that is initiated by the young child. A blending of the drive for sensation with the ability to plan the new motor actions is illustrated by Ben, who is a 9-month-old infant. This little boy generally spends his mornings at home in play with his mother. Using his newly developed mobility, he spends most of his waking hours moving in search of sensory experiences. On this day, he climbs the couch to reach the shutters, which provide a visual bonanza of light and shadow (see Fig. 7-3). As he approaches them, he becomes intrigued by the smooth texture of the wood and the rounded edges of each slat and the vertical bar that holds them together. He discovers the clicking sounds that occur as he opens and closes the slats and is intrigued with his homemade sight and sound machine, which also has an appealing feel to it. While standing on the couch to enjoy his new toy, Ben begins to bounce and sway on the cushions. A rhythm emerges blending motion with sights, sounds, and touch. Every aspect of this experience feeds his sensory drives to engage, experiment, and explore.

Whereas Ben is motivated to receive, perceive, and integrate the sensory experiences inherent in this type of activity, his basic sensory systems are also using the experience to

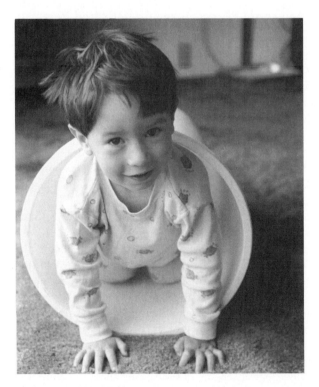

FIG. 7-2 With increasing mobility, infants begin to experiment with moving their bodies in novel ways and in novel places. (Courtesy Shay McAtee.)

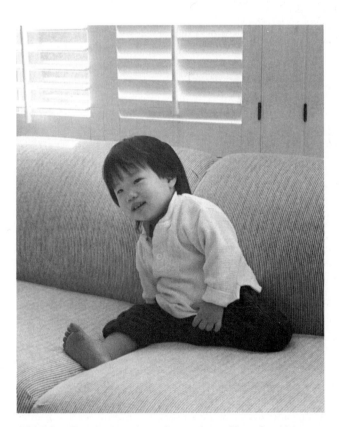

FIG. 7-3 The shutters above the couch provide a visual bonanza of light and shadow that can be manipulated by the exploring infant. (Courtesy Shay McAtee.)

lay the groundwork for more complex tasks of the future. The movement and kinesthetic experiences Ben receives through bouncing and swaying on the cushions are contributing to a fundamental sense of knowing where his body is in space. This affects his balance, his muscle tone, and the coordination of his head and eye movements, and contributes to his ability to use his hands together in a coordinated manner. His motivation to run his fingers along the wooden slats provides an opportunity to manipulate a foreign object and gain sensory information. As this occurs, he begins to integrate what he sees with what he feels, thus laying a foundation for mastering and understanding the properties of objects, how they work, and how they can be utilized with his body to experience and effectively interact with them.

The Preschool Years: A Focus on Directing Play Toward Interaction

During the preschool years, constructive play predominates, with imaginary and social play skills emerging (Caplan & Caplan, 1974). The drive for sensory experiences continues but no longer directs virtually every action the child makes in play. In this stage of development, the child continues to seek basic sensory experiences but now incorporates more complex interactions into play, with language and symbolic thought making increasingly significant contributions to the intricacies of play. The sensory integration experiences that occur within this more complex stage of play continue to provide a base for skills that are going to be needed later in life. For example, Mark, age 4, and Tricia, age 3, are next door neighbors who use play interactions that fluctuate between parallel play and an early form of cooperative play. One afternoon, their individual play with a bevy of stuffed animals flows into a cooperative experience in which they construct a deep, dark den for the animals using blankets, cushions, and pillows. The sensory aspects of the scene are found in the amount of tactile and proprioceptive sensations that are inherent in the cozy den and in being surrounded by the stuffed animals that inhabit it. But this is no longer primarily a sensory activity, as it may have been for Mark and Tricia as infants. The construction of the den becomes very important as the children concern themselves with how the cushions should be arranged. How much light should be allowed inside? How will they get to the den from across the room? Which animals belong to each child and who is in charge? As the cushions are placed, pathways are built, and negotiations take place, the sensory and motor aspects of this play experience are making a significant foundational contribution to the children's ability to make things happen. They also set in motion new neuronal models for how things work. However, and perhaps most importantly, because they occur automatically the sensory and motor functions allow more complex conceptual and social functions to emerge (Fig. 7-4).

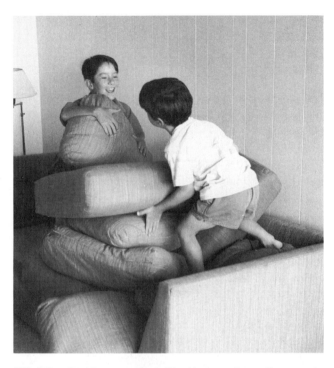

FIG. 7-4 At older ages, play with objects such as pillows, cushions, and blankets continues to provide sensory experiences, but it also carries symbolic and social meanings. Well-developed, automatic sensorimotor abilities free the child to transform the materials imaginatively into a den, a cave, a wall, or a castle without having to attend to more primitive functions such as maintaining standing balance. (Courtesy Shay McAtee.)

The School Years: More Sophisticated Play with Rules and Skills

During the school years, play in which rules and skills are important becomes more predominant (Caplan & Caplan, 1974). Motor skills that depend on efficient sensory integration and praxis become important and can influence a child's social status, motivation, and self-esteem. Although games and activities involving conceptual thought, language, and problem solving may make up a great deal of play for some children, there is clearly an emphasis on sports and skill-based play activities for this age group. Some play activities common in the school age group, such as roller blading, jump roping, playing ball sports, and constructing models with detailed patterns, require a high level of praxis, which entails timing, sequencing, and anticipatory motor skills. The very nature of many rule-generated games and sports reveals a continued emphasis on sensory and movement experiences. Most children at this age continue to enjoy spending at least some portion of their play in sensorimotor activities. The basic functions of the nervous system that ensure optimal sensory integration must be intact and efficient for a child to continue to enjoy engaging in the kinds of activities that are highly dependent on these functions, especially given that self-consciousness and peer evaluation of performance become increasingly important during this stage (Fig. 7-5). The contribution of sensory integrative functions to other developing abilities continues, but by school age, children are able to rely on alternative approaches to accomplishing a task, such as using a strategy to make an activity easier, compensating with other skills, avoiding activities that are difficult, and practicing components of skills. For example, Patrick is an 8 year old who finds balance-related activities such as bicycle riding, roller skating, ice skating, and surfboarding easy to master. He enjoys the sensory experiences they provide, as evidenced by his motivation to ride or skate fast, to turn circles, and to go up and down hills. The efficient vestibular and proprioceptive functions that are required by these play activities may also be supporting his above-average skills in academic tasks such as writing, reading, and organizing his work. His participation in these activities provides an arena for engaging in social interactions with other children. In contrast to these areas of prowess, Patrick finds ball skills and organized sports more challenging and less interesting. It is difficult for him to maintain eye–hand or eye–foot coordination needed for many of the ball skills required in these types of sports activities, and when he attempts them, he feels self-conscious about his performance. For Patrick, these skill areas are perceived as weaknesses that are uninteresting compared to his other areas of strength and enjoyment. For the most part, he is able to compensate for his limitations by practicing and developing

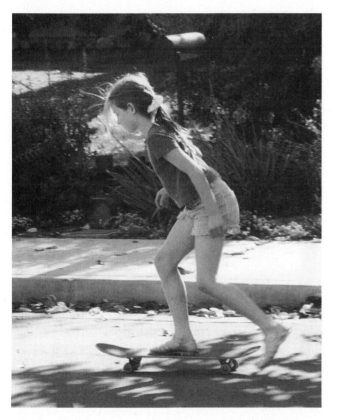

FIG. 7-5   School aged children typically spend some portion of their play in sensorimotor activities that challenge the vestibular and proprioceptive systems. (Courtesy Shay McAtee.)

strategies to improve his performance; however, he prefers to select play activities at which he excels. These provide an adequate outlet for receiving continued sensorimotor experiences appropriate to his age level.

Beyond Childhood: Play to Recreation

In older childhood, adolescence, and adulthood, sensory integrative aspects of play behavior are bound by factors such as individual skills and interests, environmental constraints, the necessity of incorporating play into more complex schedules, and associated role requirements and responsibilities (Caplan & Caplan, 1974). Although the drive for some types of movement probably decreases (Ayres, 1979), other forms of sensory experiences continue to be essential. Even at older ages, play continues to be a vehicle for experiencing sensations that are necessary for the nervous system to function well.

HOW SENSORY INTEGRATIVE DEFICITS AFFECT PLAY

An understanding of the central role that sensory integrative functions have in the development of normal play illustrates how important it is for these functions to operate in an efficient manner. When this does not occur, one of the most devastating results is a disruption in play. Parents of children who demonstrate sensory integrative dysfunction often bring these concerns to a therapist, expressing problems such as, "He doesn't know how to play with toys," "She won't play by the rules," "He breaks his toys and destroys others games," and "No one wants to play with him."

Because sensory integrative disorders are a spectrum of problems that can occur in isolation or as part of a complex of difficulties, there is a great deal of overlap in how various subsets of problems can affect play. For illustrative purposes, however, some of the most common sensory integrative disorders are discussed individually here in relation to ways in which play behavior is often affected.

Sensory Defensiveness

The term "sensory defensiveness" was first used by Knickerbocker (1980) and has been used more recently by Wilbarger & Wilbarger (1991) to describe a disorder characterized by overresponsiveness to sensory experiences that are not typically perceived as irritating or uncomfortable. Sensory defensiveness can occur in relation to one type of sensory experience or to multiple sensations. In addition, an individual's response to the sensation(s) may vary depending on the time of day, time of year, type of specific sensation, and individual state (e.g., illness, fatigue, hunger). Tactile defensiveness, auditory defensiveness, and gravitational insecurity are types of sensory defensiveness that can severely limit play behavior in children.

Tactile Defensiveness. "Tactile defensiveness" is the term Ayres (1979) used to refer to an unusual sensitivity to touch. Tactile defensiveness is commonly characterized by hypersensitivity in areas of the body, with a high concentration of tactile receptor sites, especially the hands, feet, and face.

Tactile defensiveness is a sensory integrative disorder that affects children's play behavior at a very early age and in a pervasive manner. Because early stages of play are characterized by tactile exploration, particularly through hand and mouth manipulation of objects, a tendency to avoid certain textures limits the scope of experiences the child has and the range of skills the child develops. Children with tactile defensiveness rarely put objects into their mouths during infancy; thus, this usually is not a source of worry for parents of these babies. These children often lack prerequisite skills for eating solid foods, for forming words, and for handling and manipulating toys and play materials. These early, limited sensory experiences in infancy contribute to deficiencies in visual and manipulative skills that emerge directly from early tactile experiences.

As children grow, there is a continuum of play experiences that is based on tactile play (Fig. 7-6). Play with sand, grass, mud, water, finger paints, and play dough are some of the common activities that are likely to be considered aversive by children with tactile defensiveness. Additionally, as social play emerges, tactile input from being near other children who may brush lightly against their skin when sharing materials, moving about, or bumping unexpectedly all may cause a negative reaction in children who have tactile defensiveness. Engaging in imaginary play activities such as dress-up can be disconcerting, as can participating in special event activities such as donning Halloween costumes for a school party, having one's face painted at a carnival, or visiting a petting zoo. In older grades, contact sports such as soccer, football, or baseball may create discomfort and hinder participation in these play activities, as does the need to wear uniforms and helmets.

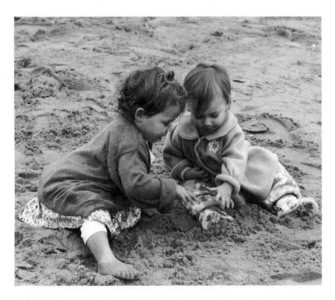

FIG. 7-6 Playing in sand at the playground or beach depends on a well-modulated tactile system. This type of play activity is usually disturbing for the child with tactile defensiveness, who will tend to avoid it. (Courtesy Shay McAtee.)

> **CASE EXAMPLE 1: TACTILE DEFENSIVENESS**
>
> Jillian's problems with tactile defensiveness illustrate the interruptions in normal play that often occur for children who experience a tactile disorder. As an outgoing, talkative 4 year old, Jillian has a lot of friends and generally enjoys spending time with them. Jillian experiences periods of extreme tactile defensiveness, often associated with changes in the weather or alterations of her daily sleeping patterns. When this occurs, Jillian starts off the day in an unstable or vulnerable state, which becomes exacerbated by the many tactile based behaviors that she needs to enact, including finding clothes and shoes that feel comfortable, getting through the morning routines of having her hair combed and her teeth brushed, and deciding on a breakfast that includes textures she finds tolerable. By the time she arrives at preschool, she is irritable and uncomfortable. Facing the challenge of sitting next to other children at play who brush lightly against her skin as they exchange toys proves unnerving, and she responds by taking her toys to her own space. Doing this makes her feel sad and confused. She would like to be playing with the other children, but simultaneously she feels the need to retreat. Over time, this kind of behavior sets Jillian apart and limits the kinds of play experiences in which she is able to participate. The impact of her tactile limitations on her ability to participate in social play is an example of how a sensory processing problem hampers further skill acquisition and satisfaction in a young life.

Auditory Defensiveness. "Auditory defensiveness" refers to an oversensitivity to sounds that are not normally disturbing or uncomfortable. The implications for difficulties in play are clearly significant since many toys, play activities, and play interactions involve some type of predictable and/or spontaneous noise.

Many toys contain inherent sound capabilities (horns, bells, and other musical instruments), are designed to use sound as an incentive for play (cause and effect toys), or use sound to teach skills (electronic games). When sound that is meant to comfort, encourage, or reward is perceived as irritating, disturbing, or frightening, a child may withdraw and refuse to participate. Equally significant is the incidental noise that arises from play interactions; children who are having a good time are typically noisy, and generate sudden bursts of intense sound that match the action of the play. Children with auditory defensiveness often withdraw from informal activities such as play in groups as well as more formal social events such as birthday parties.

Auditory defensiveness is a processing problem that limits the child's play experiences in the here and now. The concern for such curtailed activity is that in the long term there may be sequelae in more complex social, physical, and cognitive skills.

CASE EXAMPLE 2: AUDITORY DEFENSIVENESS

Derrick is a 3-year-old boy with a diagnosis of autism. He has hypersensitivity to many types of sensory input but is especially sensitive to sounds. Noises that are barely detectable to most people (e.g., an air conditioner shutting off or a horn blowing in the distance) send Derrick into a state of panic, as demonstrated by his withdrawing from the task at hand and placing his hands over his ears while rocking his body. In Derrick's case, sensory defensiveness characterized by extreme auditory hypersensitivity overrides his ability to tolerate even the most basic types of play experiences. Reactions to sounds constantly interrupt his attention to toys and drive him away from the kinds of environments in which play occurs. Derrick's oversensitivity to sound severely hinders his acquisition of skills and concepts that are part of the early play experiences from which children his age learn and gain pleasure.

Gravitational Insecurity. "Gravitational insecurity" is the term used to describe a condition in which an individual feels irrational fear, anxiety, or distress in relation to movement or a change of position (Ayres, 1979). Typically, young children derive pleasure from their experiences with movement. Because movement and using one's body to explore is such an important part of play experiences in the early years, it is easy to imagine how a disorder such as gravitational insecurity can disrupt many kinds of play experiences. Parents of children who demonstrate signs of gravitational insecurity frequently remember the early signs of distress in relation to movement when their children were small infants. Because of their reactions, these children were less likely to be swung, rocked, or otherwise moved through space, which in turn reduced the amount of vestibular sensation they received. Since stimulation of the vestibular system normally contributes to neurologically based functions such as development of muscle tone (especially of the extensor muscles), coordination of head and eye movements, balance and equilibrium reactions, and bilateral coordination (Montgomery, 1985), children who do not engage in movement activities are at risk for not developing these functions in an optimal manner. This is another example of the recursive cycle that occurs when a sensory processing problem interferes with play behavior, which in turn affects sensory processing. Finding movement unpleasant, a child engages infrequently in the kind of play that generates a great deal of movement sensation. Without this sensation, the child's nervous system does not receive the stimulation needed to develop more complex movement skills used in play and in other aspects of the child's life.

On a more generalized level, being in a state of fear or anxiety for a great deal of the time limits the desire to participate in social interactions and explore new situations (Fig. 7-7). According to Ayres (1979), "If the child-earth relationship is not secure, then all other relationships are apt to be less than optimal" (p. 85).

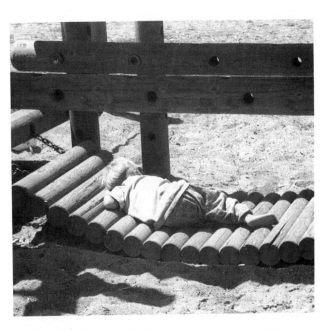

FIG. 7-7 Children with gravitational insecurity typically have limited play experiences because of anxiety in relation to movement through space. This will have a negative effect on social relationships as well as motor skills. (Courtesy Shay McAtee.)

CASE EXAMPLE 3: GRAVITATIONAL INSECURITY

Maggie is an 8-year-old girl with a learning disability. Maggie demonstrates significant signs of gravitational insecurity. As a young child, she cried if she were lifted high into the air, and she resisted climbing and swinging activities from an early age. She has always appeared distrustful and has tended to withdraw from people other than her parents. Her mother painfully recounts early play group experiences when Maggie clung to her while the other toddlers in the group scampered through the park. Now, at age 8 years, Maggie has significant difficulties maneuvering through the world. She feels uncomfortable in open spaces wherein she has less feedback about the location of her body in relation to the rest of the world. She avoids the playground and prefers to sit on a bench close to the classroom buildings during recess. Many of the activities the other girls in her class enjoy, such as bicycle riding, jumproping, and roller skating, are frightening or simply unappealing to Maggie. Her play time is limited by the sedentary nature of the activities she chooses, further compounding her already compromised base of skill. Her parents are worried about her self-consciousness and what they perceive as possible signs of depression. Maggie has the drive to engage in the play activities that would attract any girl her age, but reactions within her nervous system do not allow her to pursue them.

Vestibular–Bilateral and Sequencing Disorders

Ayres (1972, 1979, 1989) described vestibular–bilateral and sequencing disorders as characterized by poor postural mechanisms, inadequate bilateral integration, underresponsive vestibular systems, and difficulties with sequencing. Although these types of problems can severely hinder a child's ability to perform academic tasks and certain physical skills, they represent a relatively more subtle type of sensory integration disorder in comparison to other problems. Likewise, the relationship between these types of problems and play is also more subtle.

Because children with underresponsive vestibular systems probably do not receive the same type or intensity of sensation as other children unless they receive more intense motion, they often have a tendency to seek activities that involve a great deal of movement. Parents sometimes describe children with this disorder as always being in motion and not showing the usual signs of dizziness or other reactions to spinning, swinging, and turning.

This type of problem may not be as obvious in the play of young children, since refined skills are not usually required for success and it is still considered normal to seek a good deal of movement during play. In the school age years, however, difficulties such as mastering bicycle riding, roller skating, and throwing and catching a ball are more likely to emerge (see Fig. 7-8). Furthermore, confusion about directionality (right versus left) often accompanies bilateral integration problems (Ayres, 1979); therefore, situations where knowing which way to run (on the soccer field or basketball court, for example) may result in feeling embarrassed and experiencing a sense of failure. Difficulties with bilateral integration and sequencing are also likely to interfere with more construction-oriented play activities that involve cutting, pasting, folding, and building. Low muscle tone and poor extensor tone associated with this disorder may also make a child with this type of problem lethargic and sluggish in many physical activities because they have difficulty maintaining a readiness to act.

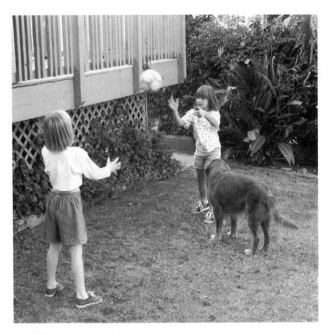

FIG. 7-8   Skill in throwing and catching a ball is dependent on vestibular–proprioceptive functions and bilateral integration. Difficulty with this kind of activity is common among children with vestibular-based bilateral integration and sequencing deficits. (Courtesy Shay McAtee.)

CASE EXAMPLE 4: VESTIBULAR–BILATERAL INTEGRATION AND SEQUENCING DISORDER

Jason is a 9-year-old boy who is representative of many children with vestibular-based bilateral and sequencing problems. From the time he was a young child, he has always loved merry-go-rounds, roller coasters, and other fast moving playground and carnival rides. At 9 years old, it is still acceptable to engage in these types of activities, but he is beginning to be aware that he craves more of this type of movement than others. He sometimes "covers up" his drive to engage in moving activities by forming themes around action play that involves motion. With limited skill for ball sports, Jason is attracted to such sports as karate and gymnastics that provide a great deal of proprioceptive feedback for his sensory needs. Jason is talented in drawing and often incorporates action figures into his artwork. However, he has trouble coordinating using his hands together in building with interlocking blocks and other construction and manipulative playthings. Although his friends spend time together playing with these types of toys, Jason does not. Overall, Jason's sensory integrative disorder interferes with some aspects of his play, but he does have other skills and opportunities that contribute to his feeling good about himself as he engages in age-appropriate play experiences.

Dyspraxia

Ayres (1985) described developmental dyspraxia as a disorder characterized by difficulty in ideation, planning, and/or execution of unfamiliar actions. Praxis is involved in enacting new and unfamiliar tasks, and children must call upon this process as they confront the many activities that are part of their day. For adults, the subroutines of daily tasks are familiar and with repetition have become automatic; therefore they do not require as much praxis. Perhaps nowhere else in the spectrum of human activity is praxis more critical than in the play of children, which involves constantly changing themes, actions, sequences, and possibilities of outcome.

Dyspraxia often occurs in conjunction with sensory processing disorders, simply because the nervous system depends on appropriate, efficient, and predictable sensory information to form action plans. If the incoming information is not perceived or processed accurately, efficiently, and effectively, acting upon it is difficult.

Praxis begins with ideation, which is an especially important aspect in enacting play behavior. Forming a notion about what to do, based on the possibilities for action that exist, is fundamental to the creative aspects of play behavior. Ideation is closely linked to the planning component of praxis, in that forming the idea of what to do leads directly to the process of knowing how to do it. Consequently, when a child has problems coming up with an idea for a plan and/or forming a plan of action, then the actual performance of the action is likely to be difficult as well (Figure 7-9).

CASE EXAMPLE 5: AUTISM WITH PRAXIS PROBLEMS

Jeremy is a 5-year-old boy with a diagnosis of autism who has significant sensory processing problems. He is often overwhelmed by his environment and tends to engage in ritualistic behaviors and routines. When he is presented with a piece of play equipment such as an inner tube swing, it appears to have no meaning to him. Whereas most 5 year olds may readily imagine sitting, lying, standing, or kneeling on the swing and compose elaborate play themes in which they star as the hero or villain sweeping through the town in flight, Jeremy merely pushes the tire away as it is swung in his direction. When he shows little interest in imitating a peer who is lying prone in a tire nearby, he is placed in this position by his therapist. Because this is something new, his first response appears to be dislike. As the tire is gently swung and bounced, he seems to enjoy the sensation. For now, this is the most complex practic interaction Jeremy can have with this piece of play equipment; he demonstrates very little ideation or planning ability in using it.

CASE EXAMPLE 6: DYSPRAXIA

Rita is an 8-year-old girl with a speech and language disorder who demonstrates low scores on tests of praxis and presents many signs of dyspraxia when she is observed trying to do something new or novel. Rita's problems with ideation are different from Jeremy's in that she often appears to be forming an idea of what she wants to do but struggles with putting a plan together. She was observed to place her rag doll on one side of a seesaw and then attempt to mount the other side. As she tried to push off from her side, her doll fell off and she tilted backward, appearing unaware of and unable to control the reduced force she needed to use to compensate for the light weight of the doll. In a subsequent attempt, she appeared frustrated when she attempted to tie the doll's legs around the seat. She was unable to master securing the doll in this way. When another child approached and asked if she could join her on the seesaw, Rita replied, "No thanks, my doll not like it." Although Rita had some concept of what she wanted to do, she could not fully put the plan together. Her poor sensory integration contributed to poor planning and execution of the intended action, and at her age, her self-consciousness about her difficulties kept her from engaging in a social play experience. Unfortunately, Rita has many similar experiences each day that make play an often frustrating and embarrassing experience.

PLAY IN THE CONTEXT OF OCCUPATIONAL THERAPY USING A SENSORY INTEGRATIVE APPROACH

The difficulties and disruptions that sensory integrative dysfunction imposes on play experience are of concern to occupational therapists working with children. Therapists using a sensory integrative approach in treatment have access to a special environment and set of tools that enable them to address the play experiences of the children with whom they work.

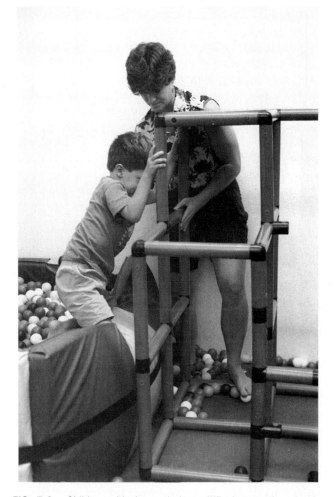

FIG. 7-9 Children with dyspraxia have difficulty enacting simple plans for action and consequently may need assistance to experience success in negotiating the physical environment. (Courtesy Shay McAtee.)

Among the fundamental principles guiding the sensory integrative approach in treatment are several notions that converge with therapists' understanding of play activity and behavior. For example, drawing on both clinical experience and the theoretical work of Mary Reilly, Florey (1985) described play as having an organizing effect on human behavior. This parallels a basic principle of sensory integration, that improved adaptive responses enhance general behavioral organization (Parham & Mailloux, 1996.) Florey (1985) also envisioned play as "a critical base for adult competence" (p. 36), which is similarly found in a major tenet of sensory integration, that "mature and complex patterns of behavior are composed of consolidations of more primitive behaviors" (Clark et al., 1989, p. 373). Consistent with the idea that intrinsic motivation is an essential component of play (Florey, 1969; Smith, 1974; White, 1971) is the sensory integration treatment concept underscoring the belief that a child who is "inner directed" will gain optimally from therapeutic activities (Parham & Mailloux, 1996).

The relationship between sensory integration and play in treatment is clearly not a simple, linear one. Knox and Mailloux (in press) described play as a means, as well as an end product, within the sensory integration approach. Bundy (1991) also highlighted the dynamic aspect of play in relation to sensory integration as she discussed the potential for both an improved ability to play through enhanced sensory integration and improved sensory integration through the incorporation of play in treatment. Recent research by Coster et al. (1995) suggests that play may give both meaning and structure to treatment utilizing a sensory integration approach. In a related study, Tickle-Degnen and Coster (1995) also noted the association between playfulness on the part of the therapist and a tendency for the child to use playful language and show signs of enjoyment and success. All of these explanations and findings on the relationship between play and sensory integration in treatment suggest a dynamic interplay that occurs between therapist and child within a therapy session.

Ideas about play in relation to the components of the treatment process are considered next, namely the preparation period, the therapy session, and the followup phase.

Getting Set for Treatment

Preparing for a treatment session is important in all types of occupational therapy. To make the most of the time spent with a patient, the therapist must have (1) a clear understanding of treatment goals, (2) a plan for what areas need to be addressed, (3) an idea of appropriate activities to achieve these goals, and (4) the supplies and materials required during the treatment session. When working with children, the preparation phase is particularly critical, since the therapist cannot rely on a child to wait while activities are set up and arranged. Preparation is especially important to allow for a natural flow that encourages the possibility of play during the treatment session.

A sensory integrative approach incorporates the role of the environment as providing an enticement to the child, allowing for imaginary themes to prosper and encouraging social interaction and challenges similar to those that may be part of games or sports. Because novelty enhances exploration and play (Bundy, 1991), selecting new or different toys and pieces of equipment, as well as unexpected combinations and arrangements, is part of preparing for a treatment session (Fig. 7-10).

In addition to readying the environment and objects within it, the pediatric therapist must prepare for the treatment session. Occupational therapists who wish to instill play in a therapy session need to be ready to play themselves. To "communicate playfulness," as suggested by Parham (1992), the therapist must check her or his own mood and state of playfulness to set the tone for the emergence of a playful situation.

Like therapists, some children require a form of preparation themselves to be ready to play. Children who have high

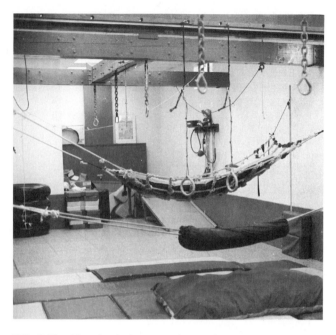

FIG. 7-10   The classical sensory integrative treatment setting is rich in objects and materials that can be set up and combined in an infinite number of novel arrangements. (Courtesy Shay McAtee.)

or low responsivity to stimuli in the environment may first need to engage in specific inhibitory or facilitory types of activities before they are ready to enter into a play experience. Lethargy, fear, anxiety, irritation, and agitation are among the feelings that are not conducive to play and therefore need to be addressed before play can occur in any setting.

CASE EXAMPLE 7: PREPARATION OF THE ENVIRONMENT AND THE THERAPIST

Emily is a 5-year-old girl who has autism. Although she scores above the average range on IQ tests, she is socially withdrawn and does not have any friends. When she plays with toys, she tends to use them in a very ritualistic manner, such as placing her dolls in specific positions and locations within a doll house. Emily has sensory defensiveness that is characterized by hypersensitivity to touch, sounds, and movement. Her occupational therapist, Mary, is hoping to encourage Emily to engage in imaginary play as a step toward her being able to interact socially with other girls her age. While observing Emily in her first few visits to the occupational therapy room at school, her therapist saw that she tended to pace around the room and avoided playing with any of the toys or equipment while delivering rambling monologues about her plans for the day. She appeared anxious and uncomfortable and unable to settle into play interactions. To provide an appropriate play experience for this child, Mary prearranged the environment, setting up an area for Emily where she could start with activities that provided calm and organizing sensory experiences. Using large pillows, dim light, and a rocking chair, Mary found she could help Emily to become relaxed and organized before other, more challenging activities were introduced. In separate areas, Mary arranged toys and equipment that encouraged imaginary play and challenged Emily to experience a greater variety of sensory experiences. For example, since Emily was extremely interested in unicorns, Mary found a stuffed unicorn and placed it atop a piece of moving equipment to serve as an enticement during vestibular challenges. Mary found that Emily first was relaxed by the initial calming stage of the therapy session and then enticed by an object of interest to her, thus becoming more open to challenging movement and touch experiences. By preparing the therapy environment and by helping Emily to become ready to accept challenging experiences in therapy, Mary found that she was able to begin to introduce dramatic and imaginary play themes into the therapy sessions. As Emily began to gain meaning from these experiences, she was also able to engage in more challenging activities for longer periods of time. Mary also found that, as a therapist, the better she prepared herself emotionally and mentally for the sessions with Emily, the more successful they were. In this case, Mary had to take time to remind herself not to become sidetracked by Emily's verbal maneuvering to avoid activity and, instead, to remember to read it as a sign that Emily needed help to become organized. By planning to avoid power struggles and by preparing for a playful experience, Mary was able to be more successful at helping Emily to reach her therapy goals.

The Session

The therapy session itself offers a broad range of opportunities for merging play with sensory integrative goals of treatment. As Bundy (1991) described it, there is an interactional effect in which the incorporation of play can enhance sensory integrative processes, and improved sensory integration allows for more elaborate play abilities.

At a basic level, incorporation of play themes can make many challenging activities more enticing and can encourage longer duration of involvement in activities for children with sensory integrative dysfunction. For example, the child who is fearful of movement may better tolerate a swinging platform if it is presented with a favorite theme of interest such as a space ship on its way to the moon. The child may be able to stay on the swing for longer periods of time if involvement in the play theme instigates the motivation for instance, to reach for a planet or catch a falling star (Fig. 7-11). At a more complex level, the dynamic relationship between sensory integrative function and play can serve the development of skills in ideation, imagination, and socialization within the context of the therapy session. Ayres (1985) describes ideation as a cognitive process that involves understanding the possibilities for actions of the self in relation to objects or other people. She states that ideation is "basic to most child's play and to many adult occupations" (Ayres, 1985, p. 20). As the key that can unlock the door of possibilities, ideation allows the child to begin to plan what to do. Ideation is almost palpable when a normal 5 year old is observed in a typical therapy room in which a sensory integrative approach is practiced. A novel piece of suspended equipment brought into the room can easily elicit a whole series of experiments that test the possibilities of interaction between the child and the toy. A child who has a sensory integrative disorder, however, may lack the basic body

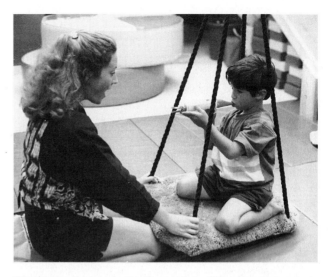

FIG. 7-11   An imaginative theme often will lead to more complex interactions and longer durations of involvement with a challenging activity. (Courtesy Shay McAtee.)

percept and awareness of the properties of objects that are vital to initiating the ideation process.

The therapy experience is designed to help a child be able to initiate ideas and plans. Although a principle of sensory integrative theory is that activity is more meaningful if it is "child directed" (Clark et al., 1989), a child who has poor ideation may not be able to self-direct his or her actions. Ayres stated, "if ideation is limited, the therapist must help the child select a simple task and help the planning and execution of it" (1985, p. 67). In most instances, choosing activities that are simple enough for a child to be successful requires more skill and attention on the part of the therapist than thinking of activities that are complex.

Helping a child to get started in a "just right" activity is likely to be initially organizing for the child, thus ensuring that a playful experience occurs. For play to continue to develop, the child needs to build on these experiences, recognizing new possibilities and generating new ideas; otherwise, actions remain limited and are likely to become rote and routinized.

CASE EXAMPLE 8: STIMULATION OF IDEATION

William is a 4-year-old who tends to move aimlessly from one piece of equipment to another. Although he occasionally stops to push a swing or knock over a bolster, he does not appear to know "what to do." At preschool, he often pushes other children and is beginning to be seen as a behavior problem. Julie, William's occupational therapist, has found that she needs to help him engage in very simple interactions with equipment. As William approaches a large inner tube and appears to get ready to kick it, Julie gently places one of his feet on the inner tube and presses it up and down, saying "jump, jump, jump." She then holds onto his hands while he stands on the mat, and she steps up into the inner tube and begins jumping herself. When William begins to move his torso up and down in a jumping motion, Julie helps him to step up onto the inner tube and they jump together. Over the next several weeks, William always goes to the inner tube first when he comes to therapy. After a few sessions, he seems to have mastered the concept of one of the things he can do on this piece of equipment. Seeing that this has occurred, Julie tries to incorporate play into the activity by saying "I'm a frog. Ribbit! Ribbit!" while jumping from a squatting position from the inner tube onto the mats. William initially needs help getting his body into a squatting position, but the idea of being a frog seems to entice him. Once he has mastered this action, he continues to be interested in playing "frog" and says, "I'm a frog, I catch flies." Julie then introduces bean bag "flies" for William to catch as he jumps through the air. For William, emerging ideation allows him to come up with new ideas of how to play. Interactions with the therapist in play, in turn, motivate him to keep trying actions that are challenging yet organizing to him.

Although imagination is a basic element of typical childhood play, it develops only after a child masters concrete understanding of the properties of his or her own body, of objects, and of people. Much of imagination is probably related to ideation, or the conceptualization of possibilities for action. Some children who have poor sensory integrative functions seem threatened by imaginary themes. This often occurs in children with autism who seem, for example, unable to cope with consideration of, say, a slide as anything other than a slide and certainly not as a drawbridge in a castle. This same tendency is also seen in some children with severe dyspraxia, who seem to have the need to deal with objects in concrete terms, with little room for experimentation or ambiguity. Therapy for these children may need to begin by helping them to feel secure enough with their own bodies to experiment with pretending that they or that some object is something that it is not. For other children, use of imaginary play in therapy can be an important motivator to try difficult or unusual movements to enact a story. Parham (1992) notes that superhuman figures are often appealing to young children and states, "The superhuman theme may be especially salient to the child with sensory integrative problems who experiences feelings of powerlessness daily" (p. 3). As discussed earlier in this chapter, imaginary play often helps a child to stick with a difficult activity and to attempt more and more challenging actions. A young girl with extreme gravitational insecurity was once observed to utilize a fantasy scenario of hanging Christmas lights for an entire treatment session. So motivated was she by the idea of decorating her imaginary house, that she hardly noticed the heights to which she was climbing or the precarious surface she stood upon while securing her decorations. Thus, helping a child be able to feel comfortable using imagination and knowing how to use imaginary play in treatment are essential parts of the sensory integrative approach.

Even the most elementary aspects of social play can be difficult for the child with a sensory integrative disorder. Tolerating another child nearby is hard for a child with sensory defensiveness, just as maneuvering through an area without knocking down another child's building may be hazardous for the dyspraxic child. The therapy environment offers a safe haven for trying out social skills under the guidance of a therapist who can help the child enter into, negotiate, and retreat from interactions with peers. This support for social interaction is facilitated by an arrangement called "tandem therapy" (Clark et al., 1989), wherein therapists work in one-to-one situations with children, while other therapist–child pairs work nearby (Fig. 7-12). This model creates a fairly unique opportunity for social interaction, where relationships can be introduced gradually, closely monitored by the therapists, and repaired or redesigned as needed. Therapist–child teams may begin by playing near each other, with one or the other therapist commenting about the other child's play or use of a piece of equipment. A natural progression includes the use of turn taking, with two or more children engaging in the same activity. Often another child can motivate a child to try something that he or she may not have otherwise been willing to attempt. Gradually, children can be encouraged to engage in cooperative, interactive play with common goals and purposes. Since each child will usually have her or his own therapist, it is possible to retreat from the interaction should one of the children become disorganized, maladaptive, or nonpurposeful.

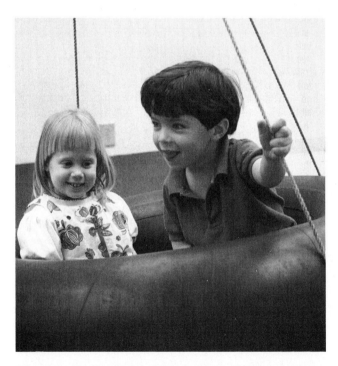

FIG. 7-12 Tandem therapy allows for close individual monitoring by a therapist; at the same time it provides opportunities for the child to develop tolerance for close proximity to other children and to build more sophisticated social skills. (Courtesy Shay McAtee.)

CASE EXAMPLE 9: WORKING ON SOCIAL PLAY

Sean and Andy provide an example of emerging social play in therapy. Sean is 6 years old and has speech and language delays as well as dyspraxia. He attends a special education class, where he works well in small groups in class but tends to play alone on the playground. Andy is an 8 year old who has some mild learning problems but attends a regular second grade. He has tactile defensiveness and signs of an underresponsive vestibular system. At school he is considered to have a behavior problem and most of the children avoid him because he tends to be a bully. Neither Sean nor Andy has experienced any true cooperative play experiences with peers. In a carefully designed effort to increase play skills in these two children, their therapy appointments were scheduled at the same time because their therapists saw the boys as having the potential for being able to play together. As the older child, Andy was at first encouraged to show Sean how to climb through an obstacle course he had constructed. Maneuvering through various textures of the pieces of equipment and keeping his balance on the unstable sections of the course were challenging for Andy, but he seemed motivated to show Sean how to do it. Sean, on the other hand, was challenged by the motor planning demands of the task but was enthusiastic about being like "the big kid." Sean and Andy played together in this way for several sessions, with Andy usually showing Sean how to do an activity. Sean had actually had generally more positive interactions with other children than Andy had and was the first to suggest that they build something together. Although he had become used to having Sean follow him through activities, Andy still seemed somewhat surprised that Sean did not appear afraid to work with him on a project, since this was the typical response he had from children at school.

The therapists planned this therapy session carefully to make sure the cooperative task was successful. Andy's therapist helped him prepare by using some calming activities that decreased his tactile defensiveness. Both therapists arranged the therapy room before the boys arrived to ensure that the materials they would need were accessible. At one point when Sean began to look frustrated because he could not express what he wanted to add to the fort structure they had decided to build, Andy's therapist asked if he had any idea about what Sean wanted, since he and Sean had all the master plans locked away in their secret hiding place. Although there were no real secret plans, Sean appeared to like this idea and readily accepted Andy's suggestion. This was one way that the therapists attempted to give the boys the message that they were capable of being successful and that it was natural for them to be able to work as a team. Experiences such as this one helped both boys to begin to have positive, cooperative play experiences, first in the therapy setting and later at home and at school.

The Therapeutic Importance of Followup

In addition to promoting play through preparation for and enactment of therapy sessions, an occupational therapist can facilitate play in the followup component of treatment. Including the family in the therapy process is one very important way this can occur. The more family members understand the difficulties a child is having and the types of activities that are helpful to the child, the better equipped they become to help the child in other settings (Fig. 7-13). Schaaf

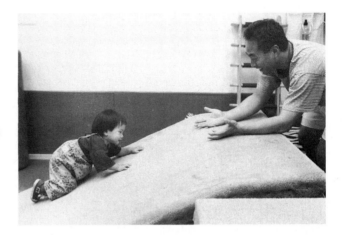

FIG. 7-13 Inclusion of family members in the therapy process helps them to gain insight into their child's sensory processing characteristics, which in turn better prepares them to solve problems concerning ways to help the child in other settings. (Courtesy Shay McAtee.)

and Burke (1992) note several ways the family can be involved in the therapy process to facilitate play, including planning activities that help the family to feel competent as caregivers, helping the family members know how to be role models for play behavior, and assisting in making environmental adaptations and suggestions for toys that can enhance sensory integration and play at home.

Including siblings is often a very productive way to ensure carryover of therapy activities at home and to make the sibling feel a part of the process. Providing home programs that are not overwhelming to a family but that involve activities which can be incorporated into everyday family experiences are most likely to be utilized than those that require something in addition to an already busy family routine. Similarly, the therapist can play an important role in helping to ensure carryover at school and in other community settings by helping those who work with the child to arrange environments and experiences that are likely to facilitate sensory integration and play.

CASE EXAMPLE 10: FOLLOWUP AT HOME

Deborah is a 3-year-old child who has a diagnosis of autism. She does not seem to know how to play with toys and tends to spend her time twirling strings. Her parents have tried to provide a variety of toys, but because she seems to like puzzles this is the most common type of toy they buy for her. Sara, Deborah's therapist, has suggested that the family consider a piece of suspended equipment for Deborah to use at home. Sara began to feel frustrated when the family continued to report that they were buying their daughter puzzles and they did not seem to be making progress on installing any suspended toy. When Sara offered to make a home visit her expectations for home intervention changed dramatically. Witnessing the hectic picture she found at home, she began to understand why the family may not have followed up on her suggestion. With a 6-month infant, a 6 year old, and a 12 year old, Deborah's mother had her hands full at home. There did not appear to be any obvious place that a swing could be hung, and although her behavior was fairly rote and nonpurposeful, Deborah did remain quietly entertained by her strings and puzzles. Sara needed to rethink the home plan in a way that was feasible for the family. Following several sessions at the home, Sara created a sensory enriched environment in Deborah's room with bean bag pillows, a quiet corner, and lots of blankets and pillows. She covered an old mattress that was in the garage and placed it in the backyard for Deborah to use for jumping. Sara also developed a plan for using a neighborhood park nearby that was within walking distance. She worked out a plan with the family whereby the 12-year-old sibling could take Deborah to the park every day after school. Here they were able to use the swings and several other pieces of moving equipment. This gave the 12-year-old sister a break before beginning her homework and allowed Deborah's mother a chance to get dinner started. This plan allowed the possibility of capitalizing on the gains Deborah was making in therapy in a way that was manageable and satisfying for her family.

CONCLUSION

Sensory integration as a normal process occurring within the nervous system is woven throughout development into a foundation from which play skills emerge. Occupational therapists can benefit from understanding how sensory integrative processes contribute to play, as well as the ways in which sensory integrative disorders hinder play. Fostering sensory integration naturally leads to enhanced play skills, just as encouraging play inherently promotes sensory integration. Application of both play and sensory integration concepts is therefore a natural and perhaps essential component in occupational therapy programs for children.

REVIEW QUESTIONS

1. Describe the development of the sensory beginnings of the play experience from infancy to adulthood.
2. During the preschool years, play becomes increasingly influenced by language, symbolism, and social relationships. How do these affect the ways that preschoolers play? In what ways do sensorimotor aspects continue to play a role?
3. During the school years, play begins to be dominated by rules and skills. How do sensory integrative components contribute to a child's success in play during these years?
4. Describe how sensory defensiveness may have an impact on the child's play development. Include issues related to tactile defensiveness, auditory defensiveness, and gravitational insecurity in your answer.
5. How do vestibular–bilateral integration difficulties typically interfere with play development?
6. How do problems with praxis typically interfere with play development?
7. In the sensory integrative approach to individual treatment, how may the therapist prepare for a treatment session in a way that encourages productive play?
8. How can play be incorporated directly into individual occupational therapy using a sensory integrative approach? Describe specific intervention strategies in your answer.

REFERENCES

Ayres, A. J. (1972). *Sensory integration and learning disorders.* Los Angeles: Western Psychological Services.

Ayres, A. J. (1979). *Sensory integration and the child.* Los Angeles: Western Psychological Services.

Ayres, A. J. (1985). *Developmental dyspraxia and adult onset apraxia.* Los Angeles: Sensory integration International.

Ayres, A. J. (1989). *Sensory integration and praxis tests.* Los Angeles: Western Psychological Services.

Bundy, A. (1991). Play theory and sensory integration. In Fisher, A., Murray, E., & Bundy, A. (Eds.). *Sensory integration—Theory and Practice.* (pp. 46-68). Philadelphia: FA Davis.

Caplan, F., & Caplan, T. (1974). *The Power of Play.* Garden City, NY: Anchor Books

Clark, F., Parham, L. D., & Mailloux, Z. (1989). Sensory integration and children with learning disabilities. In Pratt, P. N., & Allen, A. (Eds.). *Occupational therapy for children.* (pp. 457-509). St. Louis: C. V. Mosby.

Coster, W., Tickle-Degnen, L., & Armenta, (1995). Therapist-child interaction during sensory integration treatment: Development and testing of a research tool. *Occupational Therapy Journal of Research, 15,* 17-35.

Florey, L. (1969). Intrinsic motivation: The dynamics of occupational therapy theory. *American Journal of Occupational Therapy, 33,* 319-322.

Florey, L. (1985). Reilly: An explanation of play. In P.N. Clark & A. S. Allen (Eds.), *Occupational therapy for children.* (pp. 36-38). St. Louis: C. V. Mosby.

Knickerbocker, B. (1980). *A holistic approach to the treatment of learning disability.* New Jersy: Slack.

Knox, S., & Mailloux, Z. (in press). Play as treatment/treatment as play. In *Play in Occupational Therapy.* Rockville MD: American Occupational Therapy Association.

Montgomery, P. (1985). Assessment of vestibular function in children. *Physical and Occupational Therapy in Pediatrics, 5,* 43-56.

Parham, L. D. (1992). Strategies for maintaining a playful atmosphere during therapy. *Sensory Integration Special Interest Section Newsletter, 15,* 2-3.

Parham, L. D., & Mailloux, Z. (1996). Sensory integration. In J. Case-Smith, A. S. Allen, & P. N. Pratt (Eds.), *Occupational therapy for children.* (pp. 307-352). St. Louis: C. V. Mosby.

Schaaf, R., & Burke, J. P. (1992). Clinical reflections on play and sensory integration. *Sensory Integration Special Interest Section Newsletter, 15,* 1-2.

Smith, M. B. (1974). Competence and adaptation. *American Journal of Occupational Therapy, 28,* 11-15.

Tickle-Degnen, L., & Coster, W. (1995). Therapeutic interaction and the management of challenge during the beginning minutes of sensory integrative treatment. *Occupational Therapy Journal of Research 15,* 122-141.

White, R. W. (1971). The urge towards competence. *American Journal of Occupational Therapy, 25,* 271-274.

Wilbarger, P., & Wilbarger, J. (1991). *Sensory Defensiveness in Children aged 2-12.* Santa Barbara, CA: Avanti Educational Programs.

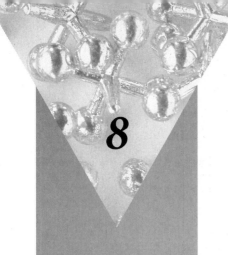

8

PLAY IN MIDDLE CHILDHOOD: A FOCUS ON CHILDREN WITH BEHAVIOR AND EMOTIONAL DISORDERS

Linda L. Florey and Sandra Greene

Clinical Vignette

An occupational therapy student with 6 weeks experience is in charge of a group of three 6-year-old boys who are impulsive and have difficulty paying attention. She has decided to have the group make animal masks in preparation for a play they are going to perform later in the week. The masks involve typical cutting, pasting, drawing, and painting activities. The goals for the group are to work together to share materials and space, to attend to the task, to persist with the activity to see it through to completion, and to encourage imaginative play. The children have been working productively for about 20 minutes. During the group, the kids begin talking about characteristics of the different animals they are making and start to get "silly." The occupational therapy student, encouraging play and creative behavior, joins in the fun asking "Does anyone know what sound a pig makes?" One child jumps from his seat and begins snorting and acting like a pig much to the delight of the other children. One by one they leave the table and begin to imitate animals. The student supports this as she believes that she is encouraging creative and imaginative play behavior based on the theme of making the masks. The children begin to escalate. The occupational therapy student attempts to calm the children down and get them back to task but the children ignore her and continue to get more and more out of control.

In this clinical vignette, the goals set by the occupational therapy student for the group were reasonable, as was the task selected and the manner in which it was introduced. The student had carefully planned the group, pacing the activity according to developmental level, providing supplies, and making the activity meaningful, relevant, and fun for the children. She thought by allowing the children to engage in imitating animals that she was encouraging creativity and imagination and that she herself was becoming more flexible in working with the group. What she did not anticipate or recognize was that this group of children did not have the skills to engage in unstructured creative play in this situation. She was unable to view and read the situation as escalating and out-of-control behavior. Children with problems in controlling impulses and focusing attention tend to be highly reactive to their settings. They have few internal controls to monitor their behavior. When they begin to act "silly," the experienced therapist begins to set limits and watches the reactions of the group. When one child leaves his or her seat and the activity, the therapist definitely intervenes to prevent the rest of the group from following. The ability of a therapist to read, interpret, and adjust therapeutic strategies in the ever-changing clinical situation is the hallmark of a seasoned therapist. In this situation, the student is demonstrating behavior of a therapist inexperienced in working with children presenting problems in focus and attention. Situations such as this are typical in clinical settings with students and new clinicians, as well as with experienced clinicians who change practice areas and begin working with children exhibiting behavior problems.

The impetus for this chapter comes from the authors' interest in the play and social interactions of children with behavior and emotional problems during the period of middle childhood. Its intent is to provide clinical information to assist in working with these children. This chapter is written with a model of clinical reasoning in mind. As such it acknowledges and is drawn from both the explicit theoretical conceptions of play and the "everyday" information gained from clinical practice. The information gained from clinical practice reflects the current interest in clinical reasoning in the work of Schön (1983), and the application of this perspective in occupational therapy guided by Mattingly (1991) and Fleming (1991). Their work details the process of identifying and analyzing the tacit or embodied knowledge that becomes part of the therapist's habitual way of doing things. This is "everyday" knowledge that practitioners acquire in the course of clinical experience, the importance and scope of which may not be readily apparent to them. There is a tendency on the part of practitioners to discount informally acquired clinical knowledge as not as important or significant as that knowledge acquired in a more formal manner; yet it is the practical reasoning based largely on clinical knowledge that guides therapists' practice. Mattingly (1991) states, "Whereas theory directs us to what is generally true, action always occurs in a unique context Given . . . the complexities and idiosyncrasies of the concrete case, any theoretical knowledge is bound to be crude and approximate, giving a starting place but not a rule book for action" (p. 982).

Clinical practice mediates conceptual and theoretical knowledge. A categorization process helps explain how this occurs; incoming information is sorted and categorized based on similarity to memories of the present situation or strict rules for interpretation of information. Barsalou (1992) describes four prominent models used in the categorization process. These are exemplar, prototype, classical, and mixed models. In the exemplar model, information is classified according to the similarity to a collection of exemplars that have been encountered in daily experience, whereas the prototype model represents a single centralized structural description. The exemplar and prototype models are both based on classifying and understanding information according to its likeness to memories similar to the present situation. Both of these models help explain how clinical knowledge is generated and how it functions to inform the practitioner. In the classical model, new information is categorized according to specific rules. It is an "all-or-none" categorization based on definitional rules and the present situation either fits or does not fit definitional rules, such as those present in the *Diagnostic and Statistical Manual for Mental Disorders, IV* (DSM IV), criteria for mental disorders. Mixed models refer to the use of all three models to categorize experience. In the clinical example of mask making with children who are impulsive and inattentive, the therapist draws on textbook descriptions of steps in activities, developmental levels of activities and impulsive behavior but she or he also draws on memories of "kids of this type" and "situations of this sort" to inform her- or himself of the possibilities inherent in the present situation as a guide to clinical intervention.

To tease out the clinical knowledge or the tacit exemplar and prototype models clinicians employ, the authors asked questions of experienced occupational therapy practitioners working with children. The therapists were asked about their experiences in clinical situations in which students and new practitioners experienced the most difficulty and asked them to speculate what piece of the puzzle the new practitioners were missing. Two major themes have emerged. One is that the new practitioners have difficulty when they are dealing with children who manifest "scattered" performance because they don't have models of hierarchical development firmly in place, particularly with respect to play activities. A child with cognitive and physical skills of a 7 year old yet the social skills of a 4 year old is difficult for them to conceptualize. Consequently, new practitioners often select and pace activities according to one set level and have problems downgrading or upgrading expectations based on individual variation. Inexperienced therapists may not know where they have been (past developmental markers) or where they are going (future markers) and often get "stuck" in having children engage in making or doing a product rather than engaging in a process. Second, they have difficulty determining how psychiatric symptoms are manifest in functional performance and they therefore miss the initial signs of behavior problems and problem identification. The authors emphasize both developmental markers in play and examples of how psychopathology is manifest in functional performance throughout the chapter sections.

This chapter is derived from knowledge acquired through theoretical constructs as mediated by clinical experience and is divided into three main sections. The first section, characteristics of play in middle childhood, addresses the developmental markers in play observed when working with children during this age period. The second section, children with behavior and emotional problems, focuses on typical symptoms of these problems and how symptoms are manifest in daily play performance. The terms "behavior" and "emotional problems" refer to the gamut of problems reflected in the behavioral manifestations children exhibit in expressing affect and in their relations with others. The third section, clinical guides to both assessment and treatment, details assessment and treatment of play in middle childhood with children exhibiting behavior and emotional problems.

PLAY IN MIDDLE CHILDHOOD

Clinical Vignette

"GaGa" is a group elimination game resembling kickball that is played in a space of about 20 × 25 feet, surrounded on four sides by a 3-foot wall. It is played with a large rubber ball and children are eliminated by being hit with the ball, by picking up a "hot" ball before it has bounced three times, or by hitting someone with the ball above the knee. A 6-year-old girl explains the rules. "There are millions of people and someone starts out and they toss up the ball. They say 'Ga, Ga, Ga' three times and you start pushing. When you get hit, you tell the counselor and you have to leave." She then goes on to explain that there are different kinds of GaGa. There is "silly face GaGa," "freeze GaGa" and "honest GaGa." Two 9-year-old girls say, "It's like this—no hits above the knee, you can block the ball with your hands but you can't touch it twice in a row, if the ball goes out, it is thrown in and it has to bounce three times before someone touches it and you say 'Ga' for each bounce, when you get down to two people, you start countdown and the last person to touch the ball loses. You can only join at the beginning and then as many as want to play join in. That's about it." A 10-year-old boy who has just been eliminated during countdown loudly says "If I've ever seen cheating at its highest rate, I've seen it here. The countdown is too fast, way too fast".

The above rules of GaGa were learned during naturalistic observation of children at a summer day camp. These rule explanations according to age level illustrate some of the changes in children's abilities to understand and process rules, which is so characteristic of changes that occur during middle childhood. To the 6-year-old girl, playing GaGa puts you in the center of a group. She describes most of the rules in general action terms—"throwing" the ball "up," saying "Ga, Ga" when others say it and "pushing." The counselor is the mediator of rules. GaGa is going with the group, yelling, and pushing until you get hit and then telling the counselor that you have been hit. You have to tell because this is the whole point of "honest GaGa." The 9 year olds can detail the main points of the game and the 10 year old not only knows the rules but is into a defense strategy. He does not refuse to obey the rule as if countdown did not apply to him, as might a child of 6 or 7, nor does he argue that he wasn't the last one hit. He has an understanding of rules and suggests that they may be manipulated by "cheaters," implying that the countdown cadence is what really has beaten him. The understanding of rules, the planning of strategy in games, the increasing complexity of the social network, and the number

and complexity of physical and social environments in which play occurs are all characteristic of changes in play that occur during middle childhood. This section reviews major changes that occur during middle childhood and characteristics of play behavior of children during this period. Suggestions for constructing a play environment are provided.

Development During Middle Childhood

Middle childhood is generally regarded as encompassing the ages of 6 to 12 years (Collins, 1984). Major theorists contributing to an understanding of development during this period include Piaget, Erikson, and Havighurst. Jean Piaget (1962) outlined the importance of middle childhood as the period in which a new form of thought is crystallized. This is the period of concrete operations, in which logic begins to structure the way children perceive relationships around them. Eric Erikson (1963) proposed eight stages in personality development, which included concern for the demands that society made on an individual at different times in the life cycle. At each stage he identified a crisis that had to be resolved, the resolution of which would add either a positive or a negative dimension to the ego. The crisis that must be resolved during middle childhood he termed industry vs inferiority. Industry involves making and doing things beside and with others and doing things well. Erikson believed that socially this is a most decisive stage because a first sense of division of labor occurs. Robert J. Havighurst (1973) identified developmental tasks that must be mastered. He characterized middle childhood as representing three major thrusts: a thrust out of the home and into the peer group, a physical thrust into games and work requiring neuromuscular skills, and a mental thrust into adult concepts, logic, symbols, and communication.

Additional information about this period of development comes from the Committee on Child Development Research and Public Policy. In 1981 they selected a panel of experts to identify significant aspects of social, emotional, cognitive, and physical development that occurred during this period (Collins, 1984). They identified three major themes. The themes stressed greater complexity in intellectual problem solving and the capacity to maintain intimate friendships, marked changes in overall capacity and behavior, and a continuity that suggested that development during this period had great significance for behavioral orientations, success, and adjustment in adolescence and adulthood (Collins, 1984). The major hallmarks of middle childhood are as follows:

1. Skills and modes of thought and behavior are characterized by *greater complexity in intellectual problem solving and the capacity to develop and maintain friendships*. Changes in cognition influence changes in social behavior. Children can keep different perspectives in mind, which in turn permits better abilities to communicate

and to consider the views of others to emerge. Children can move from a view that rules are externally imposed and governed to a view that rules are negotiated among individuals. (Collins, 1984; Piaget, 1962).

2. There are *marked changes in capacities and behavior.* Major transformations in skills and abilities take place during this period such that middle childhood cannot be viewed as a time of homogeneous functioning (Collins, 1984). Most 6 year olds function very differently from 9 year olds, who again function differently from 12 year olds. Children experience growth in the physical and neuromuscular realm and are able to use more tools and to refine their skills in hobbies, sports, and games. There is growth in the children's ability to monitor their own activities and to monitor themselves. Impulsivity decreases and capacities for regulating the child's own behavior and interactions are acquired. Children assume increasing skill in organizing tasks and in organizing time (Collins, 1984).

3. The *physical environment* becomes more complex temporally and spatially (Havighurst, 1973). During this period children spend the majority of the day engaged in activities that are conducted out of home—in school and in organized and spontaneous after-school activities. The biggest transition is in leaving home for a substantial period of the day and going to school. In addition to the classroom, there are other environments to master—the lunchroom, the playground, clubs, parks, back lots, and baseball and soccer fields.

4. The *social environment* becomes more complex with respect to adults and, most importantly, with respect to peers. Children are involved with teachers, coaches, and other adults with authority who are judging and grading them with regard to standards or outcomes such as grades or not making the team. School is the central arena for both success and failure. Academic skills and diverse social skills must be mastered (Epps & Smith, 1984). The biggest change occurs in children's allegiance to the peer group. It is estimated that children spend over 40% of their waking time with peers (Cole & Cole, 1989). In the peer group, children learn to interact with age mates, deal with hostility and dominance, relate to a leader, and be a leader. They learn to work with a group and to form best friends. They learn to cooperate and to compete (Fig. 8-1). During this period, children develop a peer culture (Corsaro & Schwarz, 1991; King, 1987). As more and more of their allegiance is transferred to the peer group, they derive their sense of self-worth and sense of being respected and valued from this group. This is the age in which children compare themselves to others and develop images of themselves based on how they "measure up" to others (Mussen et al., 1963). Among themselves, children decide who can play in a game, codes for inclusion and exclusion, how to deal with cheaters and troublemakers, and how to manipulate the situation to their own and their friends' advantage (Knapp & Knapp, 1976; Slukin, 1981).

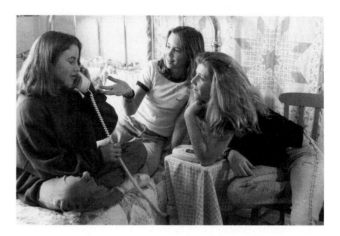

FIG. 8-1 The peer culture emerges as a prominent aspect in the lives of children during middle childhood. (Courtesy Shay McAtee.)

Middle childhood is a distinct period of development and one that reflects a range of increasing skills and abilities in the physical, social, and cognitive spheres of children. It does not represent a homogeneous period and therefore is not a homogeneous population.

Play Behavior in Middle Childhood

Play assumes major importance in middle childhood as a processor of social relatedness and relationships. Peers and peer interactions are very prominent during this time and children learn to influence one another verbally. The socialization that occurs among peers occurs largely in the context of play and games that are outside the direct supervision of an adult (Maccoby, 1984). In play, there is increasing emphasis on games and on negotiating the rules of games. Play can be conceived of as an interaction process in which socialization is learned, practiced, and mastered. Social interactions are embedded in play activities. In middle childhood, the quality of the social interactions changes, as do the play activities themselves. For purposes of highlighting differences in play behavior during this period, characteristics of play have been selected and separated and are organized according to changes in peer relationships, rules and games, and play interests. The changes in play are drawn from descriptions of children's play by Hartley and Goldenson (1963) and Gesell et al. (1977) and from clinical practice. The changes are listed in Table 8-1. They are presented in terms of differences between "younger" and "older" children. "Younger children" represent the beginning age period of middle childhood, from 6 through 8 years. "Older children" represent the end of the age period, from 9 through 11 years. These changes represent not normative changes but a progression from simple to more complex levels of behavior. The table provides not a comprehensive listing of play activities or materials during this period but simply a sampling.

In *peer relations,* the group is very important to younger children of this age period. They like to talk and look like

TABLE 8-1   Characteristics of Play During Middle Childhood

Characteristics of Younger Children	Characteristics of Older Children
Peer relationships	
■ Group very important—adjusting to group controls	■ Groups very important—join many and establish cliques
■ Learning to work with others although little cooperation	■ Clubs with passwords and secret codes
■ Leadership of group changes rapidly	■ Conformance to peer codes and competition with others
■ Help age mates, and fight with them	■ Organized activities such as scouts
■ Separation of sexes	■ Best friends
Rules and games	
■ Unable to put rules of game above need to win	■ Want to make and break rules
■ Do not understand that rules apply equally to everyone	■ Decide how rules and turns will be determined
■ Vague about how rules operate	■ Argue over what's fair and opposed to cheating
■ Like to make up own rules and go on until they win	■ More conscious of rules and of obeying them
■ Cheating, tattling common	■ Accept majority decisions
	■ Rules becoming relative not absolute
Play interests	
■ Dramatic play—details in costume and realistic emblems of roles important	■ Dramatic play—done in groups and reflects events outside of home and school
■ Collecting—quantity important, nature items popular	■ Collecting and trading—big collections, although collecting declining
■ Crafts—get bogged down in the middle and need a clear notion of sequence of steps and reassurance to finish	■ Crafts—need help with materials or procedures. Exploring many crafts and hobbies.
■ Critical of own work and work of others	■ Beginning to achieve satisfaction in making things

one another. They are not necessarily interested in one another but just enjoy being together. Being accepted as part of a group is easier with the younger children, and popularity and leadership change rapidly. With older children of this period the group is still very important, but they are becoming more selective as to who gets in (Fig. 8-2). There are often secret clubs with secret codes, and cliques are formed. Adherence to codes—in dress or behavior—established by the cliques or group is very important. Organized groups such as scouts are popular. At this same time children are beginning to pair off in smaller groups and are establishing best friends.

Rule or *game* behavior in younger children is characterized by a view that rules are externally imposed, usually by an adult. Games such as baseball are conceived of typically as action; hitting the ball and running around the bases. The number of players on the field and the number of outs in an inning are "rules" imposed by adults and children at this age have only a vague idea of how rules operate. They do not understand that rules apply equally to everyone and are often unable to put the rules of the game above the need to win. When children begin to understand that rules are agreements among the players as to how a game is to be played, they love to make up their own rules but change rules rapidly to suit their own needs. Older children during this period are more conscious of rules and of obeying them. They can decide on rules and change them to suit different occasions and different players (Fig. 8-3). For example, chil-

dren observed in a neighborhood playing a game would alter the rules depending on the age of the children playing. One of the younger children was named "Rosy" and the children in play would yell out "Rosy rules" to signal to one another that they would be playing a different and less complex version of the game. Older children spend time arguing over what is fair and allowed according to agreed upon rules (Fig. 8-4). At this age they are also able to accept majority decisions.

Play interests change during this period. An intense interest in sports begins to build. With younger children, dramatic play is still popular and details in costume and realistic emblems of roles are very important. Collecting is popular but quantity is the key. In crafts, assistance is needed in figuring out activity steps. The presence of an older child or an adult nearby is helpful. Without such guidance or instruction, younger children become frustrated and may abandon the effort. With older children, dramatic play reflects events outside of home or school. In crafts, they still need help with materials or procedures. This is a sampling age in which children try many different crafts and begin to narrow interests to form hobbies.

Constructing a Play Environment

One of the reasons for reviewing the characteristics of children and of play during this developmental period is to help the occupational therapist construct a treatment environ-

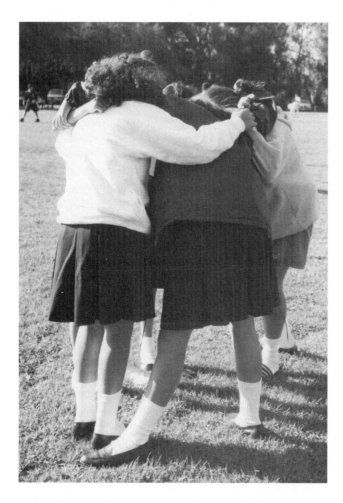

FIG. 8-2   Belonging to a group is a hallmark of middle childhood.

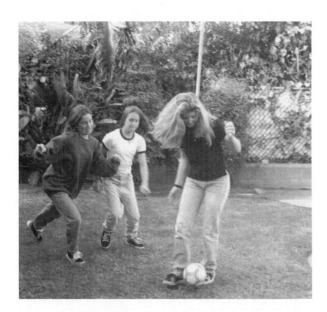

FIG. 8-3   Through the middle childhood years, children develop a growing understanding of game rules as well as a willingness to abide by them. This is reflected in the ways they engage in sports and games. (Courtesy Shay McAtee.)

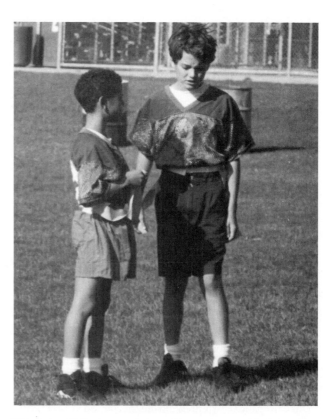

FIG. 8-4   Skills in negotiating with peers are critical in middle childhood activities, such as sports.

ment or approach based on key features of this time period. The goal is to capture the "kidlike" qualities of middle childhood and to incorporate these in treatment programs targeted to help children with identified deficits. For example, in the authors' clinical practice they teach children social skills within the context of a club. Children make club T-shirts, wear them to the club meetings, and help establish club rules. Social skills curricula or content is used within the context of the club meeting. This format provides a normalizing context for the learning of social skills and the children are eager to attend and participate. Just as the provision of dolls, doll houses, and play furniture complete with toy dishes and housekeeping equipment encourages symbolic, imaginative play with younger children, certain "props" and elements are necessary to evoke a play ambiance characteristic of middle childhood. In working with children exhibiting problems in behavior and emotional areas, other factors need to be included in developing an environment or therapeutic approach. The following are suggestions for constructing a play environment for children exhibiting behavior and emotional problems in the period of middle childhood.

1. *The play environment should be populated with peers.* The therapist may initially begin in a one-to-one situation, but as soon as is feasible a peer should be included. Peers and peer groups are dominant during middle childhood

and it is in this arena that children with emotional problems often have the most difficulty. In addition to sharing materials and equipment, children must also share space and the attention of others and it is within a small group of peers that this can be learned and practiced.

2. *Programs should be conducted within natural childhood activity models in which crafts and games are emphasized.* The occupational therapist needs to examine the process in the activity and not get stuck on the game or craft product. Crafts and games should be viewed with respect to three major dimensions so that they can be rapidly upgraded and downgraded according to the level of the children within the group. The dimensions of cognitive, motor, and social complexity of an activity need to be viewed separately with this population. *Cognitive complexity* means a mix of problem-solving processes that involve mastering steps and mastering the controls necessary to complete the steps. Activities should be examined for the number of steps they require, the sequence and complexity of the steps, and the amount of patience and persistence required in problem solving. Patience and persistence are control skills children are learning to develop. They are often very critical of their own work and become frustrated when it doesn't look like the model. Children during this period are beginning to construct projects and need to be encouraged and cajoled into following the steps to completion. In terms of *motor complexity,* an activity should be examined with regard to how much fine motor or visual motor control is required and whether the children have sufficient skills in this area. In addition to problems in the social and emotional realm, the children the authors have seen over the years often manifest deficits in visual motor integration which are identified in assessment. Learning disabilities are prominent with some psychiatric disorders of childhood (Lewis, 1991). *Social complexity* means the opportunities the situation affords for sharing and cooperating in the use of materials, space and peer and adult attention and interaction. It is often the social complexity of the situation with which children exhibiting emotional problems have the most difficulty. For that reason therapists may downgrade or make less complex the cognitive and motor components so that the social features of the situation can be learned and emphasized. For example, children often share and talk with one another more frequently when engaged in simple repetitive activities such as stringing medium size beads because they easily master the task requirements. The authors do not mean to suggest that there be no complexity with this population. Rather, therapists must have knowledge of the different processes that an activity requires so that the particular social goals they may be targeting can be addressed.

3. *Treatment should be imbedded within natural childhood activities of this age.* This includes emphasis on clubs, on scouts, or on small groups that have a distinctive identity to the children. Children of this age seek to "belong," to be a part of something, and organized groups such a scouts or the informally constructed clubs serve that need. At the University of California at Los Angeles (UCLA) Neuropsychiatric Institute and Hospital (UCLA NPI & H), we have had a Cub Scout den chartered under the Boy Scouts of America in operation since 1971. The children wear scout uniforms to the meetings, which the institute supplies; they begin the meetings with the scout oath and work on badges and activities typical of other scout troups. Social skills are emphasized in this den and are embedded within this naturally occurring childhood model. The children are registered in the scout den and we can refer the children and their caretakers to the scout program in their area. A club format is used in many groups as well, and the children have an opportunity to name the club, to decide on its special features such as "secret handshakes," "code words," or the wearing of special hats or T-shirts to the meetings. Not all of the occupational therapy programs are conducted within a club or organized group, but these "special" groups are spread throughout the week and provide a bit of novelty in the treatment situation as well as a normalizing tie to neighborhood and community activities.

4. *Rules are a major focus in middle childhood and rules should be established for each treatment session or group.* Rules for safety and for general ways of proceeding should be established by the therapist and the consequences of rule following and rule violation should be known to the children. These rules have to do with the behavioral expectations the therapist has for the way in which the group or session is to proceed. They may include such things as sitting at the table after entering the room, or not touching materials until told to do so, or taking turns. The children should also have an opportunity to construct rules and the therapist may suggest areas such as fairness, listening, and saying things nicely to others. "No fiddling with your hands" and "Feet have to stay on the floor" are examples of rules children have constructed to deal with respecting one another's personal space. Adherence to rules may be promoted by verbal praise or concrete symbols for good effort such as earning stickers. Children with behavior or emotional problems often have trouble identifying when they have done something "right" and a concrete reward of a sticker often serves this purpose. These authors ask the children to identify their positive behaviors and those they need to work on so that behavior is a matter under their control. The occupational therapist needs to have in place a behavior management system for the group. This should include behaviors that constitute rule violation and the consequences for violation.

5. *Materials and space need to be set up in advance of the group meeting.* This is particularly critical in working with a group of children who have difficulty focusing and attending to activities. This is a straightforward and simple suggestion but it is one that students and new practi-

tioners often don't consider. If the therapist is unprepared and begins gathering the necessary supplies for the activity after the children have arrived, individual children or the whole group can become unfocused and more time is spent on regaining the attention of the members than on the planned activity.

These suggestions form some parameters for establishing "structure" when working with children exhibiting problems in behavioral control. "Structure" is a term used in milieu therapy to describe social processes that affect patients therapeutically. It refers to the organization of time, space, and activity (Gibson and Richert, 1993). It is not a specifically defined process. Occupational therapists and other disciplines working in psychiatry credit structure in the environment when all goes well and refer to lack of structure or no structure in the environment when patients are unfocused or out of control. In working with children, structure has to do with capturing the attention and interest of children, and targeting the activity to the skill level of the members of the group. This is accomplished within an environment that has established temporal and spatial boundaries, in which codes of behavioral conduct are explicit.

CHILDREN WITH BEHAVIOR AND EMOTIONAL PROBLEMS

Clinical Vignette

Danielle is an 8-year-old girl attending sleepover camp for the second year in a row. She is verbal and engaging and initiates games and talk with her companions. She likes to be at the center of things and volunteers to be the walker in the dining room, the helper in the cabin, and star of the evening skit. When she doesn't get her way, she doesn't want to do anything—she says she won't eat, she won't clean her bunk in the cabin, and she won't be in the skit at all. She has a hard time obeying rules. When everyone is asked to sit, she will sit and then stands up. When asked to stand up, she stands and then sits. She accuses her peers of hitting her, of messing with her food, of taking her things. She complains of stomach aches as well. The rest of the children deny her accusations, then they pretty much ignore her. She is not well liked.

Danielle displays problems in relationships with others and in her adjustment to the rules of camp life. She may be displaying immature behavior triggered by an immediate crisis, such as homesickness or insecurity in a new situation, that which she is masking or she may be displaying behavior indicating psychopathology. Whatever the underlying cause, her behavior indicates an immediate problem in the social realm. The purpose of this section is briefly to review the different settings in which occupational therapists may encounter a population of children exhibiting behavior disorders and to describe manifestations in play typically seen in children with psychiatric disorders.

Service Settings

Children with psychopathology are identified in the mental health system, but they may be present as well in other prominent systems of care for children. These include the child welfare, juvenile justice, health care, and educational systems (National Mental Health Association Speaks, 1989). In addition to mental health settings, occupational therapists encounter these children on the pediatric wards and in the school system. On the pediatric wards, the children may have suffered bruises, fractures, or head trauma as a result of impulsive or aggressive behavior or as a result of abuse. Children with chronic medical conditions and brain damage are at high risk for developing psychiatric disorders (Offord & Fleming, 1991). Occupational therapists working within the school system are most likely to encounter this population of children. The children carry not a medical diagnosis but an educational label. Within the lexicon of special education, this group of children is referred to as seriously emotionally disturbed (SED) and this population makes up the fourth largest group of children with disabilities under Individuals with Disabilities Education Act (IDEA). It is believed that this population may be the most underserved group of students with disabilities (National Mental Health Association Speaks, 1989). The reasons for this include lack of systematic identification because of varied interpretations in definition and eligibility criteria and reluctance to label children SED because of the stigma associated with the term. New definitional criteria for this population have been proposed by the Mental Health and Special Education Coalition but have not yet been passed by the U.S. Office of Special Education. In addition to the school system and health systems, occupational therapists in private practice may encounter children with these problems.

Psychiatric Disorders and Their Manifestation in Play

It is conservatively estimated that at least 12% of children and adolescents have mental disorders that are diagnosable (Zigler & Finn-Stevenson, 1991). Incidence with respect to age and sex tends to vary with specific disorders. In general, disorders are less prevalent in preadolescence, more prevalent among boys than girls from ages 4 to 11 years, and more prevalent among girls than boys in the 12- to 16-year age range (Offord & Fleming, 1991). The causes of mental disorders are varied and include consideration of constitutional factors, physical disease and injury, temperamental and environmental factors, as well as family factors (Barker, 1988). One factor may play a lead role in the etiology of a specific disorder, but generally many biopsychosocial vulnerabilities or stressors are implicated (Garfinkel et al., 1990).

The DSM IV is one of the current systems by which psychiatric disorders are assessed. It employs a descriptive approach for mental disorders in which identification is based on identifiable behavioral signs or symptoms. The prominent disorders in middle childhood, the disorders with high incidence despite variations in epidemiologic studies, are attention-deficit hyperactivity disorder, conduct disorder, mood disorders and anxiety disorders. Specific features of these disorders are available elsewhere (American Psychiatric Association [DSM IV], 1994; Florey, 1993).

Psychiatric disorders are often "invisible" to new practitioners. Problems in the realm of "behavior" or "emotions" are not always present all of the time but are often triggered by internal or external events. In discussing what may be distinctive about psychopathology in middle childhood, Achenbach (1984) states, "Unlike major adult disorders, such as schizophrenia and manic depressive conditions, most disorders of middle childhood involve exaggerations of behavior that nearly all children show in some degree. Many disorders. . .involve a failure to develop age-appropriate behavior, rather than the decline or deviation from attained levels of functioning often seen in disorders of adolescence and adulthood" (p. 370). In some situations, the children look and act like "regular" kids, whereas in others they are extremely immature. In other childhood disability areas, such as those involving neurologic-orthopedic conditions, it is relatively easy for a new practitioner to identify or to forecast the types of problems in function children may manifest. For example, poor head, neck, and trunk control in a child with cerebral palsy is visible and the impact of this in daily play activities is clear. A problem in the realm of "behavior" is less obvious at first and the occurrence less predictable. New practitioners frequently have difficulty distinguishing behavioral difficulties from the vast repertoire of children's actions and reactions typical of play at this age and in identifying "first stages" of defiant or escalating behavior. For example, when children are demonstrating difficulty in taking turns or agreeing on rules in a game, therapists may set limits too soon or too firmly and inadvertently turn the session into one in which no disagreement at all is tolerated, or therapists may escalate the children by forcing them to dig in and defend a position. On the other hand, no "reminders" or limits at all may lead to a session in which the children begin pushing or shoving one another in their efforts to settle the dispute. The early recognition of problems and how and when to intervene are very difficult areas for new practitioners.

The following case examples have been developed in an effort to describe the effect of psychopathology on social, play, and task behaviors. They have been developed from composites of patients seen at the NPI & H and they are generalized for the purpose of illustration. The case situations portray a child with a particular psychiatric disorder playing a table game with a peer and making a simple craft project in the presence of a peer. They are presented here to assist the practitioner in recognizing problems as they are manifest in play. They are reprinted with permission from the author and publisher and are taken from Florey (1993, pp. 509-510).

CASE EXAMPLE 1: ATTENTION-DEFICIT HYPERACTIVITY DISORDER

Stevie is loud and intrusive. He can't stick with a decision about which game to play, so choices have to be narrowed down for him. He has difficulty waiting his turn in a board game and often grabs pieces of the game, such as the spinner or the dice. He does not pay attention and is constantly fidgeting. When he is sitting, he appears to be in constant motion. He is physically intrusive with his peers and does not seem aware of this. He interrupts frequently.

While doing a craft project, Stevie is unable to listen to directions. He has difficulty sequencing simple steps and becomes frustrated. He grabs at tools and materials and interferes with the work of his neighbor. He requires step-by-step instruction from a helpful adult nearby to accomplish the project. Peers often complain that Stevie "doesn't listen" and that he is intrusive.

CASE EXAMPLE 2: CONDUCT DISORDER

Tom does not give his peer a chance to respond to a choice of games and makes the choice for both of them. He is used to taking over and getting his own way. He selects the color he wishes to play in the table game, then gives his peer and the occupational therapist the remaining choices. If he is not winning, he often cheats and may attempt to cover his cheating by accusing his peer. Tom is bossy and controlling with his peers and is not liked by them. Although he understands the directions on a simple project, he becomes frustrated and stops working, labeling the project "babyish" or "stupid." He needs to be coaxed to finish his project and often doesn't show pleasure or pride in successful completion of an activity.

CASE EXAMPLE 3: MOOD DISORDER, MANIC EPISODE

Annie decides on a game and begins to open the box, but another game in the cabinet "catches her eye" and she quickly takes that game out. Choices need to be focused for her and she objects to the process, since narrowing choices interferes with her "independence." She chatters constantly. She asks questions, does not wait for the answers, and is apt to comment on various materials in the room or tell you what is on her mind. She is very easily distracted.

Annie is able to play a game with frequent reminders as to rules and taking her turn and often apologizes for needing reminders. She has better ideas for a project than the one presented to her and rattles off a list of materials she will need. She is very convincing in describing what she wants to produce but is unable to articulate a plan for accomplishing her production. She objects to completing the project given her but works quickly and makes mistakes because of her speed.

Although Annie is intrusive and demands a great deal of attention from those around her, she is not disliked by her peers. She is fun and uninhibited and her peers regard her excessive talking as something she cannot help.

CLINICAL GUIDES TO ASSESSMENT AND TREATMENT

Clinical Vignette

An occupational therapist greets Nathan, a 9-year-old boy who has been referred to her because he is having trouble keeping up on the playground with other children, often gets into fights with other boys, and is slow to complete his work at school, even though his intellectual abilities have been measured at an above-average level. The physician who referred the child wonders whether he has some "motor impairments." His parents report that Nathan often goes to his room and cries when he thinks no one is watching him and that ever since he started a new grade in school 3 months ago, he seems to be less interested in things than he used to be.

When Nathan enters the therapy room, he barely makes eye contact with the therapist. He compliantly sits in the chair that the therapist offers him but mumbles answers to questions and doesn't brighten up, even when asked about favorite toys, activities, or his pet. The therapist gives him an untimed, quick screening for eye–hand skills. He completes this in a very slow, deliberate manner, doing well on each item but making a negative comment about his abilities after each attempt. He asks the therapist repeatedly, "Did I do that right?" The therapist scores his test and finds that his score is above average. At a later time, she assesses his visual perceptual and motor skills because this has been the primary reason for referral, although she has not observed any signs of difficulty in this area. Again, she finds that Nathan is scoring at age level or a little above on everything.

The therapist continues the evaluation by interviewing Nathan, targeting areas of information about his family and where he lives, a self-report on activities of daily living (ADL) skills, chores, school, friends, and play. As the session goes on, Nathan begins to make better eye contact and converses in a less mumbling way, but the therapist notices that he often falls into a very "babyish" way of talking and that he keeps asking her for approval. Nathan answers all of the questions on the interview, with a few interesting responses that pique the therapist's interest. When asked whether he likes school, Nathan yells, "NO—I HATE IT—SCHOOL IS BORING AND THE WORK IS TOO HARD." When asked whether he has a best friend, he replies, "Yeah, I have hundreds of friends but just can't remember their names right now." In response to a question about who he likes to play with and what he likes to do when he plays, he responds, "I like to play with my dog—we go on walks." When pressed on this answer, he is unable to name any child with whom he regularly spends time after school. He also says that he comes home everyday after school and doesn't do any after-school activities. Nathan is asked whether he ever gets into fights at school. He says that he does "sometimes," but that other kids pick fights with him and that it isn't his fault.

The therapist asks Nathan to choose between two craft activities, so that she can assess the process of completing the craft: the child's ability to make a choice, follow and sequence directions, solve problems, use materials, and pay attention. She is also interested in what Nathan's reaction will be to the finished product. Instead of showing interest in the two craft projects shown to him, he goes over and picks

---

CASE EXAMPLE 4: MOOD DISORDER, DEPRESSIVE EPISODE

Mary is very compliant. She selects a game immediately but she doesn't seem interested in any of the games and is just doing what is asked of her. If her peer wants another game, she defers. She does not have difficulty with game concepts. She takes turns and is not invested in winning the game. She seems embarrassed if she wins. Mary doesn't initiate much conversation with peers or adults, but she is usually responsive when asked questions. She follows directions on craft projects and usually works slowly. At times she seems preoccupied and stares into space but can be easily directed back to the task at hand.

The most striking impression of Mary is that she seems to be going through the motions. She expresses no pleasure, seems to be having no fun, and displays little if any spontaneity. She is not disliked by her peers because she does little to provoke or annoy them. However, she is not popular with peers.

CASE EXAMPLE 5: ANXIETY DISORDER

Paul is very concerned about doing the right thing and asks for further instructions in choosing a game, for example, "Is one better than another?" He frequently asks the adult whether he is playing the game correctly and is concerned that he move game markers and manipulate game pieces properly. He is quick to point out any mistakes or instances of cheating on the part of his peers. He is the target of nicknames by his peers such as "teacher's pet" and "prissy face." His concern with correctness and neatness carries over to craft projects. Paul asks a lot of questions, although he has a grasp of the process. He needs reassurance and becomes visibly anxious when executing such "final" motions as cutting a piece of copper along the line and applying paint to paper.

Paul complains of flulike symptoms occasionally. He doesn't seem to enjoy the process of engaging in activities and doesn't seem pleased with or proud of his final product. He is not well liked by his peers because of his anxious and somewhat rigid manner.

CASE EXAMPLE 6: SCHIZOPHRENIA

Ran does not respond to the opportunity to select a game but does not object when one is brought to him. He does not initiate or direct comments to anyone, but occasionally he responds to questions asked of him. He speaks spontaneously but his speech is odd and often not related to immediate events. He obeys simple directions such as "Ran, move your marker here," but is unable to participate spontaneously in game playing. Eye contact is poor.

Ran is preoccupied with cars. He plays with cars and draws the same car the same way every time. When given a craft project of copper tooling with a mold, he disregards the mold and draws a car on the copper with a copper tool. He appears upset at the suggestion that the piece of copper on which he drew a car be placed on a mold and changed to duplicate the image on the mold. He will perform the operation when another piece of copper is placed on the mold and the process initiated by him.

Ran's looking "upset" is the closest he comes to displaying emotions. He looks neither happy nor sad but appears blank. He is neither liked nor disliked by his peers. They regard him as "weird" but they don't tease him.

up a much simpler stencil project completed by a 4 year old earlier in the day. "Can I do this one instead?" he asks and says that he likes the "easier" one better. The therapist reassures him, and tells him that she will help him with his choice of the other two projects. He finally settles on a copper tooling project and has to choose his design from about eight different tooling molds. He hesitates, and takes about 5 minutes to choose, finally settling on a lion mold. Although he is able to remember the multistep directions and doesn't need them to be repeated, he continues to ask the therapist whether he is doing the right thing, whether he should change the way he is doing the tooling, and whether she likes what he is doing. When the project is completed and framed, Nathan refuses to take the project, stating "I just want to keep it here so I can see it when I come back to this room."

During the next session, Nathan is paired with Robert, age 8 years, to assess their peer interactions. Because part of this evaluation involves observing the process the children go through in choosing and playing a game together, the occupational therapist steps back and does not intervene, only giving the boys directions to "choose a game that you like and then we'll all play it." The boys enter the room and immediately begin grabbing randomly at the many games stored in a bookshelf. They almost get into a fight over pulling on the same game box. After about 5 minutes of this kind of behavior, Robert finally chooses Candyland. Nathan retreats to the table and almost begins to cry, saying "Why did he get to choose—it isn't fair. He always gets to choose," even though this is the first time that the boys have met each other. When they sit down to play the game, they cannot organize the cards, fight over which marker they want, and don't wait their turns. Both of them are, in turn, angry when they get a "bad move" and repeatedly take themselves out of the game and then put themselves back in. When Nathan wins the game, he pumps his fists in the air and says "I won" over and over again, ignoring Robert, who is visibly angry and is on the verge of crying over losing the game.

What is happening here? Why is Nathan having such difficulty at school? Why does he keep making negative comments about himself when his physical and cognitive skills have been assessed as adequate? Why are an 8 year old and a 9 year old having such difficulty cooperating? Why did they choose Candyland, which is a game typically introduced to preschoolers as one of their first experiences with board games? Why are they having such difficulty getting organized?

The assessment and treatment of children with behavioral problems is a complex process. When working with children who have difficulty functioning with other people and doing what they should be doing at home, at school, at camp, and at soccer practice, the therapist does not have the behavioral equivalent of a precise goniometer reading to measure these problems with function. What therapists do have are keen observational skills that improve and broaden over time and the acquired experience to recognize certain behaviors as "red flags," indicating obstacles to being successful. There are many challenges these children have experienced. What is right cognitively for them sometimes isn't

right socially and emotionally. Some children with behavioral problems have learning disabilities, some do not. Some have motor and perceptual problems, and some do not. Many children with average or above-average IQs who are doing well or who have the potential to do well in school have very severe performance deficits when it comes to other life demands. The common denominator for these children is devastating social experiences that most children would not think twice about or would look forward to. This disability is often not visible, but it is a disability that severely impairs their ability to function.

When a child who is having behavioral problems is referred to occupational therapy, where does the therapist start? What are relevant areas to assess? What does the therapist do, once he or she has obtained test results? What should the therapist do if the picture is complicated by other skill deficits, such as motor or perceptual difficulties?

Clinical Guide to Assessment

The areas chosen to assess must be directly tied to the identification of a child's functional abilities, to include both areas of strengths and problems. This is old news to occupational therapists. What is proposed here is that therapists take a more comprehensive look at how children are functioning. Currently, many therapists feel tied to assessing and treating only how the motor, sensory, and perceptual skills of a child influence his or her ability to function. Certainly, these abilities critically impact upon the ways in which children are able to play, to learn, and to take part in everything children should be a part of. Yet if these areas are the therapist's only areas of concern, then he or she has taken these skills completely out of the context of a child's life. From the perspective of a child who is experiencing problems in many areas of functioning, an improvement in social abilities and experiences may be as or more important than improving gross motor skills. The normal development of skills does not take place out of context—a child develops gross motor skills by playing, often in the company of other children. The motor skills are an avenue by which play with other children can develop into a budding friendship. Therapists cannot continue to work on basic skills in isolation from their social context, hoping that the skills will transfer to real-life situations and neglecting the child's social arena in which the skills will be put to use.

Task, play and social, and perceptual–motor skills are the target areas of assessment. Equal importance is placed on standardized assessments, such as adaptive behavior scales, visual–perceptual, and motor tests, and on information gathered from an interview with the child, as well as structured observations of play, task performance, and social abilities. Children are seen individually and with a peer. They are seen individually for the administration of an interview in which they are asked to describe a "typical weekday" and "typical weekend day," for observation of task performance in a craft, and for specific testing of motor skills or adaptive behavior. Children are seen with a peer for the assessment of social behavior in a game or a task. It would be ideal if a child could be evaluated within the context of his or her own community, whether at school, at home, or on the playground. If this is not practical, the therapist can try to recreate these normal settings as nearly as possible and include other children currently being evaluated in the process. Although this is an artificially constructed peer group, common problems with peers continue to be evidenced by children with social skills deficits, even though the other children are new to them. Often the problems are stable across any group in which the child participates.

Two guides for assessing play and tasks in a social context provide ways of structuring observations of the task, play and social behaviors of children. The Activity Observation Guide in Box 8-1 was developed at the UCLA NPI & H to provide an indication of the way children approach and carry through with activities in the context of a social setting. This guide has been extremely useful to everyone from new occupational therapy students, who need help in defining what they are looking for, to experienced clinicians, who use the guide as a "jumping off place" to add more experienced clinical knowledge to the emerging picture of the child being evaluated. Although the guide can be used with a wide age range, expectations for each item should be viewed developmentally. The Social Behavior Observation Guide in Box 8-2 was also developed at the UCLA NPI & H and is adapted from Cartledge and Milburn (1985). This guide is used in conjunction with the Activity Observation Guide.

Adaptive behavior is also a crucial area to assess. There are several assessments that measure adaptive behavior, including the social–emotional portion of the Miller First Step (First Step scale) and the Vineland Adaptive Behavior Scales (Vineland scales). These assessments are usually part of a more comprehensive evaluation and are useful if the therapist wants to establish an age level of adaptive functioning for the child. The adaptive behavior checklist on the First Step scale includes the areas of daily living skills, self-management, social interactions, and functioning within the community. A social–emotional scale is also part of this screening test and includes items on task confidence, coop-

---

Box 8-1   ACTIVITY OBSERVATION GUIDE

A. TIME
1. How long does it take for the child to settle on an activity?
2. How long does the child stay engaged in the activity?
3. How does the child use structured vs unstructured (free-time) play?

B. TASKS
1. Is the child able to make decisions when given choices?
2. Is the child able to follow directions?
3. Does the child use materials and tools correctly?
4. Is the child able to tolerate frustration?
5. Does the child attempt to solve problems independently before asking for help?
6. Is the child able to ask for help when needed? Does the child ask for too much assistance?
7. Does the child participate in cleanup?
8. Is the child proud of his or her efforts?

C. STRUCTURED GAMES
1. Does the child decide which game to play?
2. Does the child know the rules?
3. Does the child know the object of the game?
4. Does the child take his or her turn in the correct sequence?
5. Does the child follow rules?
6. Is the child able to accept winning or losing?

D. PEOPLE
1. Is the child able to play alone?
2. Interaction with adults
   a. Does the child interact with adults?
   b. Is the child dependent on adult interaction?
   c. Is the child able to follow directions and rules?
   d. Is the child able to become involved in an activity through imitation and visual imitation?
   e. Is the child able to become involved in activities through verbal instructions?
   f. Is the child able to get attention from adults in an appropriate way?
   g. Does the child respond appropriately to praise?
   h. Is the child able to accept help from an adult?
3. Interaction with peers
   a. Does the child interact with other children?
   b. What type of social play does the child engage in? Onlooker play, parallel play, associate play, cooperative play? Is this developmentally what you would expect?
   c. What kinds of play themes does the child propose to other children?
   d. Does the child imitate peers? Is this appropriate or inappropriate?
   e. Is the child possessive with toys or materials?
   f. Is the child aggressive to others?
   g. Is the child able to share?
   h. If the child is old enough, does he or she compete appropriately and accept winning or losing?
4. Does the child express emotion and have fun in play?
5. Does the child pick up social cues, use feedback from others, and learn from prior interactions?

Box 8-2   SOCIAL BEHAVIOR OBSERVATION GUIDE

1. *Eye contact*
   Does the child establish eye contact when spoken to or when speaking to others?
2. *Listening*
   Does the child pay attention to the person who is talking and make an effort to understand what is being said?
3. *Conversation*
   Does the child initiate conversation? Does he or she talk to others?
4. *Asking a question*
   Does the child decide what information is needed and ask the right person for information?
5. *Asking for help*
   Does the child request assistance when he or she is having difficulty?
6. *Joining and staying in*
   Does the child have strategies for entering an ongoing group or activity?
7. *Cooperation*
   Does the child follow group rules? Does he or she comply to reasonable requests made by others? Does he or she take turns and share?
8. *Apologizing*
   Does the child tell others he or she is sorry after doing something wrong? Does the child overapologize or take responsibility for something he or she has not done?
9. *Convincing others*
   Does the child attempt to persuade others that his or her ideas are better and will be more useful than those of the other person?
10. *Expressing feelings*
    Does the child let others know how he or she is feeling?
11. *Understanding feelings*
    Does the child try to figure out what others are feeling? Does the child let others know that he or she appreciates favors?
12. *Asking permission*
    Does the child figure out when permission is needed to do something and then ask the right person?
13. *Helping others*
    Does the child give help to others who may need or want it? Does the child ask before giving help to another child?
14. *Using self-control*
    Does the child control his or her temper? Does the child respect the property of others?
15. *Responding to teasing*
    Does the child deal appropriately with being teased by others in ways that allow him or her to be in control? Is the child routinely teased by other children?
16. *Avoiding trouble*
    Does the child stay out of situations that may get him or her into trouble?
17. *Likability*
    Is the child sought out by other children to be played with?

Note: Adapted from Cartledge, G. & Milburn, J. (Eds.). (1985). *Teaching social skills to children.* New York: Pergamon Press.

---

erative mood, temperament and emotionality, uncooperative or antisocial behavior, and attention–communication difficulties. The First Step scale can be used for ages 2 years, 9 months to 6 years, 2 months. The First Step scale also includes screening items for cognitive, language, and motor abilities (Miller, 1993).

The Vineland scales assess adaptive functioning in the areas of daily living skills, communication, socialization, and motor skills. They can be used from birth through 18 years, 11 months and yield an adaptive level and age-equivalent score. The evaluation is completed by interviewing parents and/or caregivers. The Vineland scales are very useful to occupational therapists because the questions asked all examine the child's ability to function in the real world. For example, such questions as "Does the child follow community rules?" "Does the child have a preferred friend of either sex?" and "Does the child play more than one board or card game requiring skill and decision making?" are asked. Scoring criteria for each question on the Vineland scales are provided (Sparrow et al., 1984).

Although this is not the focus of this chapter, perceptual and motor skills should be thoroughly assessed as a part of any full evaluation of children who are experiencing behavioral problems, not only to rule out any deficits but also to explore whether concurrent deficits in these areas are contributing to difficulties with coping in any way. It is documented in the literature that children with learning disabilities and/or emotional–social problems have concurrent physical problems as well (Kramer et al., 1988). Clinically, therapists at UCLA NPI & H have found that at least 50% of the children admitted to the inpatient unit have deficits in visual–perceptual, visual–motor, and/or motor skills severe enough to limit that child's ability to participate in common play and work activities. In some cases, the identification of problems in these areas, subsequent intervention, and structuring activities so that the child experiences success on a consistent basis have helped children bring their behavior under control. For all children, it is important to establish whether they are having skill problems in these areas to make meaningful recommendations for them in terms of further occupational therapy intervention and for adaptations that may have to be made in community settings, including home and school. Some of the typical assessments used for this purpose include the Beery-Buktenica Developmental Test of Visual-Motor Integration (Beery, 1989), the Motor-Free Visual Perception Test (Gardner, 1982), and the Bruininks-Oseretsky Test of Motor Proficiency (Bruininks, 1978).

Case Study Evaluation. To illustrate how an evaluation of a child actually takes place, the clinical vignette presented at the beginning of this section is next used as a model to describe how the evaluation progresses and the underlying problems an occupational therapist may pick up from the child's behavior. Each evaluation area is followed by a "reasoning" section that targets some of the conclusions and further questions the therapist poses in the evaluation process. Therapists must assess and target areas for intervention quickly, and this requires prioritization of assessment strategies and interpretation and synthesis of evaluation data. This section is an attempt to tease out a portion of this clinical reasoning process that therapists use in daily practice.

Motor and perceptual motor skills. Although Nathan was referred by his physician because of a "motor impairment" question, in formal testing the occupational therapist could not find any sign of this. Visual–perceptual, fine motor, and gross motor evaluations are all at or above age level. In clinical observation, although a little slow at times, Nathan shows good skills. However, his perception of his skills is not consistent with his performance. He constantly makes negative comments about himself and constantly asks for reassurance.

Reasoning. Consider that Nathan may have anxiety about performing activities and tasks and/or that his self-confidence is poor. What is the link among his skills, his perception of his skills, and his decreased ability to engage in play activities on the playground with other children? The therapist needs more observation of this behavior in a peer group to better assess what is going on.

Task skills. Nathan initially chose a project immature for his age and one that did not match his cognitive, motor, or perceptual skills. He has some difficulty making a choice but shows good abilities in following directions and using the craft tools correctly. Again, he constantly asks for reassurance. He does not make any comments about the successful completion of his project, instead asking whether he can leave it with the therapist. He says that school is boring and that it is too hard.

Reasoning. Nathan is showing some slowed decision making and motor skills but not enough to keep him from successfully completing his project in the allotted time. He spends much of his time simultaneously working and asking for reassurance—similar to the situation with his motor skills. He is very dependent on the therapist to structure his emotional environment for him and tries to ensure structure by asking for reassurance over and over as well as by using a "babyish" voice in an effort to get and keep the therapist's at-

tention. The therapist wonders whether this kind of behavior is also present at school, thinking that he most likely does not get constant reassurance in a classroom situation and may have to be "quietly" anxious about himself in that situation. He does not outwardly show any pride in his completed project. He leaves the project with the therapist, "I just want to keep it here so I can see it when I come back to this room." Sometimes children are relieved, even in evaluation settings, that the therapist is structuring the situation and presenting challenges at their level and will leave a project, toy, or an item of clothing as a kind of insurance that they will come back to the room again for occupational therapy.

Play and social skills. Nathan's parents are concerned because he is looking sad, cries a lot, and shows less interest in things than he did previously. They wonder if this is tied to something that has happened or is happening at school. Nathan interacts socially in an odd way with the therapist. His eye contact is initially poor, he mumbles his words and shows no enjoyment when discussing activities that children usually enjoy. When he warms up in the session, he is anxious about how he is doing and speaks to the therapist in a regressed manner.

He gives the therapist cues about his social life. He cannot remember his friend's name, says he has "hundreds" of unnamed friends, likes to play with his dog more than other children, does not spend any time with children after school, and perceives that he is often picked on by other children. When he is paired with Robert, the 8-year-old boy, the social situation is disastrous. He has difficulty handling the unstructured situation presented to him, resorting to random grabbing of different games on the shelf. He is unable even to attempt to negotiate with Robert about what game they are going to play, instead giving up and going back to the table, almost crying. He objects to Robert's choosing the game but readily accepts the choice, even though it is a very immature game for him. He has a lot of difficulty waiting his turn, cannot organize the game cards, and gets upset because he has wanted the red marker, which Robert has taken. He cannot play cooperatively with Robert and shows very poor frustration tolerance when he gets a "bad move," taking himself out of the game. The concept that fortunes change in board games is not very apparent to him. He loses hope very quickly and does not persist in trying to continue with the game. When Nathan finally wins, he is a poor winner, failing to read Robert's cues of being angry and upset, continuing to gloat over winning the game.

Reasoning. With the presence of a peer, Nathan's social problems that the therapist could only imagine suddenly become reality. Nathan's social and play skills are not only immature, they are maladaptive. He is choosing easier activities in a quest for success. Unfortunately, his play and social skills are so poor that even choosing a simpler activity probably makes Nathan look even worse to other children, who by this time are playing fairly complex, competitive games with rules and teams. He does not have fun in the process of playing the game but somehow takes pleasure in winning the game, apparently oblivious to the process. He does not show any skills in cooperating, compromising, or convincing Robert of his position. Instead, he copes by giving up or by becoming irritable and angry. Nathan is immature in his relations with others, in his ability to make decisions independently, and in his selection of tasks matching his motor and cognitive skills. The therapist could give the Vineland scales to obtain an age-equivalent score, but she or he has enough information to substantiate immature and maladaptive behavior strategies in play and social situations.

Summary of the Evaluation. What is right for Nathan cognitively is not right for him socially or emotionally. His cognitive, motor and visual–perceptual skills are average or above average. His social skills are maladaptive. At 9 years of age, Nathan should be able to play a fairly complex board game in a cooperative way with a group of children. He also should be showing enjoyment over exploring new, multistep craft activities and striving to make his skills better and better. By this age, children no longer rely on adults to help them negotiate familiar social territory but have generally become quite independent. Nathan is an example of the child whose many good abilities are overshadowed by a lack of social competence. He attempts to cope with this by relying on adults, asking for reassurance, showing regressed behaviors, and withdrawing from situations when he has to compromise or cooperate with peers. As a result of this, his self-esteem has suffered and he is experiencing performance anxiety. This may have started in social situations but now is intruding on his other skills as well, such as academic skills, in which he has been previously successful. Nathan often is tearful and irritable, is motorically slowed, and does not enjoy activities as he once did. He could be suffering from depression.

Clinical Guide to Treatment

What does a therapist do with boys like Nathan and Robert? Children with behavior and emotional problems generally have very poor self-esteem, reinforced daily when their lack of coping skills and abilities makes them unable to participate in normal peer, school, and community activities with any success. In addition, many of them have very poor ability to read social cues, so feedback from the environment is impaired. Because of their behavior, their environment is often restricted and they miss out on normal daily activities that are the arena in which children learn how to interact in groups. This is the dilemma—most behaviorally disturbed children have an extremely hard time working in groups, but they have little opportunity to participate in group activities because of their behavior.

The purpose of the assessment is to identify areas of strength and weakness from which goals and treatment interventions may be developed. In targeting goals and interventions for children exhibiting behavior and emotional disorders, priority is given to the behaviors and/or situations that are causing the children the most difficulties in their social relations. Goals should be measurable, and they should address the who, what, when, and how of behavior expected in occupational therapy (Brands, 1977). The "who" and "what" identify the person and the behavior in which the person is expected to engage. The "when" and "how" identify how frequently the behavior is expected to occur and under what circumstances, such as how much assistance or prompting the therapist must give. The components of the treatment goals—the behavior, the frequency and duration, and the circumstances—all may be varied to reflect change in the child's skills and abilities.

Agrin (1987) and Schultz (1992) both wrote of models of practice for children with behavioral problems. Small group activities, with a strong emphasis on cooperation, sharing, respect for each other and for materials, and participating as a group member are recommended. In practice, this model is extremely effective. Children with social skills deficits require highly structured programs that emphasize the learning and practice of life skills in context. As the child gains more appropriate skills, he or she can be integrated into less structured activities and spend more of the day in normal play and social experiences with other children. The word "structure" is often used without explanation of what it means or why it is important. As in the case study evaluation section, a "reasoning" section is included here to uncover some of the considerations a therapist makes in constructing an approach and environment for treatment. Elements of structure are discussed in this section.

Case Study Treatment. For Nathan, the quality of his interactional skills with peers and adults was a problem, as was his dependence on adults to select activities for him. These became the target areas for setting treatment goals and selecting intervention. Initial goals for Nathan were:

1. Nathan will initiate and carry through a social interaction (e.g., asking peer to play with him, sharing materials) four times a session.
2. Nathan will interact with others using his "regular voice" instead of his "baby voice."
3. Nathan will demonstrate more independence in school, play, and home activities by persisting and sticking with an activity to completion.

Initially, all of these goals required reminders or prompts from the therapist. These formed the "start points" for intervention. Nathan was involved in the process of goal agreement and monitoring. The therapist suggested to Nathan that he needed to learn to ask his companions to share materials or to play using his regular voice and he needed to finish an activity. The therapist asked, "Do you think this is something we might work on?" and in treatment sessions would say, "Remember what we're working on." To implement the goals, Nathan was involved in an ongoing social skills club and was the therapist's helper in occupational therapy sessions with younger children. The rationale and format of these groups is stressed to provide a snapshot of "how" and "why."

Social skills club and therapist helper. The Dinosaur Club was the name given to an occupational therapy social skills group by the children. The purpose of the group was to listen to others, to include others, to express positive and negative feelings, to identify feelings in others, and to think of consequences before acting. There were currently three other children in the club, between the ages of 8 and 9 years. All members had club T-shirts that they made with their name and a Dinosaur footprint on the front. Because Nathan did not have a shirt, he was seen individually in an occupational therapy session to make his shirt and the occupational therapist also told him of the purpose and the general format of the club meetings. Each meeting had a routine format or sequence that was dependable for the children. The club meeting began with greetings to one another, followed by all members' putting on their club shirts, which were worn over their regular clothing. Following this the club rules were reviewed. Because Nathan was new, he was asked to contribute a rule to the club that could be followed by all but that would help him in working with other club members. His rule was "Talk right to others." The remainder of the club rules were read and included such things as taking turns and listening to others. The group then talked about what had happened since the last club meeting. The members were asked, "Anything going on?" and were also specifically asked about good or bad things that had happened. The club meeting then focused on an activity—a game or craft that required sharing materials with others, sequencing steps, and talking with one another. The games or crafts used were simple and initially stressed successful completion so that the social behavior could be targeted. As the group worked together, the cognitive complexity—the number of steps and independence in steps—was increased. Nathan was also involved as a helper to the therapist in a group with four younger children, ages 4 to 5 years. Nathan was responsible for providing initial verbal instruction in an activity, e.g., paper bag puppets, and for helping children share materials. In this way, he could practice some of the skills he himself needed and gain more confidence in his ability to influence others in a nurturing way.

Reasoning. Nathan is placed in a group because it is with peers that he demonstrates the most difficulty. The goals for each child must be considered, as are the goals for the group as a whole. For example, one child may be timid, one aggressive, and one impulsive. Each child has individual goals in social interactions and for participating in the activity. The goal for the timid child may be to initiate interactions with one other peer. The goal for the impulsive child may be to listen and to respond to conversations initiated by a peer, whereas the goal for the aggressive child may be to use words and not actions to make feelings and needs known. Although these three goals are different and are implemented differently for each child, the common goal everyone is working on is better social interactions, i.e., "The children will be able to play together cooperatively for 20 minutes," implementing and encouraging each individual goal to further the group goal.

In all groups, the therapist has a "game plan." This involves the selection not only of a particular activity but of a plan for how to present and pace the activity and a contingency plan if the activity is not successful. Activities should be targeted to fit the social abilities of the group, with the cognitive and motor abilities downgraded initially. The game plan also includes the anticipation of problems that may occur and a plan for intervention before things get out of hand. If children are having chronic behavioral problems, a consistent plan of action should be developed among everyone who comes in regular contact with the child, including the parents, teachers, and therapists.

The process of providing structure to children encompasses consideration of the physical, social, and activity environments within the treatment session. The process of providing structure to children encompasses several areas:

1. The therapist structures the physical environment to provide a challenging, interesting variety of toys and materials for the children. Too many items may cause the children to become disorganized and for some children, even tools such as hammers may become objects with which to test the safety rules.
2. The therapist structures the social environment as well. Rules are made and followed in the occupational therapy session. Older children can help make up their own rules, whereas younger children may need to have rules given to them. Rules help children "feel out" the boundaries of a situation and help them begin to gain independence by thinking in more positive ways of interacting and getting along with each other. Rules and consequences for transgressing rules should be consistent. Each child should have a very good understanding of what the rules of the setting are.
3. The therapist structures the activity environment by carefully analyzing the level of skill needed to participate. Choices of activities can be provided that are slightly below the child's intellectual abilities in order to give the therapist and the child more freedom to work on the social aspects of the activity. As a result, children don't become anxious about not knowing how to perform a certain task or game. As children begin to gain skills in social play, they are provided with less structure and more options to choose and carry through activities with their peers.

Children have to do the structured activity as contextually as possible. This could take the form of occupational therapy sessions during free-play time in a classroom, on classroom outings, or in after-school activities such as sports, the YMCA, or scouts.

CONCLUSION

This chapter has illustrated clinical interventions in play with children exhibiting behavior and emotional disorders informed by both theoretical perspectives and "hands on" experiences encountered by the authors. The leading construct in designing clinical interventions is play. Interventions may target a vast number of skills and behaviors in which the children are deficit, but the context is play. To embed the learning, unlearning, and relearning of skills in play is to construct a world that has meaning for the child and one in which he or she must function.

Occupational therapists are interested in improving a child's ability to function in tasks and with others in school, in the family, and in community settings. But the authors take the view that the ability to function independently in tasks and with others is immeasurably fostered, nurtured, hampered, or squelched in the peer culture during times of free play. To help children with behavior and emotional disorders understand this culture and to assist them in achieving the necessary skills to fit in is a major goal of occupational therapy practice in this area.

REVIEW QUESTIONS

1. In the first clinical vignette of this chapter, how might the occupational therapy student have tailored the group intervention to be more effective?

2. What is middle childhood? What are the major hallmarks of development in middle childhood?

3. Describe the nature of peer relations, rules, and play interests in middle childhood. Differentiate between younger and older children within middle childhood in your answer.

4. How may the occupational therapist construct play environments to enhance social skill development of children in middle childhood?

5. Discuss the impact of childhood psychiatric disorders on the development of play.

6. Describe the process of play assessment for a child in middle childhood who has a psychiatric diagnosis. What does the assessment entail, and how are data interpreted? How are assessment results then used to guide treatment?

7. The authors suggest four broad domains for guiding activity observation of children in middle childhood. What are these domains? Provide examples of questions you might ask in an assessment within each domain.

8. Discuss the variety of ways in which a therapist may provide structure to children within a treatment session.

REFERENCES

Achenbach, T. (1984). The status of research related to psychopathology. In Collins, W. (Ed.). *Development during middle childhood: the years from six to twelve* (pp. 370-397). Washington, DC: National Academy Press.

Agrin, A. (1987) Occupational therapy with emotionally disturbed children in a public elementary school. *Occupational Therapy in Mental Health, 7,* 105-113.

American Psychiatric Association. (1994). *Diagnostic and statistical manual of mental disorders* (4th ed.). Washington, DC: American Psychiatric Association.

Barker, P. (1988). *Basic child psychiatry* (5th ed.). Oxford: Blackwell Scientific Publications.

Barsalou, L. W. (1992). Categorization. In L. W. Barsalou, (Ed.). *Cognitive psychology: A review for cognitive scientists* (pp. 15-51). Hillsdale, NJ: Lawrence Erlbaum Associates.

Beery, E. (1989). *The Developmental Test of Visual-Motor Integration* (3rd ed.). Cleveland, OH: Modern Curriculum.

Brands, A. (Ed.). (1977). *Individualized treatment planning for psychiatric patients.* Rockville, MD:U.S. Department of Health and Human Services.

Bruininks, R. H. (1978). *Bruininks-Oseretsky test of motor proficiency examiner's manual.* Circle Pines, MN: American Guidance Service.

Cartledge, G., & Milburn, J. (Eds.). (1985). *Teaching social skills to children.* New York: Pergamon Press.

Cole, M., & Cole, S. (1989). *The development of children.* New York: Scientific American Books.

Collins, W. (1984). Conclusion: The status of basic research on middle childhood. In W. Collins (Ed.). *Development during middle childhood: the years from six to twelve* (pp. 398-421). Washington, DC: National Academy Press.

Corsaro, W., & Schwartz, K. (1991). Peer play and socialization in two cultures. In Scales, B., Alm, M., Nicolopoulou, A., and S. Ervin-Tripp (Eds.). *Play and the social context of development in early care and education* (pp. 243-354). New York: Teachers College.

Epps, E., & Smith, S. (1984). School and children: The middle childhood years. In W. Collins (Ed.). *Development during middle childhood: the years from six to twelve* (pp. 283-334). Washington, DC: National Academy Press.

Erikson, E. (1963). *Childhood and Society.* New York: W. W. Norton.

Fleming, M. (1991). The therapist with the three-track mind. *American Journal of Occupational Therapy, 45,* 1007-1014.

Florey, L. (1993). Psychiatric disorders in childhood and adolescence. In H. Hopkins & H. Smith (Eds.). *Willard and Spackman's occupational therapy* (8th ed., pp. 503-519). Philadelphia: J.B. Lippincott.

Gardner, M. F. (1982). *Test of visual-perceptual skills (non-motor).* San Francisco: Children's Hospital of San Francisco.

Garfinkel, B., Carlson, G., & Weller, E. (1990). Preface. In B. Garfinkel, G. Carlson & E. Weller (Eds.) *Psychiatric disorders in children and adolescents* (pp. xv-xvi). Philadelphia: W. B. Saunders.

Gesell, A., IIg, F., & Ames, L. (1977). *The child from five to ten.* New York: Harper & Row.

Gibson, D., & Richert, G. (1993). Section 1F, The therapeutic process. In H. Hopkins & H. Smith (Eds.). *Willard and Spackman's occupational therapy* (8th ed., pp. 557-566). Philadelphia: J.B. Lippincott.

Hartley, R., & Goldenson, R. (1963). *The complete book of children's play.* New York: Thomas Crowell.

Havighurst, R. (1973). *Developmental tasks and education.* New York: David McKay. Individuals with Disabilities Education Act, 1990.

King, N. (1987). Elementary school play: theory and research. In J. Block & N. King (Eds.). *School Play* (pp. 143-165). New York: Garland Publishing.

Knapp, M., & Knapp, H. (1976). *One potato, two potato…The secret education of American children.* New York: W. W. Norton.

Kramer, L., Deitz, J., & Crowe, T. (1988). A comparison of motor performance of preschoolers enrolled in mental health programs and non-mental health programs. *American Journal of Occupational Therapy, 42,* 520-525.

Lewis, D. (1991). Conduct disorder. In M. Lewis (Ed.). *Child and adolescent psychiatry: A comprehensive textbook* (pp. 561-573). Baltimore: Williams & Wilkins.

Maccoby, E. (1984). Middle childhood in the context of the family. In W. Collins (Ed.). *Development during middle childhood: the years from six to twelve* (pp. 184-239). Washington, DC: National Academy Press.

Mattingly, C. (1991). What is clinical reasoning. *American Journal of Occupational Therapy, 45,* 979-986.

Miller, L. J. (1993). *First Step Screening Test for Evaluating Preschoolers Manual.* New York: Harcourt, Brace, Jovanovich.

Mussen, P., Conger, J., & Kagan, J. (1963). *Child development and personality.* New York: Harper and Row.

National Mental Health Association Speaks. (1989). *Students with serious emotional disturbance underserved in special education.* Alexandria, VA: NMHA. (Available from NMHD, 1021 Prince Street, Alexandria, VA 22314.)

Offord, D., & Fleming, J. (1991). Epidemiology. In M. Lewis (Ed.). *Child and adolescent psychiatry: A comprehensive textbook* (pp. 1156-1168). Baltimore: Williams & Wilkins.

Piaget, J. (1962). *Play, dreams and imitation in childhood.* New York: W. W. Norton.

Schön, D. (1983). *The reflective practitioner: How professionals think in action.* New York: Basic Books.

Schultz, S. (1992). School based occupational therapy for students with behavior disorders. *Occupational Therapy in Health Care, 8,* 173-196.

Slukin, A. (1981). *Growing up in the playground.* London: Routledge and Kegan Paul.

Sparrow, S., Bolla, D., & Circhetti, D. (1984). *Vineland Adaptive Behavior Scales Manual.* Circle Pines, MN: American Guidance Service.

Zigler, E., & Finn-Stevenson, M. (1991). National policies for children, adolescents and families. In M. Lewis (Ed.). *Child and adolescent psychiatry: A comprehensive textbook* (pp. 1178-1189). Baltimore: Williams & Wilkins.

9

ELEMENTARY TO MIDDLE SCHOOL TRANSITION: USING MULTICULTURAL PLAY ACTIVITIES TO DEVELOP LIFE SKILLS

Ann Neville-Jan, Linda S. Fazio, Bonnie Kennedy, and Carolyn Snyder

KEY TERMS

Occupational Therapy Transition Program (OTTP)
curriculum-based programming
articulation activities
instrumental play
illicit play
recreational play
multiculturalism

I t is generally agreed that children spend the majority of their time in play. During play children explore, experiment, learn, and have fun. Also, play is an arena for children to develop cognitive, social, language, and motor skills. Researchers have established the importance of play for development, yet they have also documented that play in the elementary school curriculum is both undervalued and underutilized. The purpose of this chapter is to describe an innovative occupational therapy program incorporating play within the context of an elementary school curriculum used in two public school districts in Southern California.

The Occupational Therapy Transition Program (OTTP) is unique in several ways: (1) it complements the overall classroom curriculum, (2) it utilizes play as a primary means for fostering transition skill development, (3) it extends the concept of transition to the elementary school, and (4) it interjects a multicultural component. The program serves children from diverse ethnic backgrounds who are receiving special education in the public school system. Also, the program trains occupational therapy students from diverse ethnic backgrounds to be service providers.*

The overall goal of the program is to assist elementary school students (in third through fifth grade) who are in special education classes to develop the foundation skills necessary to be successful in a variety of contexts. These contexts include the student's classroom and school, home, and community. Specifically, the child acquires the skills to help him or her make the transition from elementary to middle school.

The intent of this chapter is to provide occupational therapists with a broader outlook on practice in the school system. The first part of this chapter sets the stage for the description of the OTTP. Development, factors that have an impact development, and play are concepts central to portraying the program and are highlighted within the con-

*The United States Department of Education and Rehabilitation Services, Office of Special Education and Rehabilitation Services funded the development and implementation of these programs through training grants H029F20073-93 and H029F10042-92. The authors gratefully acknowledge the assistance of Valerie Adams with this chapter.

text of the elementary age child in special education. The second part of this chapter presents the actual OTTP with the intention that the reader be able to use the description as a resource to implement a similar program. To this end a case study is also presented.

DEVELOPMENTAL ISSUES DURING MIDDLE TO LATE CHILDHOOD

Occupational therapy practice with children, within any context, must be cognizant of child development. Developmental parameters include biological, psychological, and social factors. In addition, ecological theories are important for understanding development in the context of the environments in which the child interacts, such as school and family (Bronfenbrenner, 1979). The OTTP described in this chapter concentrates primarily on the psychological and social skills that the child needs to interface with a wide range of environments.

Middle to late childhood, when the child is between 8 and 11 years old, is a somewhat tranquil period of development positioned between the early trauma of leaving home for school and the tumultuous adolescent years. In general, the child practices and refines already established physical, psychological, and social skills developed during earlier developmental stages (Havighurst, 1972). In the context of the neighborhood, school, and community the older child devotes an enormous amount of energy to the mastery of both people and tasks.

Mastery of People and Tasks

Children in the third through fifth grades are in the process of moving beyond egocentrism and are concerning themselves with others. Peers become important for developing a sense of belonging and acceptance (Maier, 1969). In the classroom students begin to work together in small groups. Outside the classroom children participate in both formal and organized clubs such as the Girl and Boy Scouts of America as well as initiate informal cliques. These child-centered subcultures may include shared passwords, secret codes, group chants, and phrases that are symbolic of a group identity. The OTTP emulates this club-type format. One class of children named their group the Rainbow Dolphins. This name reflects the multicultural focus of the activities and the school mascot. Group experiences permit and invite the child to influence a social, rule-bound environment that is a microcosm of the larger world where the child must eventually interface. School aged children extend their peer group involvement beyond the classroom to the playground, neighborhood, and the larger community. Peer relationships and the formation of friendships are a central focus of the OTTP. The typical school day presents few opportunities for the child to work in a group. This is especially true for special education classes, where the child usually works independently with one-on-one instruction by the teacher or teacher's aide. In contrast, through OTTP participation the child encounters peers in small group sessions, which increases his or her ability to communicate with a wider range of people, particularly peers. At this age peers become an extremely important network and often the barometer for evaluating success or failure in performance.

In addition to an expanding social network, third through fifth graders display an eagerness and curiosity in their interaction with a wider range of objects found within their environments. As children approach adolescence their attention spans increase. They are better able to follow complex directions and solve problems. Also, fine and gross motor skills are increased. Playing a musical instrument; participating in competitive sports; collecting objects such as cards, stamps, or stickers; playing board games; learning to use a computer; and reading books are examples of activities that engage the child during this time and foster skill development (Howe, 1993).

In learning to manage people and tasks the child demonstrates an enhanced ability to reason and a more complex conceptualization of rules, especially rules related to games. Piaget (1965) describes this as the concrete operational period. There is a new understanding of causation, rules of attribution, and the moral rules of right and wrong. According to Piaget (1965), early in the 4- to 7-year-olds' thinking, rules are absolute; later, however, from around 7 to 10 years of age, rules are not considered incontestable but are generally accepted. From ages 10 to 11 children know a bit more about the origin of rules and require a more expansive explanation before following them and, in fact, may not respect them. This is the time when the rule belief of peers is considered of more influence than that of parents or other adults in the child's environment.

An awareness of the concrete operational functions of the child and a concentrated effort to provide learning experiences appropriate to this level invite a smoother transition to the formal operational, and potentially more expansive mode of the adolescent's cognitive style. The middle school preadolescent begins to rely on reasoning as a way to conceptualize the world; however, the child in transition who is learning disabled may not move beyond the concrete operational period.

Factors That Have Impact on Development

The OTTP targets students from diverse ethnic backgrounds who are receiving special education services. Culture, language, and disability influence development and need to be considered in constructing programs for children. A critical review of studies focused on education and childrearing practices among minority groups noted a strong assumption by researchers that so-called Anglo examples were "normal" or "ideal" (Mejia, 1983). In many cases textbooks, curricula, test materials and procedures, role models, and student placements in school programs are based on white, middle-class cultural standards or norms. The multicultural nature of the program educates not only students but all school personnel concerning these biases.

Impact of Family and School Personnel. The importance of family involvement in the education of children, especially children with learning disabilities, is well documented (Turnbull & Turnbull, 1987). However, culturally diverse families with children in special education face obstacles to becoming full partners with the school in the education of their children. A variety of factors may prevent a family member from attending Individual Educational Plan (IEP) meetings. For example, some caregivers (not always the parent) may not have transportation or childcare. Time off from a job may mean lost wages. Language differences may make participation in IEP meetings difficult. Family members may not understand the jargon that is typically used in meetings and be too afraid, intimidated, or embarrassed to ask questions. Other culturally relevant factors that may affect teacher's perceptions of a student's performance or behavior include the influence of extended family members, family spiritual beliefs, nonverbal communication, and parental roles in the family (Correa, 1989; Gay, 1989; Wahab, 1973).

Professionals in classroom settings, such as teachers, are considered to be the next most important socializer of the Mexican-American child after his or her parent. The child enters school with a strong family system identity that may not fit the classroom environment and expectations. This may result in considerable stress as the child attempts to adjust to multiple, and at times conflicting, expectations for performance (Mejia, 1983). A study that compared the classroom aspirations of lower socioeconomic class African American and Hispanic children with middle-class Anglo-Americans found no differences in hopes and desires for achievement; however, the children from minority backgrounds were limited in their ability to make it happen (Phillips, 1972). Little is known about the coping strategies used by children from minority backgrounds to adapt to everyday stresses in school. Unfortunately, some children are labeled as learning disabled because of behaviors or coping strategies that are cultural rather than signs of impairment (Fradd & Hallman, 1983). Because of this mislabeling there may actually be an overrepresentation of students from minority backgrounds in special education.

Professionals in the school system have a major responsibility to develop an understanding, openness, and sensitivity regarding cultural differences. Whereas many strategies for including family members in the educational process are discussed in the literature, implementing them requires a commitment of time and money by school administrators (Correa, 1989).

Impact of a Learning Disability. A learning disability interferes with a child's potential for successful classroom performance. For example, organizational problems may be expressed by a disordered notebook or by a failure to structure time to complete homework assignments (Silver, 1989).

Visual–perceptual, sequencing, and motor coordination problems may interfere with the ability to follow directions in games, sports, or classroom activities. Further, auditory, perceptual, abstraction, and expressive language problems can have an adverse impact on relationships with peers and teachers. Teachers may perceive the child as not listening or as exhibiting a behavioral problem when he or she misinterprets requests and responds inappropriately. The child may experience difficulties working on projects with other children if communication problems are present. Frustrations encountered in meeting the demands of the classroom environment can evoke a variety of emotional responses and personality problems such as poor self-image, depression, somatic complaints, anger, or impulsive behavior (Silver, 1989).

Brier (1989) suggests that several factors, when linked with a learning disability, may increase the risk for delinquency in a child. Parental alcoholism, inconsistent disciplinary practices (overly lax or punitive), and a tendency by parents to be critical and demanding and to give less positive feedback all increase the risk for delinquency in learning disabled children. In the OTTP one child stated about her project, "My mother will think this is trash."

Some children who have a learning disability demonstrate problems in social perception skills and thus lack the ability to interpret and appropriately respond to vocal, facial, and body messages. A lack of social perception skills is an additional factor in shaping delinquent behavior. Brier (1989) proposes a multifactorial explanation for the heightened risk for delinquency in learning disabled children. As the number and intensity of factors such as those described above increases, so does the risk of delinquency.

Impact of Culture. On top of the typical problems encountered by children with learning disabilities during this stage of late childhood, children from minority backgrounds with disabilities are exposed to additional risk factors. For example, Trankina (1983) identified three groups of risk factors for Hispanic children. They included (1) family–social factors, (2) educational factors, and (3) health factors. Exposure to substance abuse through peer experimentation or from the influences of a substance abusing family member, a lack of parental monitoring after school, poor school performance, and poor nutrition and health care are factors that can place these children at risk for alcohol, marijuana, or tobacco abuse; depression; and low self-esteem.

According to Norton (1983), by approximately age 7 years " black children in the United States are aware of the social devaluation placed upon their racial group by the larger society regardless of the region in which they live or the socioeconomic status of their families" (pp. 181-82). Development of positive self-esteem rests with the significant others at home and in the immediate community. Norton (1983) notes that the "goal of the educational system, especially in the unique and diverse culture of the United States, is to respect the differences brought from the diverse environmental systems and build upon them toward aiding the child to operate in the larger sustaining society" (p. 191). A recognition and respect for diverse cultures is a functional component of the OTTP. A continuity of self-respect is encouraged from the home, to the classroom, and beyond.

The Impact of Transition. The *Random House Webster's College Dictionary* (Costello, 1991) defines *transition* as a "movement, passage, or change from one position, state, stage, etc., to another" (p. 1417). Life transitions are important areas to study because they pose both a threat to psychological wellbeing and an opportunity for growth and development (Barone et al., 1991). In the educational system "transition" broadly refers to the successful movement from school to the adult world of work. This is a central goal of education (Wehman et al., 1988). Successful transition to adult roles does not occur suddenly; instead, it is an outgrowth of skills, attitudes, and habits that cumulatively develop from birth to early adulthood.

Hirsch and Rapkin (1987) describe the transition from elementary school to middle school as a significant developmental event that only recently has received attention. This can be a difficult transition period for any child but particularly for a child who is identified as different. During middle to late childhood children make three transitions: (1) gradual increased independence at home, such as added family responsibilities; (2) a change from elementary school to middle school; and (3) increased independence and mobility in the community. Some children in special day classes also face two additional transitions: (4) a transition from special education to regular education, also known as mainstreaming, and (5) for newly immigrated students, a transition between their primary culture and the acquisition of the mainstream regional culture.

The OTTP has been developed to recognize the needs of children who are in special education and who are from minority backgrounds and to assist them to develop the foundation skills necessary to move from elementary school to the demands of the middle school environment. The program incorporates play as the context for the child to develop competence and achieve success in his or her interactions with people and tasks.

PLAY

As noted previously, children during the later stages of childhood refine and practice skills developed during earlier developmental stages. Middle to late childhood is a time for using these skills to develop a sense of competence with both people and tasks in a variety of environments. Most authors agree, despite differing theoretical perspectives, that play is an essential ingredient for a child's development (Mori, 1982). Play promotes children's cognitive, social, and emotional development. Equally important is that play is fun and enjoyable (Moyles, 1989). The overall goal of the OTTP described in this chapter is for children to become proficient in the use of their newly acquired skills. Developing a sense of

social and task competence takes place through participation in small group experiences—in the classroom, on the playground, and in the community—that are organized around the central activity of children: play.

What Is Play?

Many definitions and conceptualizations of play exist in the literature. Parham (1996), in a review of the play literature, outlines the classic work–play dichotomy in which work and play exist on opposing ends of a continuum. This dichotomy identifies work as productive, done for extrinsic rewards, and mandatory, whereas play is viewed as frivolous, engaged in for it's own sake, and freely chosen. Leisure, the adult version of play, is perceived as a respite from work with little value in itself. Individuals reward themselves with play or leisure when work is completed. A more useful and reality-based understanding views every day activities as possessing characteristics of both work and play. As Parham states "play may be enfolded in work and vice versa" (p. 6).

Play in School

The work–play dichotomy prevalent in the conceptualization of adult activities prevails in the preschool and elementary school curriculum. Rothlein and Brett (1987) interviewed parents of preschoolers and teachers about the value of play in the school curriculum. In general, many teachers and parents expressed the view that play had little value. Most parents were not interested in having their children play at school. More specifically parent's views were that academics should be emphasized, that play should be used as a rest from learning, and that children do not require much play time. A small percentage of parents and teachers surveyed did feel that play had value and was an essential component in the curriculum. Most teachers, however, described play and learning as distinct and separate activities. "Children were either playing or they were learning" (p. 51). Teachers responded that the parents' view of play influenced their decision to limit play in the curriculum. The authors recommended that teachers educate parents as well as other teachers as to the benefit of play for development in children. Although the field of early childhood education advocates the use of "child-initiated, child-directed, and teacher-supported play" (Hanline & Fox, 1993, p. 122) as the best teaching practice for young children, it is highly questionable whether this is reflected in practice at the kindergarten, preschool, or elementary level.

Although much is written about play in early childhood education, research and discussion of play in school beyond preschool has received little attention. As indicated above, even in early childhood education there is controversy over the value of play. Block and King (1987), in a comprehensive synthesis of literature and research on school play from kindergarten through high school, assert that a child's attitudes and behaviors about play are primarily formed through school. However, based on the studies cited in their review, they offer a pessimistic view of the place of play in schools today. They state "In educators' zeal to make schools excellent and equitable places for students to work, we have made them inhospitable places to play" (p. ix).

King (1987) reports on the findings of several studies of preschool and elementary school play (kindergarten through fifth grade). Researchers observed and interviewed 94 children from white middle-class families. Children were questioned about their perceptions of work and play at school. Throughout their early school years children in all grades viewed work and play as separate and distinct entities. What varied substantially were the criteria for classifying work and play. In kindergarten children were consistent in their perception of any teacher-directed activity as work regardless of how much they enjoyed it. Children in the fourth and fifth grades agreed consistently on only one activity, recess, as play. Classification of work and play becomes increasingly complex and individual as the child progresses through school. Thus, in kindergarten, children were more uniform in using social context or teacher direction as the criterion for classifying work from play. Children in the elementary grades relied more on psychological context or their mood on a particular day for determining whether an activity was work or play.

Types of Play

In a further analysis of the data, King (1987) identified three subcategories within the children's descriptions of play. These were instrumental, illicit, and recreational play. *Instrumental play* included activities that the teacher incorporated into the curriculum. These activities were controlled and organized by the teacher to include a playful component. Enjoyment is a primary component for instrumental play. Making a holiday mural, writing or listening to a story, and learning vocabulary or math through games were examples of instrumental play. Computer games that focus on varied curricular components are a recent addition to instrumental play. Children stated they enjoyed instrumental play for a variety of reasons. For example, they had contact with other children, it was interesting subject matter, they had a chance to be creative and express themselves, or they experienced the activity as undemanding.

According to King (1987) considerable research exists about instrumental play. Studies both support and refute the benefits of using play to learn academic material. Despite divergent research findings, several authors suggest that play be included in the elementary school curriculum more for fostering motivation and positive attitudes toward learning than for improving competency in academic areas.

Illicit play was the second category delineated from the children's responses. This included activities that children attempted to hide from the teacher such as passing notes, giggling, talking, and making faces. Researchers do not typically study these activities. When illicit play is examined the focus

is on controlling and eradicating it rather than on understanding it's role and value to a child's development. Teachers, parents, and researchers view illicit play as a problem.

Activities that occur during recess are examples of the third category, *recreational play*. All students in elementary school defined recess activities as play. These activities generally occurred outside the context of the curriculum and the classroom. Recess or playground activity is a category of play that provides opportunities for children to engage in spontaneous play without teacher direction or rules. Social skills are developed and practiced and friendships fostered during recess. Anthropologists and linguists tend to research this area of play. King (1987) cites studies that examined word play, games, and the children's culture on the playground. Whereas teachers tend to view recess as a time for children to expend energy or take a break from academic work, the value of this area of play, its meaning for children, and its importance for learning skills necessary for adult life are only beginning to be understood.

Play in Special Education

Special educators in elementary school appear less likely than teachers in regular education classes to use play as the context for teaching young children with disabilities. Special educators tend to organize the curriculum in terms of isolated cognitive, social, and motor skills with a focus on the student's problems and deficits. Play skills are subjected to a similar problem identification perspective (Bordner & Berkley, 1992; Shevin, 1987).

Shevin (1987), in a review of the special education literature, found several tacitly expressed uses of play in special education. The most valuable and widely used form of play was games to motivate students. Although this type of play is teacher directed, it can be translated into other play situations on the playground and after school. Another frequent use of play in special education is for behavior management or as a reinforcer for "good" behavior. For example, students receive tokens or points that they can cash in for play time or toys. Play is less frequently used as an activity to fill waiting time after work is completed. Special education teachers are reluctant to give students an opportunity to engage in behavior that may be nonnormative. The heavy emphasis in special education on a behavioral framework for learning is contrary to the types of behaviors and experimentation that occur during play. Therefore, in special education, teacher-directed models of instruction are paramount, e.g., use of worksheets, predrawn art activities, and drills as primary modalities. Practice and repetition are emphasized in the curriculum (Shevin, 1987).

The end result is that the uses of play in special education and regular education are very similar. Work is emphasized. Children are expected to learn to play in settings other than school, such as their neighborhood. However, for students in special education this unofficial arena for learning to play may not be readily accessible. One possible consequence is an inability to develop leisure skills in adulthood. Brooks and Elliot (1971) found that the play activities of childhood were predictive of psychological adjustment at age 30. Most predictive were the activities and satisfactions of children ages 8 to 11. Hanline and Fox (1993) challenge the field of special education to incorporate a play-based curriculum as the context for learning and maintaining specific skills. In a play-based curriculum the child with a disability learns skills using "... systematic instruction embedded in play activities" (p. 124).

THE OCCUPATIONAL THERAPY TRANSITION PROGRAM

With the passage of PL 94-142, the Education of the Handicapped Act, occupational therapy, physical therapy, and speech pathology therapy were defined as related services to help children in special education benefit from their educational experience. Over the years occupational therapists have struggled to fit into the educational setting and to identify specific practice models that are appropriate for this setting other than a disability or medical model perspective (Hall et al., 1992). The federal initiatives of the 1980s that focused on transition provided an impetus for a new model of practice for occupational therapy. In response to the high rate of unemployment and reliance on parental support experienced by students with disabilities in public education, the federal government amended the Education of the Handicapped Act to include a focus on the services needed by students in special education to make an effective transition from high school to a meaningful, independent and productive adult life (Wehman et al., 1988). During this time the government provided grant funding for demonstration and research projects. The United States Department of Education, Office of Special Education and Rehabilitation Services (OSERS), made transition a priority and developed a conceptual model for transition services (Wehman et al., 1988). The University of Southern California Department of Occupational Therapy was a leader in securing funding to implement transition programming. Innovative programs have been developed and continue to provide transition services to students as they make the transition from high school to community living (Jackson, 1978, 1990). The program described here builds on the earlier programs and is a novel extension of transition to the elementary school student.

Over a 3-year period, the University of Southern California Department of Occupational Therapy received two training grants from the U.S. Department of Education, OSERS, to train occupational therapy students (referred to as occupational therapy trainees) to develop and implement transition programming for elementary school children with severe disabilities. These grants included the establishment of an innovative, culturally sensitive transitional curriculum within mainstreamed school settings that contain predominantly minority populations. For ease of presenta-

tion the OTTP is discussed as a synthesis of the two grant-funded programs.

Areas of Service Delivery

The OTTP incorporates multiple areas of service delivery. These areas include student programming, parent education, interdisciplinary communication, and networking. Play, multiculturalism, and articulation–transition are the primary themes that shape the elementary school program and are integrated into all areas of service delivery.

Student Programming. The OTTP provides the children with foundation skills training that is necessary to make the transition from elementary to middle school and ultimately from high school to adult independent living. These foundation skills consist of the competencies needed for working with people and working on tasks. These skills have been presented earlier in this chapter in the discussion of the developmental needs of elementary age children. Success in the mastery of both people and tasks leads to a positive self-image. Through playful activities in the classroom, on the playground, and in the community that are centered around a multicultural theme, the children develop skills that are needed for success in middle school.

The students in the program are children from the third through the fifth grades who are enrolled in special education under the classification of communication handicap, learning handicap, severe emotional disturbance, or multiple handicap. The ethnic composition of the students in the program is approximately 43% Hispanic, 38% Caucasian, 13% African American, 5% Asian, and 1% Native American. Students spend 50% or more of their day in their special education classroom under the educational category of special day class.

Children in the program are generally seen in small groups from one to three times weekly for sessions lasting from 45 to 75 minutes. Some activity groups are held in the occupational therapy room, which is bordered on either side by two of the participating special education classrooms. Other sessions, led jointly by the occupational therapist and the teacher, are held in the special education classroom with individuals, small groups, or entire classes participating. Still other sessions are held on the playground, in the cafeteria, or in the community. The target goal of student programming is the transition of students to the middle school fortified with the skills and self-esteem necessary for success.

Parent Education. This component of service delivery was designed to build the partnership between the parents or caregivers and the elementary school and to educate parents or caregivers about the transition process. The parent component includes activities such as a monthly parent newsletter (Fig. 9-1), biannual parent meetings with guest speakers, Open House Night, Family Picture Day, coffee and

RAINBOW DOLPHIN NEWS

Welcome parents and friends!

We are delighted to bring you our first newsletter of the 1993-94 school year, introducing you to the *Rainbow Dolphins*. The *Rainbow Dolphins* is a program geared towards helping your son or daughter make a successful transition from elementary school to middle school. We feel this is an important time in your child's life because he/she is developing the skills necessary to be independent in middle school.

Meet our staff!
The *Rainbow Dolphins* is run by two supervising occupational therapists, Bonnie and Valerie, and four students, Danetta, Sandra, Chia, and Terry from the University of Southern California.

In order to work on skills needed to be independent in middle school, your child has been working on activities which expose him or her to customs and traditions from different cultures.

Upcoming Events!
Two field trips are planned to explore careers. We will be visiting a t-shirt manufacturing company and a fast-food restaurant.

We also have planned games and activities which help your child to

You are invited to participate in our Spring Culture Fair on March 29th at 6:00 p.m. The location is room 20. We will be sharing further information about our program at the fair and we will be pleased to meet you.

Thank you!

Bienvenidos padres y amigos!

Estamos complacidos en traerles las primeras noticias del ano escolar 1993-94, y presentarles le programa *Rainbow Dolphins*, (delfinesdel Arco Iris). El Rainbow Dolphins es un programa dirigido a ayudara su nino/a a hacer la transicionde la escuela elemental ala escuela media (sexto grado). Sentimos que esta es una etapa importante en la vida de su nino/aporque esta independiente en la escuela media.

Conozcan a las terapistas!
El *Rainbow Dolphins* esta dirigido por dos Terapistas Ocupacionales, Bonnie y Valerie, quienes supervisan cuatro estudiantes: Danetta, Sandra, Chia, y Terry de la Universidad del Sur de California.

Para poder trabajar en las habilidades necesarias para ser independiente en la escuela media, su nino/a ha estado trabajando en actividades que le presentan costumbres y tradiciones de otras culturas.

Eventos Venideros!
Hemos planeado dos salidas para conocer diversas ocupaciones. Vamos a visitar una compania que manufactura playeras y un restaurant de comida ligera (tipo McDonald).

Tenemos planeados juegos y actividades que ayuden a su nino/a a comunicarse efectivamente con otros.

Usted esta invitado a participar en nuestra Feria Primaveral de la Cultura que tomara lugar el 29 de Marzo a las 6:00 p.m., en el salon #20. Esa tarde les daremos mas informacion acerca de nuestro programa.

Gracias!

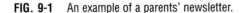

FIG. 9-1   An example of a parents' newsletter.

cookie get togethers, yearly parent conferences, home visits, a Parent Resource Manual, and parent training.

Interdisciplinary Communication. The interdisciplinary component was designed to support the special education program through sharing among special education teachers, the speech therapist, the psychologist, the adaptive physical education teacher, and the occupational therapy personnel. This strategy takes the form of joint planning and interpretation of IEP objectives and present levels of performance, sharing teaching and therapy strategies during student activities, and providing feedback regarding the effectiveness of activities. This interdisciplinary exchange contributes strongly to the ongoing development of a practical and useful curriculum.

Networking. The networking component includes identification of those services from which the students in the program may benefit. This process consists of the development of a community resource manual, developing contacts at key agencies such as the police, fire, and parks departments, and networking with transition-related service providers. Of particular importance is networking with antidrug and antigang programs, and diversity-related community agencies so as to combat potential future school failure and delinquency.

The Curriculum-Based Program

Occupational therapy in the school system is a misunderstood area of practice. Occupational therapists are typically trained to work within a medical model system of practice. This model does not adequately translate to the provision of services within the school system (Hall et al., 1992). A unique aspect of the OTTP is its organization into a curriculum with a lesson plan designed for each skill training session. A curricular framework for therapy is an alternative model of practice for occupational therapy in the school system. Box 9-1 illustrates a sample activity plan developed by the occupational therapy personnel.

Assessment. The occupational therapy trainees assessed each child's skills by using a variety of formal and informal evaluations. The trainees interviewed parents and teachers about the child's abilities and difficulties at home and in the classroom. They observed the child in the classroom and on

---

Box 9-1   SAMPLE ACTIVITY PLAN

Domain or content area: Social skills
Goal: Group cooperation
Objectives: Students will take turns, use manners (i.e., say "please," "thank you," etc.), demonstrate good sportsmanship, and engage in conversation with peers.
Time frame: Can be used for one or more sessions. *Time:* 30 to 60 minutes
Activity: Table games
Environment: Classroom, cafeteria, or outdoor picnic tables
Materials: Table games (purchased board games or homemade by students); one game for 4 to 6 students in a group.
Designer/Instructor: Bonnie Kennedy and Valerie Adams

STEPS OF ACTIVITY
1. Two small groups of students select games and set up equipment and pieces.
2. Students read directions aloud—can take turns.
3. Groups play games, learning rules.
4. Two students leave each group and join the other group.
5. Remaining students in each group teach new students how to play the game.
6. The students that left can later rejoin the original group and teach the game they have learned.

GROUP LEADER FOCUS
1. Group leader encourages using good manners, being polite to each other, sharing materials, taking turns.
2. Monitor the reading accuracy and the correct understanding of the rules.
3. Group leader may need to give verbal cues to remind students to use the communication skills they have learned in class.
4. Students may need assistance to use problem solving skills when figuring out the most effective way to teach the game to the new students in the group.

Diversity component: Use games with cultural information.
Interdisciplinary component: Teachers and speech-language pathologists consulted regarding nonverbal communication, vocabulary, language expectations, eye contact.
Postactivity review: Children learn and communicate at different rates. For example, one child completed and taught the game, whereas another child had difficulty communicating the rules of the game. Groups need to be monitored for pace and support to maintain interest and enjoyment and decrease frustration.

Note: The concept of peer instruction was drawn from: Office of Intergroup Relations (1979). *Planning for multicultural education as part of school improvement.* Sacramento, CA: California State Department of Education.

the playground using the Comprehensive Occupational Therapy Evaluation (COTE) (Brayman & Kirby, 1976) to focus their observations. The COTE distinguishes 25 behaviors that are grouped into three categories: (1) general behaviors, (2) interpersonal behaviors, and (3) task behaviors. The occupational therapy trainees rated each observed behavior on a scale from 0 (no impairment) to 4 (severe impairment). Also, the COTE was used to determine progress during the child's participation in the program. The Self-Perceived Competency Scale (Harter, 1982) provided information about what the child views as important and his or her actual competence in areas such as social, academic, and athletic performance. The child, trainee, and teacher all contribute to this assessment. Finally, the teachers completed a School Social Skills Rating Scale (S^3) (Brown et al., 1984) for each child in the program. The S^3 rating scale consists of 40 social skills that are observed in the classroom and rated by the teacher on a scale from 1 (no opportunity to observe the skill) to 6 (always uses the skill). Based on a review of the child's school record and completion of the assessments described above, the trainee and supervisor develop individual goals and objectives for each child.

Curriculum Themes. Student programming is shaped by three primary themes: play, multiculturalism, and articulation–transition to the middle school. These themes provide the framework for the activity-based curriculum focused on skill development.

Play theme. As discussed in an earlier section of this chapter, King (1987) identified three types of play based on children's descriptions of their play. They were instrumental, illicit, and recreational play. The OTTP employs instrumental and recreational play, but for different purposes from the teachers'. Teachers utilize instrumental play in the classroom to help children learn academic content. In the OTTP play is instrumental because it is used for developing skills, increasing cultural awareness, and making transitions. Likewise, time at recess and on the playground is used by the occupational therapy trainees for observing the children at play and fostering skill development, particularly social skill development.

Illicit play becomes a problem when it disrupts the group sessions. The occupational therapy trainees attempt to utilize play within a behavioral framework to manage disruptive illicit play. At the end of each group activity session the trainees give out stickers based on whether or not the student has achieved a goal that has been set at the beginning of the session. For example, one child stated that her goal was to raise her hand once in the session to ask for help, rather than yelling out her request. She accomplished her goal and therefore received stickers. The next session she stated she would raise her hand two times. The trainees and therapists attempt to shape positive behaviors rather than take away something important from the child for negative behaviors. Also, the group leaders help the children set goals that they are likely to accomplish.

The play of elementary school children differs from preschool or kindergarten play. For example, elementary school children have been described as having more obligations on their time than very young children. Also, elementary school play focuses on rule-governed games and social interaction (Knox, 1993).

In the OTTP, occupational therapy personnel guide activity sessions, providing the optimal level of challenge and structure while allowing for spontaneity and exploration. Novelty is introduced to stimulate but not overwhelm the children. Activities such as arts and crafts are fun and self-absorbing. The board games played have rules that the children learn to follow. For some games, the children assist in creating their own agreed upon set of rules.

The children develop their competence in tasks and relating to people as they play in various contexts. To be successful the play activities need to be sufficiently novel and complex, yet have enough structure, to engage the children with severe emotional disturbances and learning disabilities. Activities that are not carefully designed may set off disruptive and inappropriate behavior.

Therapists must provide the right amount of concrete visual and auditory cues during groups to encourage initiation and motivation on the part of the students at school, at recess, and on community outings. The children learn about their own strengths and limitations and define their interest areas. They are motivated to explore future careers through play. They role play adult occupations, feeling states, or troublesome situations they may soon face, such as declining a drug sale or refusing to ditch class. Through play, skills are gained to enable successful embracing of the future changes in social network, environmental complexity, body image, and daily routine associated with the middle school years.

Multicultural theme. A primary objective of the overall grant-funded training project has been to develop an awareness and understanding of diversity. This objective, a major concern of education, is applied to both the service providers (the occupational therapy students in training and the faculty) and the service receivers (the elementary students and their caregivers).

At the university level occupational therapy faculty and graduate students participated in seminars devoted to diversity issues and the curriculum. Intensive curriculum reviews focused on the inclusion of diversity issues in the classroom. Additionally, recruitment efforts in the occupational therapy department were intensified toward students from underrepresented minority groups. Those students selected for participation in the OTTP training received partial tuition remission and completed fieldwork experiences in all levels of the school system, culminating in intensive programming in the elementary school. Student service providers from similar cultural and linguistic backgrounds provided the children with positive role models. Research supports the positive effects on the therapeutic relationship when service providers are of a similar culture and language (Trankina,

1983). Anglo therapists who work with children from minority backgrounds require training related to culturally sensitive issues if effective therapeutic relationships are expected.

As discussed previously children with learning disabilities are at risk for developing a low self-image. Children with learning disabilities who are culturally and linguistically different are exposed to additional risk factors. In an effort to address these issues an appreciation for and knowledge of cultural differences was a theme that permeated the activities in the program. The focus was not limited to the cultural backgrounds of the children in the program but included a wide variety of cultural backgrounds. For example, through their participation in activities students became more aware of their own ethnic backgrounds and how these shape their choices. Cultural self-awareness also includes an awareness of self as part of a larger community, raising such questions as, "Who lives in my community?" "What ethnic and cultural groups exist in my town?" and "How does culture affect my skills and future goals?" Multiculturalism is integrated into all activities. For example, skill training sessions can focus on how various cultures celebrate holidays, the cultural origin of a variety of games, or cultural differences and similarities in cooking, clothing, and daily routines.

Articulation–transition theme. Child educators define *articulation* as the direct links developed between the students in elementary school and the middle school. The overall elementary school curriculum includes activities designed to acquaint students and teachers with the environment, structure, and activities of the middle school. Joint activities are specifically designed, whenever possible, to enable a smooth transition of fifth or sixth graders into middle school. To incorporate this theme in a relevant manner, OTTP personnel visited the middle school and made detailed lists of the behavioral settings, tasks students must complete, schedules, people, and rules of the middle school. They developed articulation activities to target these specific findings. For example, the team developed games, took photographs, planned and implemented visits to the middle school, and developed activities based on the students' visit to the school. Games, puzzles, and worksheets were developed to practice opening a combination lock, organizing papers in folders using a binder (a recommendation of the middle school teachers), and reading bell schedules and different types of clocks to prepare for changing classes.

Additional methods used to incorporate this theme involved sharing cultural activities with the middle school, creating informational career or health displays that "float" between the elementary and middle schools, inviting middle school students to speak to elementary school students about middle school, or working with them on a joint project. For example, elementary students marketed buttons from their "Badge Maker" business to clubs and organizations at the middle school.

Curriculum Activities. The program activities vary in complexity; may occur at school, on the playground, or in the community; and may span one class period, several weeks or months, or an entire semester. A sampling of activities is presented below.

A holiday boutique. Students are involved in deciding what to sell, when to hold the event, making the boutique items, pricing the items, decorating the room, advertising the boutique, holding the boutique, and spending the profits.

Middle school visit. Students plan and visit the middle school, making snacks for a class, meeting teachers and the principal, asking questions, visiting the library and cafeteria, seeing a locker, practicing a combination lock, and looking over a multiperiod notebook.

Games around the world. Students learn about games from different cultures, make their own games, play the games, and make a game poster to share with another class.

Picnic at the park. Students plan a park outing, buy snacks at the grocery store, pack a lunch, walk to the park, and play outdoor games.

Emotions game. Students play a game that requires acting out various emotions and discuss emotions they might feel as they made the transition to middle school.

International cooking activity. Students select recipes from an international cookbook for kids, determine what ingredients are needed, identify steps of the cooking process, buy the ingredients, cook, eat together, and clean up.

The Occupational Therapy Classroom Environment

The occupational therapy personnel designed the classroom environment to provide an aesthetically appealing atmosphere conducive to the development of cultural pride, responsibility, and ownership on the part of the children. The classroom was designed in bright primary colors to be pleasant and homelike with a multitable activity area, living room, and kitchen. The decor is marked by vibrant shades of blue, yellow, and green with white wicker furniture, flowered pillows and matching curtains, and a blue and white striped fabric couch and chair. A mahogany piano stands against one wall. A bulletin board was designed with pictures of famous minority leaders in politics, education, and law. The children designed another bulletin board with enlarged color pictures of themselves participating in the program. The caption reads "Be Proud Of Who You Are." At the back of the room is a triangular canvas structure holding a large green beanbag chair. This hideaway serves as a self-imposed time-out area to which students may retreat when feeling overwhelmed and disorganized. A wooden bookcase is filled with student games. An adjacent large purple chest is filled with arts and crafts supplies. A colorful framed world map is mounted on the wall. The small kitchen includes a table with

REVIEW QUESTIONS

1. Describe the general objectives and goals of an elementary to middle school occupational therapy transition program.
2. Discuss the different kinds of transitions faced by children in middle to late childhood. Consider the additional challenges posed to those who recently immigrated or have disabilities.
3. Identify cultural differences that may have an impact on the child as he or she makes the transition through elementary to middle school educational experiences.
4. Discuss the nature and functions of play for children in the elementary school environment.
5. What are the components of an elementary to middle school occupational therapy transition program?

REFERENCES

Barone, C., Aguirre-Deandreis, A. I., & Trickett, E. J. (1991). Mediators of adjustment in the normative transition to high school. *American Journal of Community Psychology, 19*(2), 207-225.

Block J. H., & King, N. R. (1987). *School play: A Source book.* New York: Garland Press.

Bordner, G. A., & Berkley, M. T. (1992). Educational play: Meeting everyone's needs in mainstreamed classrooms. *Childhood Education,* Fall, 38-40.

Brayman, S. J., & Kirby, T. (1976). Comprehensive occupational therapy evaluation. *American Journal of Occupational Therapy, 30*(2), 94-100.

Brier, N. (1989). The relationship between learning disability and delinquency: A review and reappraisal. *Journal of Learning Disability, 22,* 546-553.

Bronfenbrenner, U. (1979). *The ecology of human development.* Cambridge, MA: Harvard University Press.

Brooks, J. B., & Elliot, D. M. (1971). Prediction of psychological adjustment at age thirty from leisure time activities and satisfactions in childhood. *Human Development, 14,* 51-61.

Brown, L. J., Black, D. D., & Downs, J. C. (1984). *School social skills rating scale.* New York: Slosson.

Correa, V. I. (1989). Involving culturally diverse families in the educational process. In S. H. Fradd & M. J. Weismantel (Eds.). *Meeting the needs of culturally and linguistically different students: A handbook for educators.* TX: Pro Ed.

Costello, R. B. (1991). *Random House Webster's college dictionary.* New York: Random House.

Fradd, S., & Hallman, C. L. (1983). Implications of psychological and educational research for assessment and instruction of culturally and linguistically different students. *Learning Disability Quarterly, 6,* 468-477.

Gay, G. (1989). Ethnic minorities and educational equality. In J. A. Banks & C. A. Banks, (Eds.). *Multicultural education: Issues and perspectives.* Boston: Allyn & Bacon.

Hall, L., Robertson, W., & Turner, M. A. (1992). Clinical reasoning process for service provision in the public school. *American Journal of Occupational Therapy, 46*(10), 927-936.

Harter, S. (1982). The perceived competence scale for children. *Child Development, 53,* 87-97.

Hanline, M. F., & Fox, L. (1993). Learning within the context of play: Providing typical early childhood experiences for children with severe disabilities. *Journal of the Association for Persons with Severe Handicaps, 18,* 121-129.

Havighurst, R. J. (1972). *Developmental tasks and education* (3rd ed.). New York: David McKay.

Hirsch, B. J., & Rapkin, B. D. (1987). The transition to junior high school: A longitudinal study of self-esteem, psychological symptomatology, school life, and social support. *Child Development, 58,* 1235-1243.

Howe, F. C. (1993). The child in the elementary school. *Child Study Journal, 23*(4), 227-362.

Jackson, J. (Ed.). (1978). *Model program guidelines for occupational therapist training in delivery of high school-based transition services for students with disabilities.* Unpublished manual, University of Southern California.

Jackson, J. (1990). En route to adulthood: A high school transition program for adolescents with disabilities. *Occupational Therapy in Health Care, 6*(4), 33-45.

King, N. R. (1987). Elementary school play: Theory and research. In J. H. Block, & N. R. King (Eds.). *School play: A source book* (pp. 143-166). New York: Garland Press.

Knox, S. H. (1993). Play and leisure. In H. L. Hopkins & H. D. Smith (Eds.). *Willard and Spackman's occupational therapy* (pp. 260-268). Philadelphia: J. B. Lippincott Company.

Maier, H. (1969). *Three theories of child development.* New York: Harper & Row.

Mejia, D. (1983). The development of Mexican-American children. In G. Power (Ed.). *The psycho social development of minority group children* (pp. 77-114). New York: Brunner/Mazel.

Mori, A. (1982). Play—An elusive but important concept. *Topics in Early Childhood Special Education, 2*(3), viii.

Moyles, J. R. (1989). *Just playing? The role and status of play in early childhood education.* Philadelphia: Open University.

Myers, H., & King, L. (1983). Mental health issues in the development of the Black American child. In G. Power (Ed.). *The psycho social development of minority group children* (pp. 275-306). New York: Brunner/Mazel.

Norton, D. (1983). Black family life patterns, the development of self and cognitive development of black children. In G. Power (Ed.). *The psycho social development of minority group children* (pp. 181-193). New York: Brunner/Mazel.

Parham, D. (1996). Perspectives on play. In R. Zemke & F. Clark (Eds.). *Occupational science: The evolving discipline* (Chapter 8). Philadelphia: F. A. Davis.

Phillips, B. N. (1972). School-related aspirations of children with different socio-cultural backgrounds. *Journal of Negro Education, 41,* 48-52.

Piaget, J. (1965). *The moral judgment of the child.* New York: Free Press. (Original work published 1932.)

Rothlein, L., & Brett, A. (1987). Children's, teachers', and parents' perceptions of play. *Early Childhood Research Quarterly, 2,* 45-53.

Shevin, M. (1987). Play in special education settings. In J. H. Block & N. R. King (Eds.). *School play: A source book* (pp. 219-251). New York: Garland Press.

Silver, L. B. (1989). Psychological and family problems associated with learning disabilities: Assessment and intervention. *Journal of the American Academy of Child and Adolescent Psychiatry, 28,* 319-325.

Trankina, F. (1983). Clinical issues and techniques in working with Hispanic children and their families. In G. Powell (Ed.). *The psycho social development of minority group children* (pp. 307-329). New York: Brunner/Mazel.

Turnbull, A. P., & Turnbull, H. R. (1987). *Families, professionals, and exceptionality: A special partnership.* Columbus, OH: Merrill.

Wahab, Z. (1973, November). Barrio School: White school in a brown community. Paper presented at the Annual Convention of the American Anthropological Association, New Orleans, LA.

Wehman, P., Moon, M. D., Everson, J. M., et al., (1988). *Transition from school to work.* Baltimore: Paul Brookes.

Additional Resources

Derman-Sparks, L. (1989). *Anti-bias curriculum: Tool for empowering young children.* Washington DC: National Association for the Education of Young Children.

Fradd, S., & Hallman, C. L. (1983). Implications of psychological and educational research for assessment and instruction of culturally and linguistically different students. *Learning Disability Quarterly, 6,* 468-477.

Fradd, S. M., & Weismantel, M. J. (1989). *Meeting the needs of culturally and linguistically different students: A handbook for educators.* Austin, TX: Pro-Ed.

Kavanagh, K. H., & Kennedy, P. H. (1992). *Promoting cultural diversity: Strategies for health care professionals.* Newbury Park, CA: Sage Publications.

Kuykendall, C. (1992). *From rage to hope: Strategies for reclaiming Black & Hispanic students.* Bloomington, IN: National Education Service.

Lamport, N. K., Coffey, M. D., & Hersch, G. I. (1993). *Activity analysis handbook* (2nd ed.). New Jersey: Slack.

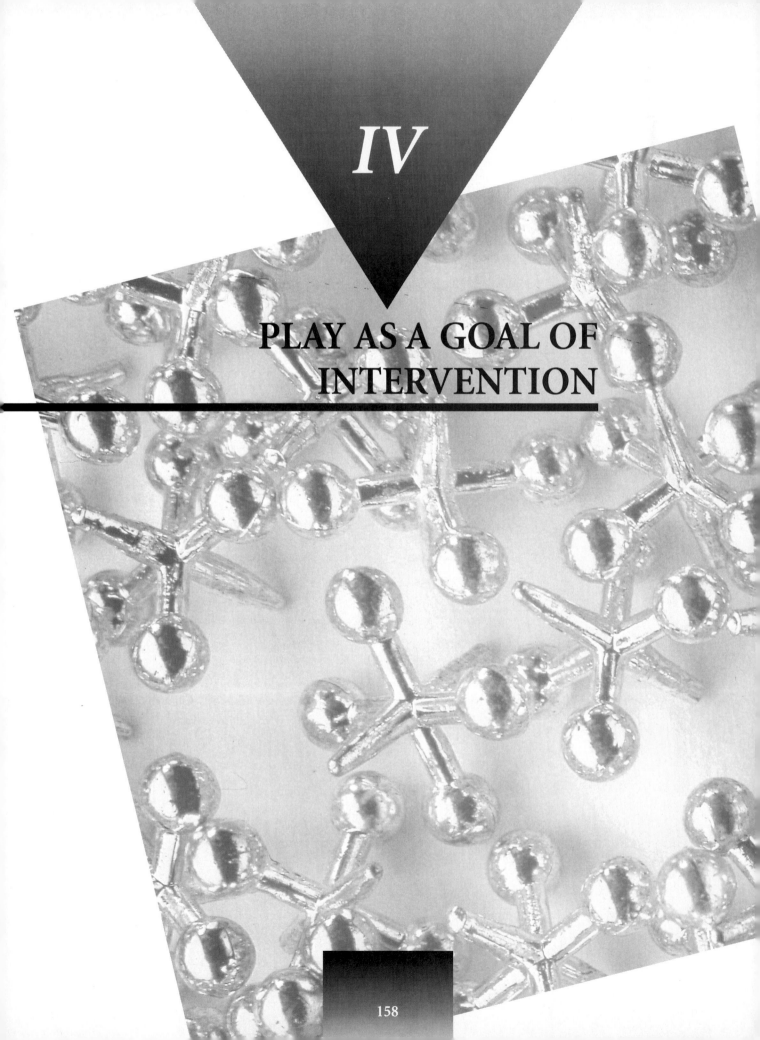

IV

PLAY AS A GOAL OF INTERVENTION

10

INTEGRATING CHILDREN WITH DISABILITIES INTO FAMILY PLAY

Jim Hinojosa and Paula Kramer

Several concerns arose in the conceptualizing and writing of this chapter. The first is that play differs greatly among individual children, whether the child has a disability or not. Play is strongly affected by the child's environment including culture, family, and setting. What is considered play by one child may seem totally inappropriate and even distasteful to another child based on his or her prior experiences and personal preferences. The second concern is defining "family" in a manner that reflects the diversity of families as they exist in society today, without overtones of discrimination or bias. Family is a complex concept that has to be defined broadly to include the many variations that occur. The third concern relates to the occupational therapist's perspective on the use of play as a therapeutic medium as opposed to play purely for the sake of pleasure. An important extension of the therapeutic intervention with the child is to guide family members toward integrating the child with disabilities into the family's play routines.

For the purposes of this chapter, play is any activity that is engaged in for its own sake. It may involve action on or with nonhuman objects or interaction with other people. Play entails a freedom of choice in the activity as well as a sense of enjoyment (Anderson et al., 1987; Missiuna & Pollack, 1992). Children play because it is fun; however, when engaged in play activities children develop life skills without even realizing it. Thus play facilitates their ability to function effectively within their environment. Children with disabilities do not always have the same access to play, and therefore their play may not have the same inner direction of children without disabilities. Children develop play skills through experience and interaction with other children. Children who have disabilities spend much of their formative time in medical and therapy environments and not in playgrounds or play groups. Additionally, physical, cognitive, or behavioral disabilities can be restrictive in play situations, and other children frequently reject or avoid those who seem different from themselves.

The primary function of the family is to provide a supportive and nurturing environment for the child's development while meeting and recognizing the needs of all family members. A family is a group of two or more individuals who provide the environment within which the child physically develops, matures, and learns. Families usually include parents and children and may include other significant people. Nuclear, extended, expanded, and single-parent households are all typical configurations of the family in current American society. Families play and devote time to leisure activities. The range of activities and the level of participation of the individual members may vary. Families and individual members operate in their own unique ways (Hinojosa & Kramer, 1993). The presence of a child with a disability within the family may have a strong influence on the family's play styles and practices.

Play is a major modality for pediatric occupational therapists. Occupational therapists traditionally use play as a therapeutic modality toward a specific goal. Therapists are highly skilled in the analysis, adaptation, and synthesis of play activities. Their focus on the therapeutic use of an activity may preclude the use of an activity for play's sake. Therapists tend to use play as a means of reaching a specific goal. However, another important role of the therapist is to provide guidance and suggestions to parents in the family's use of play both as an enhancement to therapy and as a means of strengthening their interaction with their child to provide a typical childhood experience. The latter therapeutic role—to assist family members to engage in play with the child who has a disability—is more unusual because it is a role to which therapists are less accustomed; it is the focus of this chapter.

DEFINING PLAY AS IT RELATES TO THE FAMILY

Play within the context of the family is different from typical childhood play that takes place in a playground or in school. Whether family play is organized, such as a family football game, or spontaneous, such as tickling a child during dressing, it is always influenced by the family's values, culture, and setting (Fig. 10-1, *A, B*). For example, building a doll house may be considered a play activity within one family, whereas it is considered work within another family. In reviewing theories of play, Florey (1981) concluded that there were six characteristics of play common to many theorists. These six characteristics include play as: (1) being a complex set of behavior characterized by fun and spontaneity; (2) being sensory, neuromuscular, mental, or a combination of these; (3) involving repetition of experience, exploration, experimentation, and imitation of the child's surroundings; (4) integrating the child's internal and external world; (5) allowing the child to rehearse his or her interpretation of reality and fantasy; and (6) following a sequential, developmental progression. These characteristics do not, however, take into account the context of play and how that context may influence play.

The nature of play within a family is strongly influenced by the family's collective values. If the family values activity and physical fitness, then the play may be more physically oriented. If the values are more intellectually oriented, then activities involving learning may be more prevalent (Fig. 10-2, *A, B*). Moreover, because children tend to emulate their adult role models, their family play may be geared toward

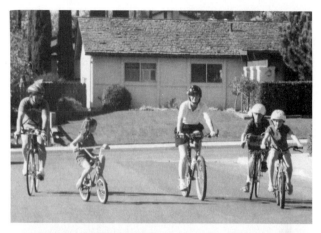

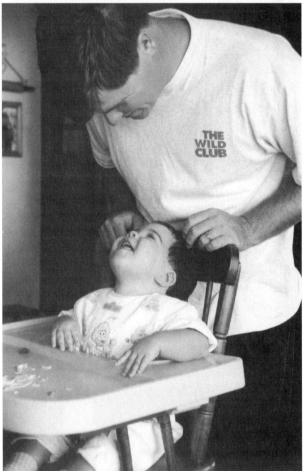

FIG. 10-1 Play in the family context **(A)** may be preplanned and organized, or **(B)** may arise spontaneously in the course of daily routines. (Courtesy Shay McAtee.)

the values and preferences of the adult participants. It is not possible to impose play on a family, because play arises out of the context of that particular family. If particular play activities are imposed from the outside, those activities may not be relevant to that family and may no longer be play. Children's concepts of what constitutes play are also influenced by their physical environments, their experiences individually and with other children, their cultures and the cultures to which they are exposed, and their ages and genders. They are also influenced by their experiences with the families of their peers; however, often the families that interact together are fairly homogeneous.

The family with a child who has a disability is a family first. Parents still have the same values and responsibilities as other parents, but they now also have increased responsibilities toward this particular child. Sometimes these increased responsibilities cause play and pleasure-oriented activities to be placed on hold or cause them to fall toward the bottom of a list of priorities. There is also a tendency for the family to become child centered. In a child-centered family, the child with special needs becomes the focus of the family and may dominate the family activities (Featherstone, 1980; Hamner & Turner, 1985). As a result of the impact on the family of the child's disabilities, the recreational needs of other family members may not be addressed. Examples of such recreational needs may be parents not taking time to go out by themselves to a movie, siblings not going to a sports event, and grandparents not taking the children out camping. Because recreation is an important need for all families, it should be a priority both on an individual level and for the family group as a whole.

For all families, developing and enjoying activities together helps encourage family cohesion. A family planning a trip to visit Grandma out of town can start with a discussion of how they will get there, what routes will they take, and also what each family member wants to do when he or she arrives. When all members of the family have an opportunity to contribute ideas for the activities and feel that their personal desires are included, they can become invested in the activity. This breeds a sense of consideration, respect, and inclusion of all members and the task then truly becomes a group project. Through

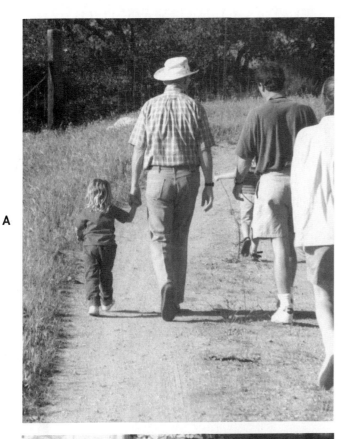

A

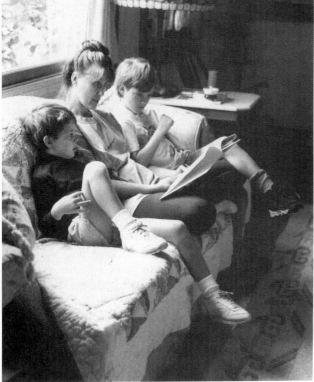

B

FIG. 10-2 The collective values of a family influence their choices of play activities. Physical and outdoor activities are prominent among families that value physical activity and fitness **(A)**, whereas literacy-oriented activities are emphasized among families that value intellectual and verbal pursuits **(B)**. (Courtesy Shay McAtee.)

CASE EXAMPLE 1: THE CASEY FAMILY

The Casey family made a tradition of Sunday dinner. They viewed this Sunday dinner as part of their family recreational time. They enjoyed having a meal together and interacting with all the children and extended family around. Everyone was able to have fun together and talk about the things that had happened to each of them during the week. The table was always set with china and crystal because the family liked this time to be special. They needed to rethink this when they realized that Billy, age 6, who had cerebral palsy, might break the china and crystal accidently because of his poor coordination when eating. The choice became whether to abandon the family tradition of Sunday dinner, modify the type of plates and glasses used, or continue in the same manner and accept the consequence of broken tableware. Their decision was to maintain the tradition by simply changing the type of dishes and glassware that everyone used. Maintaining a longstanding family tradition with the inclusion of Billy as part of that tradition became the important issue rather than the table service used. The family's time together could still be special without particular dishes and glassware. Everyone continued to enjoy Sunday dinner, with no one excluded or made to feel different. This family found a way to continue their tradition and develop family cohesion with the inclusion of Billy.

this type of process, the family matures and functions as a unit.

Although a child with a disability should not preclude the development of family cohesion, the disability may influence the types of activities that the family chooses to do. The child with a disability should be included to the extent that it is possible; however, the family needs to come to terms with the fact that activities may need to be modified.

At times, the child with a disability becomes the central focus of the family and cohesion develops around the child's needs rather than the development of the family as a group (Featherstone, 1980; Hamner & Turner, 1985). To counteract this tendency, the family's leisure activities can provide opportunities for focusing on the needs of the group rather than allowing the child's needs to take precedence.

Obviously, the degree and type of disability that the child has is going to affect his or her ability to engage in specific recreational or play activity. In other words, the disability affects the type of activities in which the child can participate and the degree to which the child can participate. The disability may also determine the satisfaction that a child receives from an activity. Congruent with this perspective, a child does not need to engage in an activity physically to enjoy it; he or she may be able to participate as a spectator (Fig. 10-3). Although it is recognized that there is the potential for the child to feel like an outsider in this type of situation, the inclusion of the child in the activity to the extent that it is possible should be the focus rather than the child's inability to participate fully. Enjoyment happens in varying degrees of participation. Sometimes simply being part of the family experience brings its own pleasure.

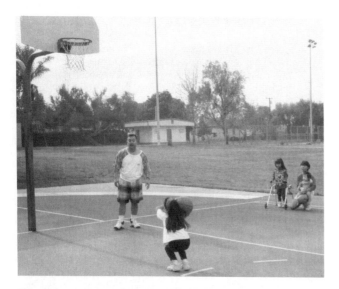

FIG. 10-3 Being a spectator is a legitimate way that a child can participate in a family play experience, even if the presence of a disability precludes physical engagement. (Courtesy Shay McAtee.)

PLAY AS A LEGITIMATE TOOL

Occupational therapists tend to use play in a singular manner as a legitimate tool for practice. As a legitimate tool, it is an acceptable medium to use during intervention to address specific performance deficits (Kramer & Hinojosa, 1993; Mosey, 1986). The performance deficits addressed fall within the domain of concern of the profession and are categorized into the performance components. These performance components are an arbitrary division of function into parts, such as sensorimotor components, cognitive integration and cognitive components, and psychosocial skills and psychological components (American Occupational Therapy Association, 1989).

In the treatment of children, play is a natural medium for facilitating the development of important skills. For example, a 3-year-old boy who lacks fine motor skills may work with a therapist on building a block tower. Whereas the child is willing to play with the blocks because this age-appropriate toy is attractive to him, the therapist is focused on the development of fine motor skills. The activity has been selected because it is age appropriate and has a therapeutic value for skill development. It attracts the child because it is fun, but that is not the primary reason that it was chosen by the therapist.

PLAY AS AN ASPECT OF THE PERFORMANCE AREA OF PLAY OR LEISURE

Occupational therapists also have the potential to view play as an aspect of the performance area of play or leisure, which is a classification of the purposeful activities that people engage in for enjoyment. Viewing play as a performance area rather than as a legitimate tool is challenging, because the therapist must now look beyond specific performance deficits that require intervention. This broader perspective compels the therapist to view play in the context of the child's life as a whole being, instead of using play more narrowly as a means to achieve change in one specific aspect of performance. Concerning the previous example of the 3-year-old child, in this broader perspective the therapist would provide the child with blocks without working on the development of fine motor skills and the expectation of building a tower. Instead, the therapist would allow the child to be self-directed in the activity. Whether the child builds a tower, hits the blocks together, handles the blocks, or throws the blocks, the blocks are being used by the child to derive pleasure and simultaneously allow the child to develop creativity and spontaneity in play.

Occupational therapists can also provide suggestions about play as an aspect of a performance area of the family. This process involves numerous stages for the therapist. The Family Observation Guide has been developed (Box 10-1) to assist therapists in obtaining pertinent information related to family play. First, the therapist needs to become familiar

Box 10-1   **FAMILY OBSERVATION GUIDE**

BECOMING FAMILIAR WITH THE FAMILY
- Who are the family members?
- What is each family member's role within the family structure?
- What are each family member's values?
- What do the members enjoy doing alone or as a family?
- How does the family's culture influence its choice of activities?
- What are the occupations of each family member and for the family as a whole?
- What are the family's resources?
- Does the family have any limitations that should be considered?
- How does the family react to the child's disabilities, impairments, or handicaps?

OBSERVING THE CHILD WITH A DISABILITY WITHIN THE FAMILY CONTEXT
- What role does that child take in the family?
- What is the child capable of doing?
- What does the child enjoy doing?
- What does the child do spontaneously, without prompting from others?
- Which family members does the child interact with and how does he or she interact with them?
- Who does the child interact with in the daily context and who does he or she seek out for interaction?
- What are the child's specific limitations in play and in activities in general?

INFORMATION ABOUT THE ENVIRONMENT OF THE FAMILY
- Where does play take place for this family?
- What objects, such as games, toys, and other materials, are available in the environment?
- Are there space limitations?
- Does the majority of family play take place within the home or outside of the home?
- Are there other environments where family play takes place that the therapist should know more about?

MATCHING THE INFORMATION ABOUT THE FAMILY AND THE CHILD WITH DISABILITIES
- Based on the activities that the family enjoys, how can the child with his or her abilities, limitations, and interests be incorporated into these activities?
- Does the child's limitations preclude involvement in any of these activities?
- If the child is unable to participate in these activities, is he or she able to observe them and still feel included as part of the family?

with the family. The therapist may reflect on such questions as, Who are the family members? What are each family member's roles within the family structure? What are each family member's values? What do they enjoy doing alone or as a family? How does the family culture influence its choice of activities? What are the occupations of each family member and of the family as a whole? What are the family's resources? Does the family have any limitations that should be considered? How does the family react to the child's disabilities, impairments, or handicaps? Because the family is the essential unit, it is the initial focus. From an occupational performance perspective, the child is not viewed as the core to which the family unit needs to adapt.

The second stage involves observing the child with a disability within the family context. Questions may include, What role does that child take in the family? What is the child capable of doing? What does the child enjoy doing? What does the child do spontaneously, without prompting from others? With which family members does the child interact and how does he or she interact with them? With whom does the child interact in the daily life context and who does he or she seek out for interaction? What are the child's specific limitations in play and in activities in general? This information provides the basis for considering how the therapist can best facilitate play as occupational performance within the family (Fig. 10-4).

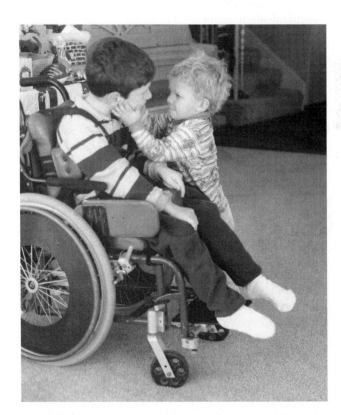

FIG. 10-4   Sibling relationships are an important consideration when evaluating a child within the family context. Such relationships may be an important resource for facilitating play within the family. (Courtesy Shay McAtee.)

Another important aspect that the therapist needs to obtain is information about the environment of this family. The third stage is answering such questions as the following: Where does play take place for this family? What objects, such as games, toys, and other materials, are available in the environment? Are there space limitations? Does the majority of family play take place within the home or outside of the home? Are there other environments where family play takes place that the therapist should know more about? This information provides the circumstances and settings where play takes place so that the therapist can obtain a full picture of play for this family within its context.

In viewing play as an area of occupational performance, all this information should be obtained as an integral part of a comprehensive assessment of a child with a disability and the child's family. This type of assessment is necessary to construct a total picture of the child and his or her family. Viewing play as an aspect of occupational performance precludes focusing only on specific areas of strengths and limitations. Information about play within the context of the family can be obtained in several ways during a comprehensive evaluation.

One way to obtain information about play is through observation of the child within the home. If the family is amenable, group discussions can be an additional means of gathering information about the ways in which a family engages in play. However, because play is typically natural, spontaneous, fun, and at times fleeting, it may be difficult to observe or to talk about.

If family members see therapists in their traditional roles of therapists, they may think and talk in terms of what is therapeutic and therefore "good" for the child with disabilities. Because of a possible tendency of the family to give what is perceived as a therapeutically acceptable answer, therapists need to give family members permission to talk about activities that are fun for each of them, activities that they like to do by themselves and with the child with a disability, and activities that the child enjoys doing alone or with each family member, without the burden of thinking of these activities in relation to whether they are therapeutic. Therapists need to convey to the family that just by being fun some activities can be beneficial to the child with disabilities and to the family as a whole.

After the information about play within the context of the family has been gathered, the next step involves matching the information about the family and the child with disabilities, so that the child can be integrated into the routine play of the family. Several questions can be asked: How can the child with his or her abilities, limitations, and interests be incorporated into the activities that the family enjoys? Do the child's limitations preclude involvement in any of these activities? If the child is unable to participate in these activities, is he or she able to observe them and still feel included as part of the family?

When occupational therapists work on guiding families to think of activities in terms of their play benefit, they need to take into consideration the family's values, needs, and resources. Attention is given to each family member's age, interests, and desires. Possible suggestions are activities that the family may enjoy doing together. Going to the beach, visiting the zoo, camping, or having a picnic are examples of activities that the family may enjoy together. Although the therapist may make activity suggestions, strategies for doing the activities need to come from the family. The suggestions need to be individualized by the family, taking into account the physical and emotional setting in which the activity is going to take place. This perspective views the child as part of the family and not as an isolated person within the family. If therapists devise the strategies instead of the family, the suggestions and strategies may become burdens on the family, and the family members may feel compelled to comply with the suggestions for therapeutic reasons instead of enjoying the natural play that has been intended (Fig. 10-5).

Although this area of performance is essential to occupational therapy, evaluation and possible intervention related

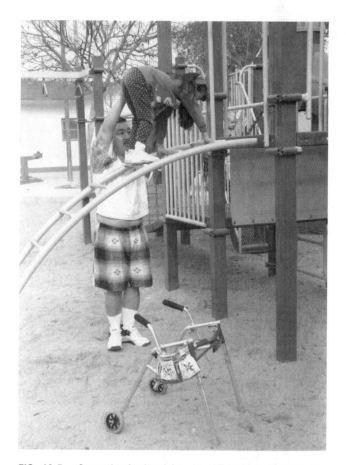

FIG. 10-5 Strategies for involving the child with a disability in a family activity, such as going to the park, should be generated by the family rather than the therapist. Otherwise, the activity may be transformed into a chore that is done solely for therapeutic reasons instead of for fun. (Courtesy Shay McAtee.)

to family play needs to be handled with skill and delicacy. Families require a balance of play wherein the interests of all parties involved are addressed. The family may view the questions and observations of the therapist as being intrusive, and if they are already actively involved in playing with their children this focus may upset their natural balance of family play. However, this line of questioning may facilitate the development of play within the family. The following

CASE EXAMPLE 2: THE JONES FAMILY

The Jones family consists of a single mother, her 15-year-old son, Tom, and her 12-year-old daughter, Valerie, with cerebral palsy, athetoid type. They live in a two-bedroom apartment in New York City. Tom is a typical adolescent boy who enjoys riding his bike and playing with other children. Valerie has significantly delayed developmental milestones.

Valerie currently attends a center-based program where she receives occupational therapy, physical therapy, and speech therapy. Progress is slow because she is wheelchair bound and dependent in all aspects of activities of daily living (ADL). Psychological testing before she entered kindergarten revealed that she appeared to be mentally retarded, but the psychologist was unable to determine a specific score because of Valerie's extensive motor impairment and limited speech. Furthermore, Valerie was found to have a significant bilateral hearing loss and was fitted with hearing aids.

Tom attends high school. He is an average student who enjoys team sports and is on the school basketball team. He is protective of his sister and, with the exception of very close friends, does not often bring friends home because he is concerned about how they may react to her. In general, he is social and outgoing.

The family is warm and loving. Mrs. Jones and Tom are actively involved in Valerie's intervention programs. Mrs. Jones is very active, attending most of Valerie's treatment sessions. She initially educated herself about Valerie's disability and was active in obtaining proper medical and therapeutic services for her. She explained Valerie's disability to Tom, who is very protective of Valerie, especially in social situations.

Until recently, family life revolved around Valerie and the various interventions that she needed. They tried to follow home programs and were involved in outings with other families who had children with disabilities. Mrs. Jones described how the home program activities often resulted in frustration for both her and Valerie when a goal was not reached or when Valerie did not want to cooperate. Gradually these sessions developed into playtime, using materials, suggested by the therapists, that could be used to have fun together. For example, while using playing cards to teach Valerie about sorting colors and shapes, Mrs. Jones tried to teach her how to play Go-Fish and War. Over time, she found that Valerie was able to understand these games and she started spending time playing the games with her rather than doing the prescribed home activities. Whereas Mrs. Jones was very attached to Valerie's therapists, she felt that the therapists generally did not understand the need for a typical home life.

Mrs. Jones described an incident during one summer when Valerie was a toddler that helped to change her perspective on her family life. It was a very hot day and she didn't have any air conditioning in her apartment. Her automatic response was to take the children to the beach, but she wondered whether this was appropriate for Valerie. Tom, who was 7 years old at this time, and his best friend really wanted to go to the beach, where Mrs. Jones knew that they would play together. Despite her hesitancy, she decided to go, planning to place Valerie on a blanket under an umbrella. Once she got to the beach she found that Valerie had other ideas. She rolled off the blanket toward the water and spontaneously began playing in the sand. Mrs. Jones talked about this as an enlightening experience, when she first realized that Valerie had the ability to adapt to her environment and had the natural capacity to find her own way to play like any other child.

Mrs. Jones recalls that she then began thinking that their family life was not typical, and she became concerned about whether the focus on Valerie was fair to Tom. After this incident, she got him involved with Little League, and outings became more family centered, rather than "Valerie centered."

case study demonstrates how a family has developed an appreciation of its own balance of play, almost by accident, without intervention.

This case example illustrates the natural process that takes place in some families. This mother followed her instincts and the needs of the whole family and she was able to integrate the child with a disability into family play activities. Mrs. Jones did not feel supported by the occupational therapist in developing family play because the therapeutic focus was on Valerie's skill development. This occupational therapist did not facilitate family play and missed the potential to address an important occupational performance area. The next section illustrates the role of a therapist in this domain, facilitating the development of family play as part of the therapeutic process.

FAMILY PLAY AS PART OF THE THERAPEUTIC PROCESS

Whereas some families naturally develop in a manner that allows them to integrate children with handicapping conditions into their play, other families may need assistance to achieve this. Occupational therapists can help families to develop their own strategies for integrating play into the life of the whole family so that the needs of all members can be met. Instead of providing direct treatment, the therapist may suggest changes in the family activity to promote enjoyment for its own sake within the family group. This type of intervention is not directly aimed at meeting specific treatment goals for the child but intended to promote play or leisure for the child and family. The interventions that occupational therapists may suggest fall into six major categories of concern: (1) the process of play, (2) the people engaging in play, (3) the environment where play takes place, (4) the materials used in play, (5) the imaginary and symbolic nature of play, and (6) the cognitive and physical aspects of play.

The Process of Play

The process of play starts with an activity that spontaneously elicits pleasurable reactions. Moreover, the process of play follows a natural sequence of play development. The play sequence begins with mutual and reciprocal interactions between infant and parent. As development proceeds, solitary play becomes important and children are able to play alone and amuse themselves. Next, children tend to become involved with parallel play, playing side by side with other children without interacting. Later, they begin to take toys from each other while playing in a parallel manner, which signifies the beginning of cooperative play, when children actually begin to play together. Older children subsequently get pleasure from formal game play, where group play involves formalized rules and patterns (Olson, 1993; Pratt, 1989).

As an example, consider a 4-year-old child with mental retardation playing with blocks by banging them together. The child is using spontaneous sensorimotor play, banging the blocks together for fun. This is solitary play, which is typical of younger children; however, children with mental retardation often engage in play behaviors typical of younger children (Hellendoorn & Hoekman, 1992). Frequently, when parents realize that such behaviors are typical of younger children, they attempt to prevent the immature play from occurring. For example, in the case of the 4-year-old child banging blocks, the parents may react by taking the blocks away, thus interrupting their child's play process. Therapists may intervene by educating the parents about the value of such play and by guiding the parents to become involved in the child's play. For example, therapists may suggest that the parents of the 4-year-old respond by encouraging the child with a smile as they imitate the banging. They may suggest that parents interact with the child using the blocks to experiment with different types of block play. In this manner, the parents are becoming involved in the play process starting from the level at which the child is functioning, in an activity that the child has initiated, to increase the child's repertoires of behavior to include social interaction and imitation. However, if the parents were to move to a level of play complexity that was beyond the child's capability, such as stacking the blocks to build a tower, the potential exists to distort the activity or interactions in such a way that it would no longer be play or fun.

The People Engaging in Play

The social dimension of play ranges from solitary activities to interacting with one or more individuals. Usually, children spontaneously interact with people around them, finding or creating play experiences wherever they are. Children with disabilities, however, are often limited in their opportunities to interact freely with other children or adults, and their lives tend to be more controlled by what they are unable to do or by what they are not expected to do because of their disabilities. Further, activities of daily living may take them longer, and they need to spend time in therapy sessions and at medical appointments. Therefore, time is often limited to interacting with adults instead of playing freely with other children. In addition to adults stimulating the child's development, children tend to develop relationships with peers who are physically similar, further placing children with handicapping conditions at a disadvantage (Short-DeGraff, 1988). This potentially limits the child's experience with children without disabilities.

Because the adults who surround children with disabilities often are concerned with stimulating the child's development, they tend to be directive in their play with the child instead of encouraging spontaneous play. Adults generally want to assist the child to reach optimal performance; this focus tends to preclude their attention to play and having fun with the child. At times, this may be the result of a therapeutic recommendation, wherein the therapist has suggested particular activities or toys to parents or caretakers and they follow through in a contrived or artificial manner, concentrating on these activities rather than interacting spontaneously with the child as they would with any child.

Imagine a 5-year-old girl, Ginny, with spina bifida, who is mobile only with a wheelchair. Although Ginny is mainstreamed in school, her opportunities to interact freely with children are limited because the wheelchair acts as a barrier to other children. Ginny is restricted in playground activities and cannot freely engage in imaginative play activities such as "playing house" or dressup games. To intervene, an occupational therapist may show Ginny ways in which she can engage in some of these activities. She may engage Ginny in pretend cooking followed by cleanup. Although this would help to serve a therapeutic goal of developing a positive self-concept, it would also serve to demonstrate that Ginny could engage in imaginative play and see herself in different roles. Additionally, the occupational therapist may suggest to the family that Ginny invite other children with whom she feels comfortable to their house for a tea party. Therapists need to be sensitive to the family's concerns about gender and cultural issues and not impose their views on the family.

The Environment Where Play Takes Place

The environment is complex because it includes both the physical and psychological contexts of the activity. The characteristics of both of these contexts equally affect play behavior. The physical environment has a strong influence on the types of activities that a person does. Children are active on a playground and sedentary in a movie theater. Children typically have experiences in many types of environments and they tend to be creative in play within those environments. A revolving door may suddenly become a time capsule or part of an obstacle course. But these spontaneous experiences in the physical environment may not be possible for some children with disabilities. Children with disabilities tend to spend most of their time at home, at school, and in the places where they receive therapy.

Occupational therapists may explore with parents the various physical environments where their child spends time, suggesting how play can be incorporated into these physical environments and how the environments may be modified. Alternative environments can also be suggested. Creative play may have to be role modeled for the child to imitate so that it can become spontaneous, because the child with a disability may have been guided into structured therapeutic activities without having the opportunity to develop a natural childhood sense of fun.

The psychological context of the child's environment is more complex and therefore more difficult for therapists to ascertain. This environment includes a broad realm of moods and feelings that surround the child and may change from person to person in his or her surroundings.

In addition to the moods and feelings that surround the child, attitudinal barriers in our society continue to be restrictive to children with disabilities. Occupational therapists need to explore the parents' attitudes about their child, particularly attitudes about the role of play for a child with a disability. They can help parents to reframe unhelpful attitudes. Once parents are aware of how attitudes may influence their child's play, they may be better able to provide alternative opportunities in which their child with disabilities can play.

The Materials Used in Play

Play materials vary depending upon the activity, environment, and resources of the family. Any person, object, or material may become part of play. Although children typically play with toys and household objects, when family play is considered, objects may not be of primary importance. They may take a back seat to the interaction or the activity. For example, infants often begin to babble to the figures in their cribs. This spontaneous play is augmented by parents who interact with the child by imitating the babbling sounds, picking up and tickling the child. The play materials in this example are the crib figures, the parent, and the bodies of the parent and child. When the child is younger, the interaction between the people involved is very important; however, as the child gets older the nature of play tends to focus more on the activity, the game, or the setting for enjoyment.

As noted earlier, other aspects of the therapeutic process include adapting the materials in the environment or providing alternative strategies for incorporating play into the family. Whereas therapists typically focus on adapting materials for the child, in family play situations the adaptations or alternate strategies need to be developed so that the family as a whole can become involved in play (see Fig. 10-6). Simple adaptations of a specific toy are not the focus, but complex strategies that take into account the players, their personalities, and the activities they enjoy. When therapists work with children with motor impairments, they frequently adapt equipment to best meet the child's physical needs from a therapeutic perspective. In play situations, the therapist may need to concentrate on removing materials that interfere

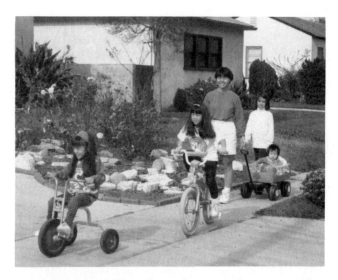

FIG. 10-6   Families may have to make accommodations in their play routines, materials, or equipment to include a child with a disability while at the same time retaining the valued family activity so that all parties can enjoy it. (Courtesy Shay McAtee.)

with play rather than attending solely to proper positioning and adaptive devices.

The Symbolic Nature of Play

Play has a symbolic nature for all people, whether or not they have disabilities. The occupational therapist needs to understand the child and the family well enough to know the meanings of play activities to them, whether they are specific to the culture, to the region, or to the individuals involved. The therapist cannot change the personal meanings of play to the participants but must work with that information. When facilitating play within the family group, the activities have to be consistent with the meaning and values of the family involved. Gender, roles, ethnicity, and related beliefs may determine appropriate activities for the family. For example, if having the whole family involved in cooking activities is not acceptable within this family, then the therapist should refrain from suggesting such an activity. In some cultures, males would not be expected to participate in most cooking activities, or girls would not participate in building or constructional tasks (see Fig. 10-7).

The Cognitive and Physical Aspects of Play

Play is widely recognized to be an enhancer of physical and cognitive development in children (Piers, 1972; Wehman & Abramson, 1976). When parents or therapists choose toys or activities, it is important that they be at an appropriate cognitive and physical level for the child so that he or she can play and gain enjoyment without feeling frustrated. Therapists usually look at the child's developmental levels in terms of cognitive and physical capa-

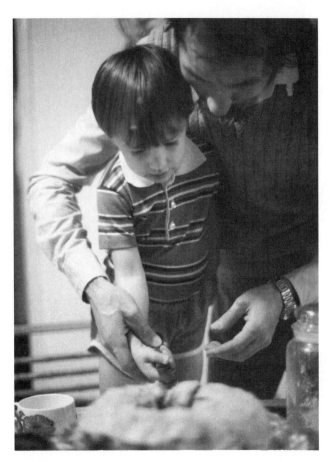

FIG. 10-7 In this family, males are involved in serving food, an activity that many children experience as play when allowed to help. This scene would not be commonplace in all cultural groups because serving food is not an acceptable activity for males in some cultures. (Courtesy Shay McAtee.)

bilities when choosing toys. This often leads to a focus on the therapeutic properties of the toy rather than focusing on the play properties of the toy. However, when the activity centers exclusively in the enhancement of learning or development, the fun aspects of play can be lost. Highlighting the therapeutic goal of the activity may interfere with the enjoyment of the activity or the play aspect of the activity (Procter, 1989).

The following example highlights the difficulties in balancing the suitability of a toy for play vis-à-vis therapeutic purposes. Daniel is an 8 year old boy with mild cerebral palsy, spastic diplegia type. He frequently engages in independent play and has told his mother that for his birthday he wants a building set. His mother was concerned about his choice of this toy because, although this might be helpful in developing his fine motor coordination, it would not necessarily enhance his social interactive skills and foster playing with other children, a goal suggested by his therapist. She finally decided to buy it for him because it was what he wanted and was something that he would enjoy.

THERAPEUTIC INTERVENTION TO FACILITATE ADAPTATION

Although some families adapt naturally, as in the case example of the Jones family, others require intervention to facilitate adaptations to develop family play. The following case example describes a family who required intervention to develop play activities that would include the whole family.

CASE EXAMPLE 3: THE WAYNE FAMILY

Andrew Wayne, a 10-year-old boy, suffered anoxia following surgery when he was an infant, resulting in brain damage. He walks independently but has cognitive and motoric delays. Andrew comes from an upper middle class background. He lives in a large house with his parents and two sisters, Janet, who is older and Carey, who is younger.

Andrew's mother has taken most of the responsibility for his medical care and treatment because his father works long hours as a partner in a law firm. Andrew went to a therapeutic nursery school program, followed by special education in private schools. Additionally, he has received occupational therapy and speech therapy, both inside and outside school. Progress has been slow, with periodic plateauing.

Currently, Andrew is independent in most tasks, including ADL with supervision, but does not have good social skills. He is still very dependent on his mother. He has very few friends. Andrew has many toys but tends to play alone in his room most of the time. When family members are playing with Andrew, they let him choose the activity and frequently let him win games. Going to the zoo with his mother is a favorite activity, and she also takes him to movies and shows that she thinks he will enjoy. His sisters join them occasionally. They are very loving toward Andrew. Janet will also take him to the playground periodically. The family tries to eat together most nights, but Mr. Wayne frequently comes home late. Sunday dinner is a time for the whole family to get together.

The Wayne family lives near the city and enjoys going to many cultural events, such as museums and the theater. Often, Andrew is not included in these outings because the family believes that he would not enjoy them.

The occupational therapist who was working with Andrew at home was concerned about his poor play and social skills. Using the Family Observation Guide, the therapist gained some insight into the family situation. Information about how the family interacted and played with Andrew gave her the basis for an appropriate intervention plan. She encouraged the family to spend more time playing with Andrew but suggested that they should be involved in choosing the activities rather than always letting Andrew control the play situation. It was a gradual process to get the family accustomed to playing with Andrew and including him without focusing on him and treating him specially. Family members were included in some intervention sessions so that the therapist could role model play with Andrew, without focusing on the skill-building aspects of intervention activities.

The therapist also suggested that Andrew be included in the family cultural activities. Although some initial resistance was apparent, the family tried taking Andrew to a museum. He enjoyed being included, although he needed some limits set on his behavior. The therapist reminded the family that all children need to learn how to behave in different situations and that in this situation Andrew was no different from other children. It was also suggested that other family members become involved in Andrew's chosen activities. Everyone could enjoy going to the zoo and the playground. The family members found that they enjoyed watching Andrew's delight in these trips and soon became involved in the activities themselves.

Facilitating these changes in the family activities took time and effort for all involved. It required them to look at their styles of play and how they functioned as a family unit. The family loved Andrew but viewed his care as part of Mrs. Wayne's role. He was treated differently from other family members because of his limitations. The Waynes had "Andrew activities" and "family activities," which they enjoyed but which often did not include Andrew. Through suggestions and gentle guidance from the occupational therapist, they were able to develop an awareness of family play and incorporate it into their lifestyle.

The intervention designed by the therapist facilitated several family adaptations. The process of play for this family included trips to the city and going to museums and plays; however, Andrew was excluded from many of these activities. In addition, Mrs. Wayne took Andrew to the playground and the zoo but did not include Janet and Carey in these trips. The only time the family consistently was together was during Sunday dinner. Based on this information, the therapist realized that she needed to suggest strategies to get the family to include Andrew in their activities. By including the whole family in the trips to the museum or plays, all of them could gain new experiences and enjoy these activities together.

The people involved in play were the whole family as well as the dyadic groups of Andrew and his mother and Andrew and Janet. The therapist reinforced the aspect that Andrew's special times with his mother and sister were an important part of his play time but suggested that it would also help Andrew to see himself as a member of the family if he were also included in family outings. Whereas all family members needed time to pursue their own activities, the exclusion of Andrew alone from some family activities was not sensitive to Andrew's needs. The therapist also guided the family to understand that each family member needs to have his or her own activities, as well as family activities, and that each family should play a role in choosing activities that are done as a family group.

The family was initially resistant to including Andrew because the family members seemed to feel that a museum environment was not suitable for him. The therapist helped them to understand that all children needed to learn how to act in different settings and that Andrew would not develop appropriate museum or theater behaviors unless he was given the opportunities or the experiences. Similarly, trips to the zoo or playground could also be viewed as family outings instead of something just for Andrew to enjoy. As the family tried new activities as a group, its members became more comfortable with each other and in trying new things with Andrew. This also resulted in a change in the parents' attitude toward trying new things with their daughters.

The materials of play were not as relevant to this family, since they had many resources and preferred family outings to games or toys. Symbolically, the therapist was sensitive to the family's culture in choosing to stay with activities in which they were already involved and that suited their upper middle class stature. Additionally, Andrew's inclusion in the family trips contributed to his developing an understanding of himself as a family member.

This family's priorities focused on the cognitive nature of the activities they did together. The therapist helped them to develop an understanding that Andrew would enjoy some aspects of these trips and that, as with any child of this age, a museum which was interactive might be more enjoyable to him and his sisters. In suggesting family outings to the playground, the therapist pointed out that all of the children would enjoy the physical activities inherent in that setting.

CONCLUSION

Play is an activity that is engaged in for the sake of pleasure. Family play is the involvement of the various members in pleasurable activities individually and in groups. The family who has a child with a disability has many priorities to deal with because of the child's special needs and may not view family play as important in their daily activities. Attention needs to be given to the essential role of play in family life.

Occupational therapists have a unique contribution to the role of play in the family of a child with a handicapping condition. Whereas play is used as a modality for intervention to facilitate the child's development of functional skills, play or leisure is also an occupational performance area. The role of the therapist in facilitating this performance area is subtle and often overlooked. This requires the therapist to have a broader perspective in viewing the child within the context of the family rather than focusing on the child in isolation.

The Family Observation Guide is suggested as a format for gaining information about the family and play preferences. This view includes the child as a member of the family and not as a focal point with more importance than any other member. Based on the information obtained, the occupational therapist can then guide the family to develop activities in terms of their play benefit to the family and within the context of the family's culture and values. The therapist's role is to introduce strategies so that the needs of all family members are met. Intervention is directly aimed not at treatment goals for the child but at the play needs of the family as a whole. There are six major categories of concern that occupational therapist address: the process of play, the people engaging in play, the environment where play takes place, the materials used in play, the imaginary and symbolic nature of play, and the cognitive and physical aspects of play. Intervention is not focused on the child's developmental issues but involves suggesting changes to promote the integration of the child with a disability into family play as activity for its own pleasurable sake.

REVIEW QUESTIONS

1. Consider how play may be viewed as an aspect of the performance area of play or leisure.
2. How is family play influenced by values, culture, and setting? Provide specific examples of each.
3. How do play and leisure activities contribute to family cohesion?
4. How may the presence of a child with a disability affect family play? When a member of the family is a child with a disability, what are the strategies a family can use to maintain a satisfying family play life? How can the therapist facilitate family adaptation using play?
5. What is a "child-centered" family? How may overfocusing on the child with a disability have a negative effect on family play?
6. What are the four domains in the Family Observation Guide? Provide examples of the kinds of questions you might ask within each domain.
7. Describe how play may be viewed as a process and how this view may be incorporated into family play.
8. Discuss how the presence of a disability may affect the social dimension of a child's play.
9. Describe how physical and psychological contexts integrate to form the environment where play takes place.

REFERENCES

American Occupational Therapy Association. (1989). *Uniform terminology or occupational therapy* (2nd ed.). Rockville, MD: AOTA.

Anderson, J., Hinojosa, J., & Strauch, C. (1987). Integrating play in clinical practice. *American Journal of Occupational Therapy, 35,* 519-528.

Featherstone, H. (1980). *A difference in the family: Life with a disabled child.* New York: Basic Books.

Florey, L. L. (1981). Studies of play: implications for growth, development and for clinical practice. *American Journal of Occupational Therapy, 35,* 519-528.

Hamner, T. J., & Turner, P. H. (1985). *Parenting in contemporary society.* Englewood Cliffs, NJ: Prentice-Hall.

Hellendoorn, J., & Hoekman, J. (1992). Imaginative play in children with mental retardation. *Mental Retardation, 30,* 255-263.

Hinojosa, J., & Kramer, P. (1993). Influence of the human context on the application of frames of reference. In P. Kramer & J. Hinojosa (Eds.). *Frames of reference for pediatric occupational therapy* (pp. 475-482). Baltimore, MD: Williams & Wilkins.

Kramer, P., & Hinojosa, J. (1993). Domain of concern of occupational therapy relevant to pediatric practice. In P. Kramer & J. Hinojosa (Eds.). *Frames of reference for pediatric occupational therapy* (pp. 9-23). Baltimore, MD: Williams & Wilkins.

Missiuna, C., & Pollack, N. (1992). Play deprivation in children with physical disabilities: the role of occupational therapy in preventing secondary disability. *American Journal of Occupational Therapy, 45,* 882-888.

Mosey, A. C. (1986). *Psychosocial components of occupational therapy.* New York: Raven Press.

Olson, L. (1993). Psychosocial frame of reference. In P. Kramer, & J. Hinojosa (Eds.). *Frames of reference for pediatric occupational therapy* (pp. 351-394). Baltimore, MD: Williams & Wilkins.

Piers, M. W. (1972). *Play and development.* New York: W. W. Norton.

Pratt, P. N. (1989). Play and recreational activities. In P. N. Pratt & A. S. Allen (Eds.). *Occupational therapy for children* (2nd ed.). St. Louis: C. V. Mosby.

Procter, S. A. (1989). Play and recreational activities. In P. N. Pratt & A. S. Allen (Eds.). *Occupational therapy for children* (2nd ed.), St. Louis: C. V. Mosby.

Short-DeGraff, M. A. (1988). *Human development for occupational and physical therapists.* Baltimore, MD: Williams & Wilkins.

Wehman, P., & Abramson, M. (1976). Three theoretical approaches to play: applications for exceptional children. *American Journal of Occupational Therapy, 30,* 551-559.

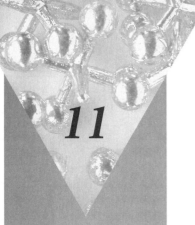

11

FOSTERING PARENT–INFANT PLAYFULNESS IN THE NEONATAL INTENSIVE CARE UNIT

Elise Holloway

The neonatal intensive care unit (NICU) is an acute care environment that focuses primarily on the medical needs rather than the social and developmental needs of its patients. The NICU staff is highly trained to care for preterm and sick full-term newborns during the most critical phases of their hospital care. In fact, neonatology and neonatal nursing have been called emergency medicine specialties because of the critical nature of the care they give (Gilkerson et al., 1990). Recent advances in the care of these immature and critically ill newborns have resulted in improved survival rates and a growing interest in their cognitive, neuromotor, and social–emotional outcomes (Als et al., 1989; Hack et al., 1991). Occupational therapy is one of many health and development disciplines to show this interest (Gorga, 1994).

This chapter addresses parent–infant play within the context of the NICU. Before this is discussed, however, an overview of relevant play theories and concepts of neonatal developmental care is reviewed. This information can then help to frame the question regarding the role of play in parent–infant relations within the neonatal intensive care environment.

APPROACHES TO PLAY

As is apparent from the various chapters in this book alone, there are many theories and perspectives regarding the purposes of play. Solnit and Cohen (1993) view play from a child-centered psychotherapeutic perspective in describing the multiple roles that play has for children: Play expresses and represents to the child and others the child's life experiences. Children may use it to learn about and cope with unhappiness, conflict, and trauma. In this view, play becomes a window into the child's cognitive and emotional functioning. Psychotherapists suggest that play can be an intermediary process between acting and thinking and between acting and emoting and so help us to understand the child's internal processes (Solnit, 1993).

The evolutionary perspective on parent–child play suggests that behavior as common as play must have an evolutionary function and that it represents a very important adaptation. Play is conceptualized as an "environment-engagement device" (MacDonald,

1993, p. 117) with the purpose of providing stimulation for the child to assist in the development of neural structures that aid the child in adapting to his or her environment. Play and neurologic development are thus viewed as being intimately connected to each other.

Cultural–ecological theories suggest that children's play varies depending on the ecological characteristics of the play setting. Whereas parent–infant play has a unique species-typical character of rhythm, tempo, synchrony, and body and eye contact, broader cultural norms, values, and beliefs define children's play contexts and the type of play activity. This type of sociocultural interaction theory recognizes that social interaction is embedded within family routines and that culture is transmitted via active participation in daily activities. There is an assumption that children have an intrinsic interest in their world and that they have the skills to participate in it. They are viewed as active and motivated participants because they have internalized species-specific and culture-specific behavior; this behavior is elaborated on by experience (Bloch & Pellegrini, 1989; Fogel et al., 1993).

It has been suggested that even though parent–child play is species and culture specific, it cannot be explained solely by genetics or infant maturation and learning. Fogel et al. (1993) suggest that "parent–child play is a creative process, emergent from the dynamics of social discourse between two different individuals in a particular cultural and physical context" (p. 45). They suggest that other theories which rely on internal schemes to account for play and interactive behavior are inadequate to account for the spontaneity, variability, and creativity that is seen within an interaction. Instead, these interactive rules may be the results of the dynamics of interaction between parent and infant. This two-person system is thought to be self-organizing and process oriented. As a result, a wide variability is seen in parent–infant play even within one cultural setting. Furthermore, a change in the dynamics of the interaction results in a change in patterns of parent–infant social play. An example of this process is provided by Tronick and Cohn's still-face paradigm (Cohn, 1993; Cohn & Tronick, 1983). During face-to-face play, mothers were asked to simulate depression with a flattened affect while continuing to look at their babies. Initially the infants attempted to sustain play, but they then reduced their smiling and gazing after just a few minutes.

Occupational therapists have various perspectives on play as well. Play, to many occupational therapists, is a tool, much in the same way that neurofacilitation techniques or adaptive equipment are tools. Play has been used as a motivator to accomplish a specific motor act or to "learn" spatial relationships, for example. It also has been used by therapists to engage the child in environmental exploration (Bundy, 1991; Burke, 1993). Although occupational therapists may emphasize the role of intrinsic motivation in play behavior, they usually tie it to the rationale of using play to support the development of skills or role behavior. It is rare that an outcome of occupational therapy treatment is play for its own sake, that is, for the process as described by Fogel rather than the outcome of skill development (Burke, 1993; Fogel et al.

1993). Play has been defined as self-initiated, self-directed, and flexible, and yet occupational therapists frequently choose to direct a child's play activity to achieve a therapist-driven goal.

Sutton-Smith (1993) warns that play has become more supervised and controlled by adult interests as it has been shown to be a means of improving academic competence. He suggests that influencing play to improve developmental outcomes can be a device to justify the socialization of one cultural group according to the standards of another group. An occupational behavior-based view of play is that if the child is successful in the player role, he or she experiences feelings associated with productivity, satisfactory quality of life, meaningfulness, and value (Burke, 1993). Although these are qualities that the dominant culture of the United States generally values, occupational therapists must be careful not to project them onto families whose own cultures may not value play and these types of outcomes (MacDonald, 1993). When therapists overgeneralize the values of the dominant culture, they themselves fall into the trap to which Sutton-Smith (1993) refers.

THE SOCIAL CONTEXT OF INFANCY

Infants develop in a social context. From the moment of birth they are involved in social interactions with adults in their environment. Infants have been shown to respond differentially to adults with slower extremity movements and more alert facial expressions than they do to objects. Some interactions meet infants' daily care needs, but other interchanges are more playful, with mutual engagement and synchronized exchanges of smiles, sounds, and gazes; enjoyment is the only purpose (Brazelton et al., 1979; Whaley, 1990). In addition, infants need adequate support from the caregiving environment to master their social, interactive, and exploratory skills. How parents engage with their newborn plays a critical role in facilitating or interfering with their infant's ability to master these skills and to experience pleasure in the process (Beeghly, 1993; Greenspan, 1990).

Beeghly (1993) describes organizational developmental psychopathology's perspective of early infant development and parent–infant play. In her view, behavioral systems such as cognition, social-communicative behavior, affect, and self-regulation are organized hierarchically and are all interrelated. In each stage of development, a child must negotiate a series of cognitive, social, and affective tasks. Accomplishing a certain developmental task helps the child adapt to the environment and readies him or her for developing competence in a more complex task. Establishing competence via play promotes later age-appropriate adaptation by integrating earlier competencies in the social, emotional, and cognitive realms into later function. This organizational perspective, when applied to parent–infant play, implies a multidimensional approach that takes into consideration the child's unique characteristics, his or her age and developmental level, the interrelationships among the various developmental realms, and the unique characteristics of the caregiving and sociocultural environment (Beeghly, 1993).

The organizational approach describes major tasks of infancy that occur in a developmental sequence that must be mastered to function adaptively. For each task infants must use their full range of social, affective, cognitive, and self-regulatory capacities, enabling their current level of behavioral competence to be observed. The major tasks for the birth to 3-month period are regulatory ones. These are to stabilize sleep–wake cycling, patterns of feeding and elimination, and state organization. If this is achieved, the infant is able to interact more consistently with the caregiver within his or her environment and begin to establish a reliable early signaling system. How well infants accomplish one task has an impact on their accomplishment of future tasks. For example, a newborn's difficulty regulating his or her state of arousal may interfere with this infant's ability to engage in a social task such as face-to-face interaction with a parent. Biologically at-risk infants may have difficulty with state organization or regulation and mastery of social-interactive and exploratory skills that are crucial for negotiating the next developmental task successfully (Als et al., 1982).

The Parents' Contribution

One significant task of parenting in the newborn period is establishing parent–infant interaction and patterns of communication. These interactions are often embedded within other aspects of parenting such as child-care activities and nurturance (Patteson & Barnard, 1990). Newborns are viewed as active participants in any interchange, social organisms that are innately predisposed to interact with their environment. These interactions have been noted to be bidirectional, i.e., involving communication from parent to infant and from infant to parent (Gianino & Tronick, 1988). Because of both external and internal feedback processes, this interchange cannot be predicted solely by a linear model but must include the dynamic process between parent and child (Nugent & Brazelton, 1989; Nugent et al., 1993). The infant's development takes place in a particular cultural context or niche: his or her family. The family structure provides the social resources to help organize the infant's niche so as to provide nurturance and stimulation to engage in this parent–infant dance of interaction (Nugent et al., 1993).

Parents attribute intention and motives to infants. Frequently, infants are viewed as individuals with subjective experiences, social awareness, and a sense of self from birth (Brazelton & Cramer, 1990). Meanings that parents attribute to their infant's behavior may arise from the parents' personal histories and memories as well as from their infant's unique characteristics. This provides parents with a set of internal rules for interpreting their infant's behaviors. Parental perceptions of their newborn's interactive behaviors guide their interactions with the baby (Brazelton & Cramer, 1990; Cardone & Gilkerson, 1990; 1992).

Cross-cultural research has shown significant variability in parent–infant interaction patterns, with the range and form of adaptations shaped by both the demands of culture and the dynamics occurring between parent and infant. Patterns of feeding, diapering, swaddling, holding, touching, and looking are all mediated by these processes. So it is important, then, to focus not on the "*what* of behavior but the *how* of behavioral responsivity" (Nugent & Brazelton, 1989, p. 94) of both partners in understanding early parent–infant play.

It is during the newborn period that both parents and infant are in a state of heightened readiness for exploratory interaction to assist in reorganizing the family niche (Nugent & Brazelton, 1989). In addition to the cultural context, the infant's social responsivity and communication cues may determine the amount of caregiving that he or she elicits from parents. Research has shown that a certain degree of unpredictability or variability in the infant's state behavior may elicit more parental caregiving involvement (Nugent et al., 1993).

This variability in infant behavior, parent attributes, and varying cultural values about the nature of infant care and development necessitates a "nonprescriptive stance" (Nugent & Brazelton, 1989, p. 93) when engaging with parents and newborns. This nonprescriptive stance is one that sensitizes parents to their infant's unique adaptive abilities and communication cues without adding a label or value to those capacities. In this way, the therapist may initiate a positive cycle of mutually rewarding interactions, essentially defined by the parent–infant dyad itself, which may result in positive long-term influences on parent–infant relations (Brazelton & Cramer, 1990; Nugent & Brazelton, 1989; Patteson & Barnard, 1990).

This approach is an important consideration when working with high-risk populations, such as infants who are biologically at risk. However, definitions of risk are cultural constructions, so what constitutes risk status in one setting, for example the hospital, may not in another, such as the community (Nugent et al., 1993). Thus it is even more important that the therapist integrate this "nonprescriptive stance" into her or his work with infants and families in the NICU. This strategy is discussed further in the following sections.

DEVELOPMENTAL CARE IN THE NICU

With the advent of specialized neonatal intensive care units in the late 1960s and early 1970s, survival rates of preterm and critically ill newborns improved significantly. Research emphasis in the new field of neonatology began to shift from mortality to neurodevelopmental morbidity. Outcome studies indicated that many infants had cognitive and neuromotor deficits (Gottfried & Gaiter, 1985). During this time, researchers in development postulated that the isolating and sensorially depriving hospital environment contributed to these poor outcomes. Accordingly, intervention studies that offered packages of sensory stimulation, most frequently tactile, vestibular and kinesthetic–proprioceptive, were initiated (Gregg et al., 1976; Leib et al., 1980; Powell, 1974; Rice,

1977; Scarr-Salapatek & Williams, 1973; Solkoff & Matuszak, 1975; Solkoff et al., 1969; White & LaBarba, 1976). Although almost all of these studies reported positive outcomes in terms of improved weight gain, feeding abilities, state regulation, motor development, and visual attention, there were clear methodologic problems that limited their applicability.

These intervention programs varied in timing, type, and intensity of stimulation. Some were applied to infants of one gestational age, whereas others were used with infants of varying ages. In general, these studies did not report baseline environmental conditions before, during, or after their intervention, complicating even further the analysis of the effects of these supplemental stimulation programs (Cornell & Gottfried, 1976). Another significant limitation was the lack of understanding of the preterm infant's central nervous system (CNS) organization; there was little knowledge about CNS regulation of heart rate, respiration, or arousal (Gilkerson et al., 1990). In addition, these studies were carried out with a relatively low-risk, stable infant population. Today's NICU sees a much more fragile, gestationally immature infant, whose nervous system is more vulnerable to environmental demands and who may indeed be compromised physiologically by caregiving activities that are appropriate for robust full-term infants and even more stable preterm infants (American Occupational Therapy Association, 1993; Gilkerson et al., 1990).

When the NICU sensory environment was examined in research, it was not found to be consistently sensorially depriving. In fact, at times it was noted to be overwhelming to some infants. In general, stimulation levels did not appear to match the states of arousal or behavioral readiness of the infants and appeared to affect them physiologically. For example, ambient noise levels often were quite high and correlated with decreases in infant blood oxygen levels and increases in intracranial pressure (Bess et al., 1979; Long et al., 1980a; Speidel, 1978). Routine caregiving procedures that were standard for all infants were also found to result in physiologic changes (Long et al., 1980b). Little diurnal variation in activity or lighting levels was noted; the nursery's schedule was based on caregiver needs rather than infant needs. Handling or talking usually was not related to the infant's state of arousal. Infants showed both immediate and delayed, subtle and gross signs of distress related to caregiving and other environmental events (Gaiter, 1985; Gottfried et al., 1981; Linn et al., 1985; Newman, 1981).

The recent trend in NICU developmental intervention research is directed toward understanding the immature and sick infant's neuroregulatory abilities and then letting this guide developmentally supportive interventions. This trend first began with the characterization of the healthy full-term newborn as competent, capable of responding to the environment, and able to elicit responsive behaviors from the caretaker to receive the kind of interaction and caregiving it needs (Nugent & Brazelton, 1989). The infant was viewed as effectively communicating via behavioral cues to indicate his or her readiness for stimulation, stress, and need for rest.

With this perspective in mind, researchers such as Als, Gorski, and Barnard began to describe behaviors of sick and immature newborns in attempts to understand these infants' thresholds of stress and stability and to then design supportive intervention programs in which the infant's behavior guided the caregivers' actions. This approach recognizes and treats infants as individuals and consequently individualizes each infant's intervention program (Als, 1986; Barnard & Bee, 1984; Gorski et al., 1990).

The work of Als and her associates is one example of this intervention trend. Als conceptualized a model termed the Synactive Theory of Newborn Neurobehavioral Organization. This model describes the newborn's emerging behavioral organization and how development proceeds via a continuous balancing of infant–environment interactions and the continuous interplay between five neurobehavioral subsystems within the infant (Als, 1983, 1986; Als et al., 1982, 1986, 1989). These five subsystems are:

1. *Autonomic system:* The newborn's primary task is to stabilize and integrate autonomic functions such as heart rate, respiration, thermoregulation, and digestion.
2. *Motor system:* The newborn demonstrates varying degrees of postural adjustments and modulation of muscle tone.
3. *State organizational system:* The newborn demonstrates differentiation of states of arousal with emerging sleep, wake, and crying states; distinctness versus diffuseness of states and patterns of state transition are observed.
4. *Attention–interaction system:* The infant shows ability to modulate arousal and attention to interact with and elicit input from the world.
5. *Regulatory system:* The infant demonstrates ability to maintain or regain a stable, well-modulated subsystem balance. This includes the facilitation that the infant requires from his or her environment to achieve and sustain this balance.

Each of these subsystems matures sequentially, and all are interdependent. Autonomic system instability can be observed in changes in respiratory patterns, skin color, and various visceral signs. Motoric organization is seen via muscle tone, posture, and movement. The range of availability of the infant's states of arousal and transitions between states, i.e., sleep to drowsy to alert, influences both motoric stability and the infant's attentional–interactional system. Once able to achieve and maintain an alert state, the infant's interactive responses demonstrate his or her ability to orient and attend to visual and auditory stimuli without becoming fatigued. In the healthy, term newborn, these subsystems function smoothly and in synchrony via the regulatory system. The less mature or ill newborn shows a less organized interplay of subsystems, with lower thresholds for stimulation and relatively fewer self-regulatory abilities. Therefore, routine caregiving and interactive demands can be stressful and cause physiologic instability in the infant.

This work examining neuroregulatory abilities emphasizes the individualized caregiving needs of preterm and sick newborns. Infant readiness for environmental demands and ability to cope with the potential mismatch between infant capabilities and the environment continues to be at the heart of developmental intervention research. This model is one that "focuses on the way individual infants handle the experience of the world around them rather than on skills" (Als et al., 1989, p. 6).

Gilkerson et al. (1990) appropriately remind us that there is still a very limited understanding of these infant regulatory functions. They question whether intervention efforts should be focused on changing or shaping behaviors that are not well understood. For example, they ask whether it is appropriate at any given point in an infant's neuromaturation to attempt to change the amount of time that an infant is in awake states, possibly at the expense of other states; they suggest that there may be as yet unknown consequences of losing time in other arousal states that "might serve some less obvious but equally vital purpose during a particular stage of maturation" (Gilkerson et al., 1990, p. 460). This perspective regarding the current limited knowledge of newborn infant neuroregulatory abilities, along with the better understood organ system fragility of these infants, must underlie any discussion of occupational therapy intervention in the NICU.

Parental Experience in the NICU

Parents' assumptions about themselves, the world, and how their family is going to function can be violated by having a preterm or critically ill newborn hospitalized in the NICU (Affleck & Tennen, 1991). This experience can pose a significant threat to the parents' psychological well-being; emotional distress is common. Throughout the infant's hospitalization, parents show a range of emotional reactions in a "rollercoaster ride" (Hughes & McCollum, 1993, p. 57) that follows the ups and downs of their infant's hospital course. Emotional stressors reported by parents include separation from the infant, concern regarding the infant's health, disruption in family routines, not feeling like a parent, ambivalence regarding their emotional investment in the infant, and anxiety concerning the infant's future development (Hughes & McCollum, 1993; McGrath & Myer, 1992). Coping strategies are linked to each individual's perception of personal stressors. To cope, parents report that they have sought out social support, information regarding their child's problem, a meaning to the whole perinatal–neonatal experience, and escape (Able-Boone & Stevens, 1994; Affleck & Tennen, 1991; Affleck et al., 1990; Hughes et al., 1994). Parental coping efforts could influence the nature of their current and future interactions with their infant and must be considered when attempting to foster a mutual interchange between parent and infant.

PLAYFULNESS IN THE NICU

As mentioned earlier, infants develop in a social context. They are born adapted to their family niche. They have innate abilities to organize their physiologic, motoric, state,

and interactional systems to elicit caregiving and nurturance from their parents. Parents, for their part, bring their own contributions to the dynamic interchange that forms the basis of parent–infant play. Their values, beliefs, and memories assist them in reading and interpreting their infant's communications. This process supports the infant in achieving an early primary task: feeling calm and alert and ready to develop a consistent, refined signaling system by which to engage with the parent.

Infants in the NICU are not necessarily adapted to extrauterine life and its demands because of either immaturity or illness. They may be inconsistently able to organize smooth functioning of their neurobehavioral subsystems. Their efforts to do so, especially in the face of the environment's social and physical demands, may be physiologically destabilizing, causing apnea, bradycardia, and hypoxia. As preterm infants mature, they begin to achieve a balance in these subsystems. However, any extra demand can threaten that fragile balance.

The fragility of the hospitalized infant creates stress for parents. Additionally, the NICU experience imposes stress on parents as they attempt to establish a relationship with their infant. When a parent enters the NICU, she or he sees a high-tech, unfamiliar environment with monitors and equipment evident visually and auditorally. Even the location of the infant in that environment may not be obvious, at first (Fig. 11-1). The sense of being overwhelmed may

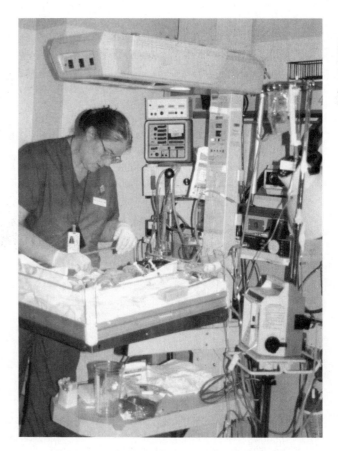

FIG. 11-1 The overwhelming NICU environment.

grow as the parent draws near to the infant's bed and sees his or her baby (Fig. 11-2). Parents have reported that it can take weeks or even months, watching their infant grow and recover, before they are comfortable touching or holding their infant (Holloway, 1994). With this in mind, occupational therapists must seek to determine at what point a parent may feel comfortable and relaxed enough to feel playful.

Als et al. (1982) suggest that preterm and sick infants communicate their needs via their behaviors. They can be overstimulated easily but may be able to indicate this, as well as their readiness for interaction, to their caregivers. These behavioral cues become more evident as the infant grows and matures, as he or she becomes more physiologically stable. The infant in this process is working on the first major developmental task of infancy, according to the organizational perspective. However, the developing signaling system may be inconsistent or difficult to read at first. If a young infant is struggling to establish his or her neurobehavioral balance within the environment and has just begun signaling, the infant is not yet ready to engage in play. The nature of play and the attributes and skills needed by both partners for a successful, playful interchange suggest that often preterm or acutely ill infants and often their parents are not ready for play during most of their hospitalization.

Occupational therapists practicing in the NICU can support the precursors of play by assisting parents in reading their infant's communication signals, in assigning their own meaning to these signals, and in feeling comfortable with the actions that they do and don't take with their baby. Infant signals can be subtle or very obvious to a parent. For example, an infant who is overaroused (Fig. 11-3) is as unavailable for a positive interchange at that moment as one who is underaroused (Fig. 11-4). Likewise, an infant who is grimacing, splaying her or his fingers or yawning may be saying that she

or he needs a break in the interaction (Fig. 11-5, *A* and *B*). Parents may learn that just sitting quietly, looking at their infant or possibly touching her or him may be providing just the right amount of sensory information to match their infant's arousal threshold (Fig. 11-6, *A* and *B*).

Occupational therapists may support parents in learning alternative ways of engaging with their infant. The father in Fig. 11-7 discovered early on that his daughter loved to suck on his little finger and he expressed great pleasure in this. Amanda's act of sucking on his finger symbolized to him her acceptance and responsiveness to him. This became the basis for their growing signaling and engagement system. The positive meaning that he attached to his infant's sucking encouraged him to try to engage with her in other ways and at other times, such as during dressing (Fig. 11-8, *A*). Figure 11-8, *B*, shows another instance of parent–infant engagement occurring spontaneously within the context of a daily care activity, bathtime. These moments cannot be taught via parent education but can be facilitated and supported by the occupational therapist as she or he seeks to understand what is meaningful to a parent and how that may relate to the infant's neurobehavioral capacities.

These parent–infant interchanges, which become more active and frequent as the infant becomes more medically stable, mature, and closer to going home, can help to establish the beginning of playfulness between parent and infant. As the parent learns to read the infant's rhythms and subsequently adapts his or her behavioral tempo, and as the infant matures in self-regulation, their mutually positive experience is prolonged. By focusing on the "how" of parent–infant responses and engagement, the occupational therapist can help to create an emotional space for a creative, playful process to emerge from the growing dynamic between parent and infant as they go home together.

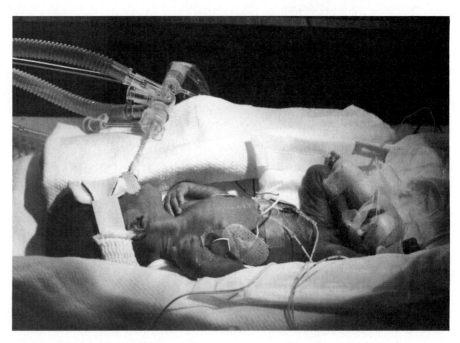

FIG. 11-2 Initially, the fragile infant struggles with physiologic stability.

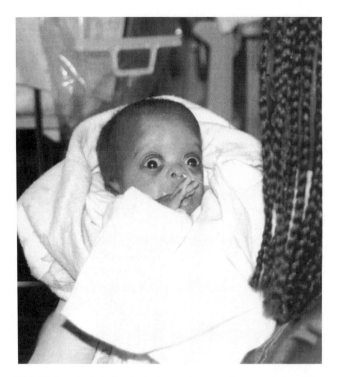

FIG. 11-3   An infant who is hyperalert may be overwhelmed by social interaction.

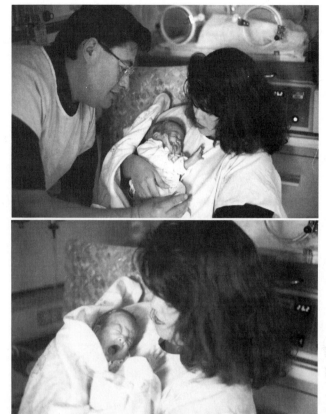

FIG. 11-5   **A** and **B,** Parents may adjust their interaction styles based on infant communication signals. (Courtesy Shay McAtee.)

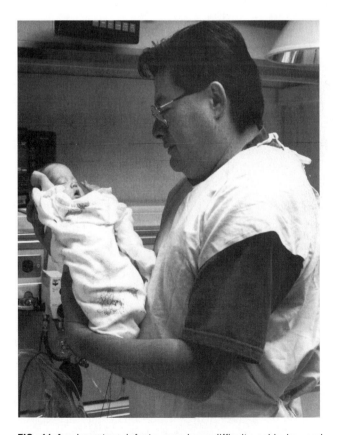

FIG. 11-4   Immature infants may have difficulty achieving and maintaining an alert state. (Courtesy Shay McAtee.)

Some infants hospitalized in the NICU develop chronic health conditions that necessitate more prolonged hospitalization (Gottfried & Gaiter, 1985). Frequently, there continues to be a mismatch between the infant's neurobehavioral capabilities and the environment's demands. Whether it is based on the evolutionary perspective, that the infant uses play to engage the environment so as to get the stimulation necessary for neural structure development, or upon Fogel's contention that play is important for its own sake, the occupational therapist's challenge becomes threefold: facilitating the infant's ongoing development, learning the meaning of play for the parent, and adapting the environment to encourage both infant and parent readiness so as to provide opportunities for play.

First, the occupational therapist must return not only to examining the infant's developmental skills, for example, reaching for a toy, but also to the "how" of accomplishing those skills. How does the infant process the environment's sensory input? How and in what way does he or she engage? Does the infant behave differently when he or she is having difficulty with feedings or when having respiratory distress? In other words, understanding all of the infant's interrelated physiologic, sensory, neuromotor, and social–emotional processes provides the foundation for developing therapy

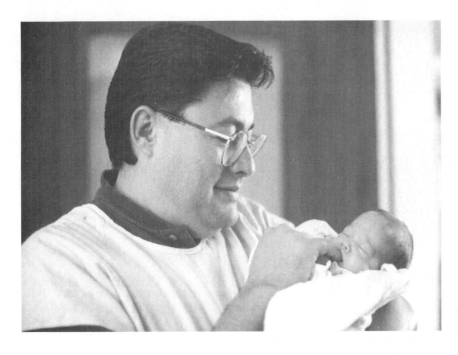

FIG. 11-6 **A,** Quietly looking at each other can be a mutually rewarding interchange. **B,** At other times, the infant may be able to respond to her parents' voices. (Courtesy Shay McAtee.)

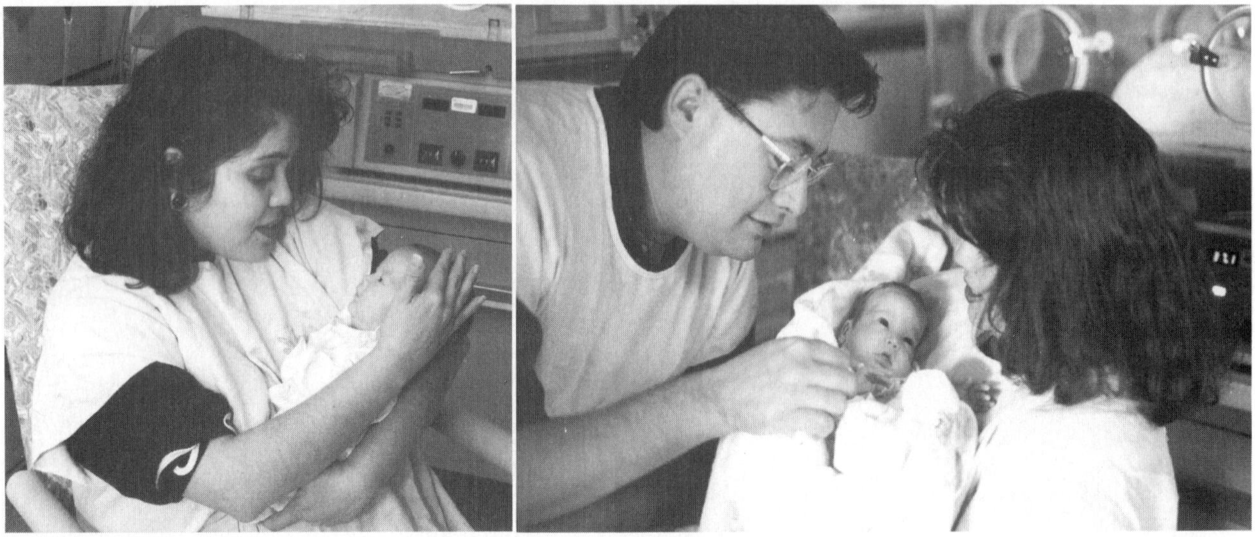

FIG. 11-7 Touch can be as meaningful as looking and listening. (Courtesy Shay McAtee.)

interventions that promote play. This understanding comes about from direct interaction with the infant, in addition to observing him during nursing care procedures and parent interactions.

In some instances, one-to-one therapy with the infant may be appropriate, focusing on strengthening, for example. One reason for strengthening may be to improve head control in supported sit. However, another may be to promote postures that support the infant's engagement with the therapist. The goal of strengthening activities may be to enable the infant to hold his or her head up during playtime with the mother. Alternatively, direct intervention may seek to assist the infant to remain available for interaction in the face

of environmental demands or to answer how the infant indicates his or her needs and what events interfere with his or her signaling efforts.

Since parents and infants work toward a dance of give and take in interaction and play (Nugent et al., 1993), therapy time can be devoted to facilitating the infant's ability to participate in two-way communication and in stringing several behaviors together. The occupational therapist can plan to wait and watch for infant responses and then act in a manner that is contingent upon the infant's behavior to facilitate his or her portion of the "dance." Additionally, the therapist needs to be able to tap into her or his own sense of playfulness and express that to the infant in a

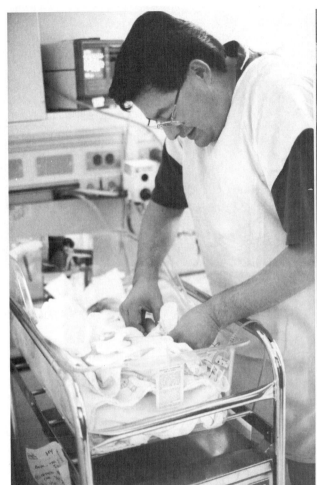

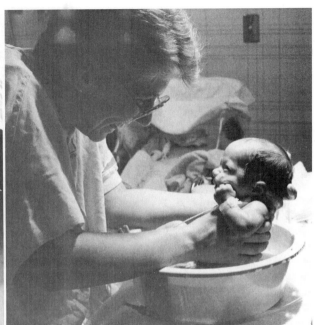

FIG. 11-8   **A** and **B**, Parent–infant engagement occurs within the context of daily care activities. (**A**, Courtesy Shay McAtee.)

well-modulated way, matching the infant's own tempo and rhythms, to elicit the infant's playfulness.

Environmental adaptations are not only physical in nature (e.g., turning down bright hospital lights) but are also social. As play often occurs within the context of daily activities, the older chronically ill infant may benefit from having a daily schedule with built-in routines. Consistency of caregivers and caregiving approaches promotes the infant's sense of predictability and assists the caregiver in getting to know the infant. This may allow the infant's subtle or fleeting efforts at signaling to emerge and to be responded to appropriately. Daily routines and schedules can be arranged so that an infant is "ready" for his or her parents, if possible. In this way, the infant may be at his or her rested and responsive best for play with dad, even if it is at 10:00 pm when the father gets off of work.

With the understanding that each individual family's cultural norms, values, and beliefs define for it where one plays and how one plays, the therapist must seek to learn the parents' view of playfulness and play. The only assumption regarding this definition that the therapist may safely make is that very few parents idealize the NICU as a play environment! Information to be elicited from parents includes: What needs to happen for the parent to feel comfortable in the NICU? How would the parent like to act with his or her baby if no one were around? Does the parent wish for one-on-one time or for the whole family to be together? If there were no rules, where would the parent like to be with his or her baby: in a chair, in bed, on the floor? When does the parent feel most at ease in the NICU? Is the parent a morning or night person? How does the parent characterize his or her current coping? Does the parent feel like playing?

This type of information can assist the occupational therapist in facilitating a play dynamic between parent and infant. Together therapist and parent can discover the types of activities and infant responses that have meaning to them, that may be perceived as fun or playful. Although sharing what has worked between the therapist and the infant during their therapy sessions may be helpful, the goal is to encourage the parents' vision of play and nurturing, to take that nonprescriptive stance (Nugent & Brazelton, 1989). Play may mean smiling face to face (Fig. 11-9, *A*), feeling the baby holding onto one's shoulder as one "dances" (Fig. 11-9, *B*), or something that baby, mother, and father do together (Fig. 11-9, *C*).

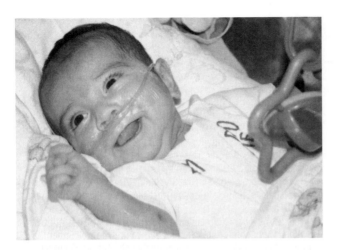

FIG. 11-10 Regardless of posture, a playful interchange can take place.

The therapist adapts the environment and play activities to account for the infant's medical fragility and the parents' definition of play. Using Nugent's "nonprescriptive stance," therapist, infant, and parent elaborate upon their current successful engagement and other early play experiences. At these times, the infant's posture may not be optimal, the hand splints may need to be foregone temporarily, or the opportunity to teach a therapy technique may be postponed (Fig. 11-10). Knowledge of each infant's physiology and neurobehavioral maturation along with an understanding of parents' dreams, fears, and beliefs about play is necessary for the therapist to support the creative, dynamic process that most often occurs spontaneously for other families.

REVIEW QUESTIONS

1. Consider the relevant play theories discussed by the author. Describe how these relate to the infant in the NICU.
2. Describe the social context of the infant. How does the environment of the NICU alter this social context?
3. How does the infant's stay in the NICU alter the development of parent–infant communication and play?
4. What are neuroregulatory abilities, and how do they influence parent–infant interactions, including play?

5. The presence of a preterm or critically ill newborn hospitalized in the NICU can have tremendous impact on the parents. Describe parental experiences in the NICU and indicate how occupational therapy can intervene to enhance parental coping.
6. Describe some of the ways occupational therapists practicing in the NICU may assist parents in supporting the precursors of play.

REFERENCES

Able-Boone, H., & Stevens, E. (1994). After the intensive care nursery experience: Families' perceptions of their well-being. *Children's Health Care, 23*(2), 99-114.

Affleck, G., & Tennen, H. (1991). The effect of newborn intensive care on parents' psychological well-being. *Children's Health Care, 20*(1), 6-14.

Affleck, G., Tennen, H., & Rowe J. (1990). Mothers, fathers and the crisis of newborn intensive care. *Infant Mental Health Journal, 11*(1), 12-25.

Als, H. (1983). Infant individuality: Assessing patterns of very early development. In J. Call, E. Galenson, & R. Tyson (Eds.). *Frontiers of infant psychiatry* (pp. 363-378). New York: Basic Books.

Als, H. (1986). A synactive model of neonatal behavioral organization: Framework for the assessment of neurobehavioral development in the premature infant and for the support of infants and parents in the neonatal intensive care environment. *Physical and Occupational Therapy in Pediatrics, 6*(3/4), 3-53.

Als, H., Duffy, F. H., McAnulty, G. B., and Badian, N. (1989). Continuity of neurobehavioral functioning in pre-term and full-term newborns. In M. H. Bornstein & N. A. Krasnegor (Eds.). *Stability and continuity in mental development: Behavioral and biological perspectives* (pp. 3-28). Hillsdale, NJ: LEA Publishers.

Als, H., Lawhon, G., Brown, E., Jibes, R., Duffy, F. H., McAnulty, G., and Blickman, J. G. (1986). Individualized behavioral and environmental care for the very low birth weight pre-term infant at risk for bronchopulmonary dysplasia: NICU and developmental outcome. *Pediatrics, 78*, 1123-132.

Als, H., Lester, B. M., Tronick, E. Z., and Brazelton, T. B. (1982). Assessment of pre-term infant behavior (APIB). In H.E. Fitzgerald & M. Yogman (Eds.). *Theory and research in behavioral pediatrics* (pp. 64-133). New York: Plenum Press.

American Occupational Therapy Association (1993). Knowledge and skills for occupational therapy practice in the neonatal intensive care unit. *American Journal of Occupational Therapy, 47*(12), 1100-1105.

Barnard, K. E., & Bee, H. L. (1984). The assessment of parent–infant interaction by observation of feeding and teaching. In T.B. Brazelton & B. Lester (Eds.). *New approaches to developmental screening in infants.* New York: Elsevier.

Beeghly, M. (1993). Parent–infant play as a window on infant competence: An organizational approach to assessment. In K. MacDonald (Ed.). *Parent-child play: Descriptions and implications* (pp. 71-111). New York: State University of New York Press.

Bess, F. H., Peck, B. F., & Chapman, J. J. (1979). Further observations on noise levels in infant incubators. *Pediatrics, 63*(1), 100-106.

Bloch, M. N., & Pellegrini, A. (1989). Introduction. In M. N. Bloch and A. Pellegrini (Eds.). *The ecological context of children's play.* (pp. 1-5). Norwood, NJ: Ablex Publishing.

Brazelton, T. B. & Cramer, B. G. (1990). *The earliest relationship.* Reading, MA: Addison-Wesley.

Brazelton, T. B., Koslowski, B., & Main, M. (1979). The origins of reciprocity: The early infant-mother interaction. In M. Lewis & L. A. Rosenblum

The purpo...
apists and ot...
they struggle...
gin with a b...
mental and...
drug exposu...
the remainde...
strategies. So...
garding inter...
natal drug ex...
with prenatal...
by case exam...
program. Fin...
deemed succe...
gram are deli...

EFFECTS...
DRUG E...

Does in utero...
caine, amphe...
long-term lea...
ing child? Ma...
so. After all, t...
nervous syste...
cross the plac...
1980). Howev...
posure to illi...
mental risk, t...
long-term effe...

To provide...
known—and...
effects of pren...
research is pro...
periods in infa...
infancy and to...

Neonatal Pe...

A large body of...
ternal drug ab...
exposed to co...
utero, where p...
constriction, t...
mations (Bing...
1989). Cocaine...
birth and othe...
weight, small...
tory patterns (...
1988; Oro & D...
cle tone, feedi...
also be seen in...

Infants pre...
tend also to be...
perinatal medi...
fants born to o...

(Eds.). *The Effects of the Infant on the Caregiver.* New York: Wiley and Sons.

Bundy, A. C. (1991). Play theory and sensory integration. In A. G. Fisher, E. A. Murray, & A. C. Bundy (Eds.). *Sensory integration: Theory and practice* (pp. 46-68). Philadelphia: F. A. Davis.

Burke, J. P. (1993). Play: The life role of the infant and young child. In J. C. Smith (Ed.). *Pediatric occupational therapy and early intervention* (pp. 198-224). Andover MA: Andover Medical Publishers.

Cardone, I. A., & Gilkerson, L. (1990). Family administered neonatal activities: An exploratory method for the integration of parental perceptions and newborn behavior. *Infant Mental Health Journal, 11*(2), 127-141.

Cardone, I. A., & Gilkerson, L. (1992). Family administered neonatal activities: An adaptation for parents of infants born with Down syndrome. *Infants and Young Children, 5*(1), 40-48.

Cohn, J. F. (1993). Mother-infant play and maternal depression. In K. Mac-Donald (Ed.). *Parent-child play: Descriptions and implications* (pp. 239-256). New York: State University of New York Press.

Cohn, J. F. & Tronick, E. Z. (1983). Three month-old infants' reaction to simulated maternal depression. *Child Development, 54,* 185-193.

Cornell, E. H., & Gottfried, A. W. (1976). Intervention with premature infants. *Child Development, 47,* 32-39.

Fogel, A., Nwokah, E., & Karns, J. (1993). Parent-infant games as dynamic social systems. In K. MacDonald (Ed.). *Parent-child play: Descriptions and implications* (pp. 43-69). New York: State University of New York Press.

Gaiter, J. L. (1985). Nursery environments. In A. W. Gottfried and J. L. Gaiter (Eds.). *Infant stress under intensive care* (pp. 55-82). University Park, MD: University Park Press.

Gianino, A., & Tronick, E. Z. (1988). The mutual regulation model: The infant's self regulation and coping and defensive capacities. In T. M. Field, P. M. McCabe, & R. Schneiderman (Eds.). *Stress and coping across development.* Hillsdale, NJ: Lawrence Erlbaum.

Gilkerson, L., Gorski, P., & Panitz, P. (1990). Hospital-based intervention for pre-term infants and their families. In S. J. Meisels & J. P. Shonkoff (Eds.). *Handbook of early childhood intervention.* New York: University of Cambridge.

Gorga, D. (1994). The evolution of occupational therapy practice for infants in the neonatal intensive care unit. *American Journal of Occupational Therapy, 48*(6), 487-489.

Gorski, P. A., Leonard, C. H., Sweet, D. M., Martin, J. A., and Sehring, S. A. (1990). Caregiver-infant interaction and the immature nervous system: A touchy subject. In K. E. Barnard & T. B. Brazelton (Eds.). *Touch: The foundation of experience* (pp. 229-251). Madison, WI: International Universities Press.

Gottfried, A. W., & Gaiter, J. (1985). *Infant stress under intensive care.* Baltimore: University Park Press.

Gottfried, A. W., Lande, P. W., Brown, S. S., King, J., Coen, C., and Hodgman, J. E. (1981). Physical and social environment of newborn infants in special care units. *Science, 214,* 673-675.

Gregg, C. L., Haffner, M. E., & Korner, A. F. (1976). The relative efficacy of vestibular-proprioceptive stimulation and the upright position in enhancing visual pursuits in neonates. *Child Development, 47,* 309-314.

Greenspan, S. I. (1990). *Infancy and early childhood: The practice of clinical assessment and intervention with emotional and developmental challenges.* Madison, WI: International Universities Press.

Hack, M., Horbar, J. D., Malloy, M. H., Tyson, J. E., Wright, E., and Wright, L. (1991). Very low-birth weight outcomes of the National Institute of Child Health and Human Development neonatal network. *Pediatrics, 87,* 587-597.

Holloway, E. (1994). Parent and occupational therapist collaboration in the neonatal intensive care unit. *American Journal of Occupational Therapy, 48*(6), 535-538.

Hughes, M., & McCollum, J. (1993). Maternal stress and coping in the NICU: An exploratory study. *ACCH Advocate, 1*(1), 57-61.

Hughes, M., McCollum, J., Sheftel, D., and Sanchez, G. (1994). How parents cope with the experience of neonatal intensive care. *Children's Health Care, 23*(1), 1-14.

Leib, S. A., Benfield, G., & Guidubaldi, J. (1980). Effects of early intervention and stimulation on the pre-term infant. *Pediatrics, 66,* 83-90.

Linn, L., Horowitz, F. D., & Fox, H. A. (1985). Stimulation in the NICU: Is more necessarily better? *Clinics in Perinatology, 12*(2), 407-422.

Long, J. G., Lucey, J. F., & Philip, A. G. (1980a). Noise and hypoxemia in the intensive care nursery. *Pediatrics, 65*(1), 143-145.

Long, J. G., Philip, A. G., and Lucey, J. F. (1980b). Excessive handling as a cause of hypoxemia. *Pediatrics, 65,* 203-207.

MacDonald, K. (1993). Parent-child play: An evolutionary perspective. In K. McDonald (Ed.). *Parent-child play: Descriptions and implications* (pp. 113-143). New York: State University of New York Press.

McGrath, M. M., & Myer, E. C. (1992). Maternal self-esteem: From theory to clinical practice in a special care nursery. *Children's Health Care, 21*(4), 199-205.

Newman, L. F. (1981). Social and sensory environment of low-birth weight infants in a special care nursery: An anthropological investigation. *Journal of Nerve and Mental Disability, 169*(4), 448-455.

Nugent, J. K., & Brazelton T. B. (1989). Preventive intervention with infants and families: The NBAS Model. *Infant Mental Health Journal, 10*(2), 84-99.

Nugent, J. K., Greene, S., Deering, D. W., Mazor, K. M., Hendler, J., and Bombardier, C. (1993). The cultural context of mother-infant play in the newborn. In K. McDonald (Ed.). *Parent-child play: Descriptions and implications* (pp. 367-386). New York: State University of New York Press.

Patteson, D. M., & Barnard, K. E. (1990). Parenting of low-birth weight infants: A review of issues and interventions. *Infant Mental Health Journal, 11*(11), 37-56.

Powell, L. F. (1974). The effect of extra stimulation and maternal involvement on the development of low-birth weight infants and on maternal behavior. *Child Development, 45,* 106-113.

Rice, R. D. (1977). Neurophysiological development in premature infants following stimulation. *Developmental Psychology, 13,* 69-76.

Scarr-Salapatek, S., & Williams, M. L. (1973). The effects of early stimulation on low-birth weight infants. *Child Development, 44,* 94-101.

Sheikh, L., O'Brien, M., & McCluskey-Fawcett, K. (1993). Parent preparation for the NICU to home transition: Staff and parent perceptions. *Childrens Health Care, 22*(3), 227-239.

Solkoff, N., & Matuszak, D. (1975). Tactile stimulation and behavioral development among low-birth weight infants. *Child Psychiatry and Human Development, 6,* 33-37.

Solkoff, N., Yaffe, S., Weintraub, D., and Blase, B. (1969). Effects of handling on the subsequent development of premature infants. *Developmental Psychology, 1,* 765-768.

Solnit, A. J. (1993). From play to playfulness in children and adults. In A. J. Solnit & D. J. Cohen (Eds.). *The many meanings of play: A psychoanalytic perspective* (pp 27-53). New Haven: Yale University Press.

Solnit, A. J., & Cohen, D. J. (1993). Introduction. In A. J. Solnit & D. J. Cohen (Eds.). *The many meanings of play: A psychoanalytic perspective.* New Haven: Yale University Press.

Speidel, B. D. (1978). Adverse effects of routine procedures on pre-term infants. *Lancet, 1,* 864-865.

Sutton-Smith, B. (1993). Dilemmas in adult play with children. In K. Mac-Donald (Ed.). *Parent-child play: Descriptions and implications* (pp 15-42). Albany, NY: SUNY Press.

Whaley, K. K. (1990). The emergence of social play in infancy: A proposed developmental sequence of infant-adult social play. *Early Childhood Research Quarterly, 5,* 347-358.

White, J. L., & LaBarba, R. C. (1976). The effects of tactile and kinesthetic stimulation on neonatal development in the premature infant. *Developmental Psychology, 9,* 569-577.

Kaltenbach et al., 1979; Wilson, 1989). The phenomenon of declining infant cognitive test scores is typical of economically disadvantaged populations and cannot be attributed to in utero drug exposure.

There is some evidence that when differences between drug-exposed and socioeconomically matched non–drug exposed infants are found, they tend to be in the area of motor development (Hans, 1989; Johnson et al., 1984; Mayes et al., 1995; Rosen & Johnson, 1982; Schneider et al., 1989; Strauss et al., 1976; Wilson et al., 1981). However, it is important to note that the average motor development scores of the drug-exposed children in these studies fall within normal limits. Moreover, motor development may be affected primarily in those drug-exposed children with the most serious social risk factors (Hans, 1989).

Some researchers have observed qualities that may be precursors of behavioral or learning problems. These include short attention span, hypersensitivity, high activity level, and lack of refinement in fine motor skills (Lodge, 1976; Wilson et al., 1973; 1981). However, most of these observations have been incidental or anecdotal rather than a primary focus of study. An exception is a recent study by Mayes et al. (1995), who found that cocaine-exposed 3-month-old infants were more likely than matched non–drug exposed infants to react with irritability and crying during a habituation procedure. Cognitive test scores of the two groups did not differ. These researchers suggested that prenatal cocaine exposure might affect arousal and attention regulation rather than cognition. The young age of these infants must be considered, however; it may be that the tendency toward irritability is outgrown as the infants mature.

One interesting study addressed the play of drug-exposed children (Rodning et al., 1989). These researchers observed a small group of 18-month-old drug-exposed toddlers and a group of matched control children in free play and in interactions with their caregivers. They found evidence that the drug-exposed children had insecure attachments to their caregivers and that their play was more immature and disorganized than the comparison children. Specifically, the drug-exposed children engaged in pretend play (such as stirring a pot or combing a doll's hair) less frequently and for much briefer periods. They tended to scatter, bat, and drop toys instead of combining, exploring, or fantasizing with them. The researchers noted that these children seemed unable to initiate and organize complex behavior in unstructured situations. Such indicators of impulsive and disorganized behavior were found even in the drug-exposed toddlers with very high cognitive scores.

Within the field of occupational therapy, Hyde and Trautman (1989) have suggested, based on their clinical experiences, that drug-exposed infants appear to have sensory integrative difficulties. A few researchers in the profession have begun systematically to explore whether drug-exposed infants have identifiable sensory processing problems. Master's thesis research conducted by Michelle Robert at the University of Southern California addressed this issue

(Robert, 1992). Robert administered the Test of Sensory Functions in Infants (TSFI) (DeGangi & Greenspan, 1989) to seven drug-exposed and seven non–drug exposed infants, aged 10 to 12 months, all of whom came from socioeconomically disadvantaged families in the same geographic area. No differences were found between the two groups; six of the seven drug-exposed infants scored within normal limits. These very preliminary findings do not support the presence of sensory processing problems among these infants. However, these results may be influenced by the very small numbers of children in the study and the restricted range of ages. Perhaps sensory processing problems are evident in drug-exposed children during some other age period, or perhaps the TSFI is not sensitive in detecting sensory processing problems within the narrow age band of 10 to 12 months.

Another occupational therapist, Shelly Lane, has reported on pilot data using the TSFI with cocaine-exposed infants (Lane, 1992). Her preliminary data suggest that these infants have heightened sensitivity to vestibular stimulation at 8 months and at 18 months of age. These results do not clearly indicate sensory processing difficulties, however, because at 8 months of age the TSFI's reliability is weak, and at 18 months the score may be influenced by the infant's desire to be unrestrained (Lane, 1992).

Taken together, the studies on infants and toddlers who have been prenatally drug exposed do not reveal cognitive delays beyond what is typically seen among children from socioeconomically disadvantaged families. Typically, these infants and toddlers score within the low average range on tests such as the Bayley. Research results are inconclusive as to whether sensory and motor development is affected. Some evidence suggests that as infants and toddlers these children may have difficulty with attention regulation and impulse control and that this may be manifested in their play. Perhaps what some clinicians and researchers are noticing is an emerging difficulty with self-regulation that places the infants at risk for learning or behavior disorders.

The Preschool Years

Relatively few researchers have examined developmental outcomes of prenatally drug-exposed children during the preschool years (from approximately 2½ through 5 years of age). With respect to cognitive development, results of these studies show patterns similar to what has been found in infants and toddlers: drug-exposed children tend to score lower than non–drug exposed children, but the differences are not always significant and, even when they are significant, the drug-exposed children's average IQ and perceptual scores fall within low normal limits (Bauman & Dougherty, 1983; Griffith et al., 1994; Kaltenbach & Finnegan, 1989; Lifschitz et al., 1985; Strauss et al., 1979; van Baar & de Graaff, 1994; Wilson et al., 1979).

Fine motor coordination has been noted anecdotally by some observers to be an area of concern with respect to drug-exposed preschoolers. However, few studies have addressed this domain, and those that have typically have not used well-developed measures of fine motor skill (e.g., Strauss et al., 1979).

An exception is the research of an occupational therapist, Linda Adintori (1995). In her Master's thesis at the University of Southern California, she used the Fine Motor Scale of the Peabody Developmental Motor Scales (PDMS) (Folio & Fewell, 1983) to compare eight cocaine-exposed and amphetamine-exposed children with eight non–drug exposed children. In this study, the drug-exposed children had been identified and followed from birth at a hospital-based clinic but were not receiving special services. Children with known developmental disorders were excluded from both groups. The two groups lived in the same geographic area and were carefully matched for age, gender, ethnicity, and socioeconomic status. All were 2 or 3 years old. Matching of comparison groups is critical in a study such as this because it minimizes the possibility of children in the two groups having dramatically different experiences because of culture, gender, or age. In Adintori's study, a significant difference between groups was found only on the Eye–Hand Coordination subscale of the PDMS. Scores for this scale were significantly lower in the drug-exposed preschoolers and, furthermore, the mean score for this group fell below age expectations (z score of -1.74). This subtest involves the greatest complexity with respect to visually guided action and places the heaviest demands on praxis, compared to the other subscales. The tasks on this scale also require focused attention.

In another study conducted as Master's thesis research by an occupational therapist, Angela Persic (1995) compared six prenatally drug-exposed to six non–drug exposed preschoolers using the Miller Assessment for Preschoolers (MAP) (Miller, 1988). The groups were closely matched for age, gender, ethnicity, and socioeconomic status. Persic found significant group differences on the verbal, complex tasks, and total MAP scores. It is important to note that, in her study, the drug-exposed children all were in a special preschool and had been referred to occupational therapy services, so they did not represent drug-exposed children in general. Instead, they were likely to be among the more developmentally compromised drug-exposed children because they already had been identified as needing special services. With this in mind, it still is interesting to note the areas in which the children had the most severe problems. The results suggest that verbal skills are often affected in a clinic population, as well as complex skills requiring organization, planning, and sustained attention.

In studies that have addressed qualitative aspects of behavior, nearly all have found evidence of such factors as impulsivity, poor attention, high activity level, behavior problems, and other socioemotional risk indicators (Azuma & Chasnoff; 1993 Bauman & Levine, 1986; Strauss et al., 1979; van Baar & de Graaff, 1994; Wilson et al., 1979). This evidence suggests that, although drug-exposed preschoolers typically score within normal limits on standardized tests, they may exhibit behavioral and emotional qualities indicative of poor self-regulation. This, in turn, may place them at risk for later academic and social problems.

Anecdotal reports from teachers working with prenatally drug-exposed preschoolers tend to confirm the impression that these children are likely to experience difficulties with the preacademic and social demands of the preschool classroom. In a special preschool program for prenatally drug-exposed children in Los Angeles, difficulties were noted with attention, problem solving, imaginative and social play, communication, motor skills, and perception, despite age-appropriate intelligence. In addition, disturbances in emotional expression were described, such as extreme aggression or passivity, excessive trust or fearfulness of others, apathy, problems with attachment, or generally unpredictable behavior (Los Angeles Unified School District, 1989).

These anecdotal reports are corroborated by the Master's thesis research of Julie Ewald at the University of Southern California (Ewald, 1993). She conducted a qualitative study that involved description of the play characteristics of three preschoolers who attended a 30-session pilot group program for drug-exposed children. The three target children initially seemed to be overwhelmed in this play-oriented group setting, perhaps because of sensory overload. Imaginative play was rarely observed. Instead, the children tended to become absorbed in solitary stimulus-bound play. Many of the children had developmental weaknesses that made it difficult for them to participate successfully in certain play activities. Some commonly observed areas of difficulty included following verbal directions, eye–hand coordination, and two-dimensional and three-dimensional constructional praxis (Fig. 12-1, *A, B*, and *C*). Over the 15 weeks of the program, improvements were noted in the children's abilities to organize themselves, to initiate and persist with challenging activities, to play independently and successfully, and to interact with others. Additionally, the children seemed better able to make use of adult assistance that was directed toward problem solving, imagination, and social interactions in play. The apparent responsiveness of these children to intervention suggests that environmental factors have a powerful influence on the play of drug-exposed children.

The collective results of other research studies indicate that environmental influences are extremely important contributors to the developmental outcomes of prenatally drug-exposed children. When home environment variables are considered, they almost invariably are strongly related to cognitive performance and other outcome measures (Bauman & Daugherty, 1983; Griffith et al., 1994; Johnson et al., 1991; Lifschitz et al., 1985; Strauss et al., 1979). The typically "low normal" test scores of these children are not surprising when one considers that the lives of many prenatally drug-exposed children may be exceptionally stressful because of such factors as the chaotic lifestyle of the drug-abusing parent, violence in the home or neighborhood, or the instability of moving from one foster home to another.

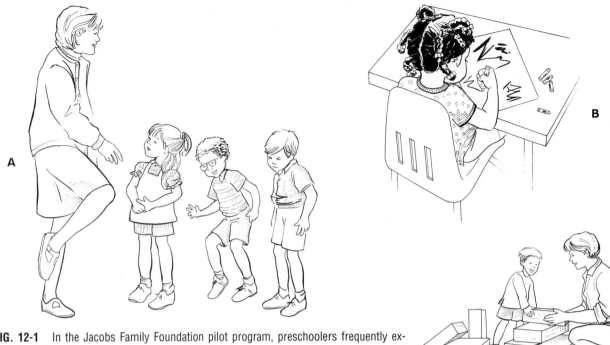

FIG. 12-1 In the Jacobs Family Foundation pilot program, preschoolers frequently experienced difficulty participating in play activities because of underlying developmental problems. **A,** Following and responding to verbal directions was problematic for many of the children. **B,** Eye–hand coordination was poor in many of the children, interfering with coloring and drawing. **C,** Constructional activities, such as building a structure with blocks, requires well-developed praxis. This ability was weak for many of the children. (Illustrations by Jeanne Robertson.)

What has been surprising to many observers of these children is their resilience (e.g., Johnson et al., 1991). Most drug-exposed preschoolers are not developmentally delayed; many are above average in intelligence. They certainly are not the hopeless cases that the media have often portrayed them to be. Given nurturing and stable environments, there is reason for optimism that the biological disadvantages present at birth need not pose permanent barriers to a happy, productive life. The remaining sections of this chapter build on the authors' optimism that intervention programs have the potential to make a positive contribution to the lives of children with prenatal drug exposure.

GENERAL CONSIDERATIONS ABOUT INTERVENTION

When a professional introduces intervention into the life of a child who has experienced prenatal drug exposure, a number of considerations should be borne in mind. A knowledge of developmental characteristics of children with drug exposure is important, but perhaps more critical is an awareness of the potentially damaging effects of labeling the child as drug exposed. Public misperceptions of "drug babies" usually assume that the unfortunate start in life condemns these children to a future of crime or helplessness. Pejorative labeling of these children is dangerous because it may generate a self fulfilling prophecy (Howard & O'Donnell, 1995; Neuspiel, 1993). It is

imperative that the individual needs of drug-exposed children be supported through intervention when appropriate, but the history of drug exposure in most cases is a matter of utmost confidentiality. The child's family needs to know that there is good reason to believe that positive changes in the environment will lead to benefits for the child.

The intervenor needs to approach these children and their families with respect and sensitivity. If a parent who is actively abusing drugs is involved, she or he has special needs that must be considered. These parents will need a great deal of support and specific suggestions for strategies on how to manage the child. Children living with drug-abusing parents should be monitored for signs of abuse and neglect, and if any are detected the family should be referred to a child welfare agency for intervention (Hawley, 1994). If he or she is involved in a drug rehabilitation program, a great deal of support should be given to the parent to stay involved with it.

The foster parent or adoptive parent has special needs too. Often these parents are not prepared for the challenges of handling a difficult infant or child. The professional can help by giving them support as well as specific suggestions for management strategies.

Traditionally, occupational therapists have worked within the context of individual, clinic-based therapy to influence the child's engagement in daily occupations. Many have used a sensory integrative approach in working directly with the child, but sensory integrative principles are also used to guide recommendations to parents regarding the sensory aspects of handling the child and organizing the environment (Hyde & Trautman, 1989).

Because the family's orchestration of occupations in the home is very influential on the young child, the occupational therapist may support the child's development by focusing on the way the parent organizes and enacts caregiving and household tasks. An important alternative or supplement to individual, clinic-based therapy is therefore providing caregiver support and guidance via home-based intervention. Provision of occupational therapy within the context of a drug rehabilitation program for mothers is another promising approach that tackles the caregiving environment.

Intervention using a small group format provides a useful context for helping children develop their play skills, particularly the social aspects of play. In the following section, a group program designed to develop therapeutic strategies for enhancing the play experiences of prenatally drug-exposed preschoolers is described in detail.

A GROUP PROGRAM FOR PRESCHOOLERS WITH PRENATAL DRUG EXPOSURE

The qualitative study conducted by Ewald (1993) was designed, first, to describe the play characteristics of preschoolers with prenatal drug exposure and, second, to begin to identify therapeutic strategies that are useful in facilitating the play experiences of these children. The research involved in-depth study of three children who participated in a 30-session pilot group program for children with prenatal exposure to drugs. Videotapes of the target children participating in the group sessions were transcribed and coded. In addition, detailed field notes were recorded for each child following each session and for the program as a whole each week. These were also reviewed, coded, and integrated with the videotape-based data to describe the play characteristics of the children and the therapeutic strategies employed by staff with these and other children who participated in the program.

It is important to note that the inclusion of drug-exposed children in the group program was done for investigative purposes only. The authors do not recommend that special group programs be set up solely for drug-exposed children. The dangers inherent in labeling children as drug exposed are too serious to justify doing so. Moreover, many children without a history of drug exposure have difficulties with attention, imaginative play, and social skills that are similar to the problems these authors have observed in the children in this group program and may benefit from the therapeutic strategies that have been employed here.

The group pilot program was funded by the Jacobs Family Foundation and was developed by staff at the Ayres Clinic in Torrance, California. It was designed to develop intervention strategies appropriate for prenatally drug-exposed children aged 3 to 6 years. The program was based on

sensory integration principles as well as concepts of play development.

The group met twice a week for 90 minutes in a total of 30 sessions. The program was directed by an occupational therapist with the assistance of an educational specialist. Staff who participated in the program also included one aide and a group of five volunteers who attended on a rotating basis. The staff were educated about the program purpose and format and additionally received some background information on sensory integration, prenatal drug exposure, and play development during one orientation meeting and a series of informal meetings conducted before and following each group session.

Initially 10 children attended the program, but because of changes in residence, the number of children attending lowered to seven after several weeks. All of the children had histories of prenatal exposure to illicit drugs (such as cocaine, heroin, and PCP) according to maternal self-report of drug abuse during pregnancy or medical records indicating positive toxicology results for birth mother and/or infant. Children with a diagnosis of fetal alcohol syndrome were excluded; however, it is likely that many of the children in the program had been exposed to multiple toxic substances, including alcohol, in utero.

The philosophy of the program was to provide a variety of opportunities for development of play skills via age-appropriate activities that included sensorimotor and imaginative components. The initial session opened, according to the original plan, with free play time, offering a wide variety of toys and sensorimotor activities. This was conducted in one large room while the children arrived. Free play was immediately followed by a group activity based upon the *Movement Is Fun* curriculum by Susan Young (1988), which was conducted in an adjacent area within the same room. The program concluded with more free play time.

It quickly became apparent that the original plan for the program was too loosely structured for the children who participated because it made too many demands on their limited capacity for self-regulation. The program was soon reorganized to better meet the needs of the children. The revised program began on the third day that the group met. It commenced with a free-play time, as in the original plan; however, the sessions became more structured spatially and temporally.

Niches were established around the large play room for specific play stations, including areas for fine motor and visual–perceptual tabletop tasks, tactile exploration, imaginary play, and music and reading. A gross motor area was established in an entirely separate room. This gross motor room was part of a sensory integration–style treatment area, so it permitted closely guided use of suspended equipment as well as other activities providing a variety of vestibular, proprioceptive, and tactile experiences in the context of gross motor play.

The program structure was further revised to allow for much closer monitoring and structuring by the staff. During the free-play time, the children were divided into two groups that alternated playing in the gross motor and large free-play areas. This meant that only half of the total group was in a particular area at a given time. Additionally, staff and volunteers were stationed as guides in each play area, allowing for closer support to individual children.

A group movement activity based on the *Movement Is Fun* program (Young, 1988) was maintained as circle time in the schedule and continued to take place in the adjacent area designated specifically for it. The area was more clearly delineated spatially to provide additional structuring for the children. The protocol of the program was modified to increase structure and adult assistance and to decrease praxis demands and expectation of time engaged in activities. For example, the adult–child ratio was increased to one adult for every one to two children to allow for more individualized attention. The original *Movement Is Fun* program was designed for typically developing preschoolers and relied heavily on verbal instruction and demonstration by the adult leader (Young, 1988). This format posed auditory-language, ideational, motor planning, and attentional challenges that were too great for the children in the program. To enhance active participation and sustained attention during the movement activities, props were added that provided visible and tangible cues. Favorite songs and activities were frequently repeated from session to session to build the children's involvement and acquisition of skills.

Circle time was followed by a snack and story time. Snack time provided a break from sensorimotor play and provided opportunities to develop social and self-care skills in the context of a daily occupation. Story time was designed as a quiet group time to decrease arousal level and assist the children with the transition to leaving at the session's end. This consisted of quiet stories, rhymes, songs, and routine goodbyes. Special attention was made to choreographing transitions between all of the program sections because this appeared to be a particular problem area for the children.

The program revisions appeared to increase its effectiveness dramatically in promoting the play experiences of the children. Furthermore, staff were able to devote more attention to individual children and so could refine their intervention strategies. The strategies that appeared to be most helpful in promoting play that was more sustained and more complex are described in detail later in this chapter. Before a discussion of specific strategies, two cases are presented to provide the reader with a feeling for the children who participated in the program and for the context in which therapeutic strategies have been implemented.

CASE EXAMPLES

The following cases are drawn from Ewald's (1993) study of several preschoolers who participated in the pilot program described in the preceding section. The first case was a child with minor areas of deficit, and the second was more extensively involved. Each case example consists of a section on the child's background followed by one on strengths and weaknesses as noted by primary caregivers and program staff members. Because these children participated in a study utilizing the *Sensory Integration and Praxis Tests* (SIPT) (Ayres, 1989) during the year of the group program, their sensory integration profiles are integrated into the section on strengths and weaknesses. Next, their characteristic play patterns are described, and progress throughout the program is discussed, including specific therapeutic strategies used and outcomes. Pseudonyms are used to protect the identities of the children.

CASE EXAMPLE 1: JACKIE

Background
Jackie is a cheerful, outgoing little girl of African-American ancestry. She was 3 years and 4 months old when the program commenced.

Jackie had a rough start in life. She had been born prematurely at 30 weeks gestational age with a birth weight of 3 pounds, 3 ounces. According to her adoptive parents, toxicology reports were positive for cocaine exposure at birth.

She had resided with her white adoptive family since they took her home from the hospital at the age of 25 days, when she was released from the prenatal nursery. Her adoptive mother reported that, as a young infant, Jackie slept 24 hours a day and was not interested in eating; neither did she appear to have a drive to survive. She was identified as an infant with failure to thrive and irregular sleep patterns.

Jackie also had a history of hearing problems associated with otitis media. Around the age of 2 years she wore a hearing aid for 5 months.

Jackie had received early intervention in the form of speech therapy for 2 years. She first attended a clinic for 6 months where she received speech therapy twice a week combined with parent conferences and attendance at a preschool that placed children with hearing problems back in the mainstream. This intervention was funded through the local regional center, a California state-funded agency that serves children who have developmental disabilities or infants and toddlers who are at risk for developmental problems. Jackie then received in-home speech therapy for 1 hour twice a week through the local school district. After the age of 2 years, Jackie was discharged from the regional center because she no longer demonstrated enough evidence of developmental delay to qualify for ongoing services.

Early motor milestones were acquired within the normal age ranges, although Jackie reportedly walked on her toes. When the Jacobs Family Foundation group program began at the Ayres Clinic, she did not attend school reportedly because she was not completely toilet trained. By the end of the 15-week program Jackie had begun attending a preschool 4 days a week for 2½ hours a day.

Strengths and Weaknesses
Jackie's strengths included motor-free visual perception, ability to imitate demonstrated motor actions, ability to make friends as reported by her adoptive mother, and general engagement in age-appropriate self-care activities. Jackie was generally a happy, cheerful child who enjoyed attending program sessions and engaging in a variety of the play activities offered.

Particular areas of weakness included difficulty following verbal directions, poor fine motor skills, distractibility, difficulty separating from her adoptive mother, and delayed acquisition of toileting skills. Jackie's adoptive mother described her as being restless, stubborn, and overreactive at times. In addition, she said that Jackie possessed nervous habits and sometimes objected to being touched, especially unexpectedly. She also described a tendency for Jackie to isolate herself from other children.

Jackie was administered the SIPT (Ayres, 1989) at 4 years, 2 months of age. All but two of her SIPT scores were within the average range, indicating generally good sensory integrative abilities. On the Praxis on Verbal Command and Design Copying tests, however, her scores, respectively, fell much below and below average in relation to other children her age. These scores indicate weaknesses in ability to use verbal instructions to plan action and in visual–motor ability.

Play Patterns

When Jackie began attending the Jacobs Family Foundation program at the Ayres Clinic, she had some difficulty with play and group activities that involved following verbal instructions or motor planning using her hands. Jackie sometimes had problems with integrating pieces of play equipment and manipulating tools to accomplish play tasks, such as making a structure or cutting with scissors, on her own. In addition, she required physical demonstration for assistance since she had difficulty following verbal directions. This is illustrated by the following transcript from a session during the third week of the program:

> As she is emptying the box, I ask her if she can build a tower with the pegs. She looks at me without answering. I attempt to clarify my question by saying "Remember how we built a tower with the blocks the other day? Can you build a tower with the pegs?" She puts all the pegs away—and needs direction and clarification from her adoptive mother to build by putting one peg on top of the other instead of next to it. Jackie also needed additional verbal and physical cues to complete the activity successfully.

In this and in many other situations, Jackie required adult demonstration and support during constructional play activities.

Jackie's problems with language and praxis were perhaps related to the observed paucity of Jackie's imaginative and dramatic role play. In order to initiate and engage in this type of play a child needs to attain a certain level of ideation and planning. In addition, the expression of imagination during other tasks, such as drawing or coloring, was precluded by her strong need to explore the sensorimotor properties of tools and media.

Social difficulties included a lack of knowhow when required to respond to others' play overtures and to initiate and sustain thematic cooperative play. Often such situations require the ability to negotiate with other children. During the fifteenth group session it was noted that Jackie had not yet initiated play with another child during the program, even when in the same play space. Field notes from that same session comment that Jackie "steps back while Annie plays with some of the toys on the counter in front of Jackie. Jackie looks bewildered and does not know what to do or say to Annie who has invaded her play space."

During free play Jackie frequently shifted from one activity to another before she had the chance to explore the equipment or materials fully and develop a strategy or imaginative theme. She was easily distracted and overwhelmed by group situations. Furthermore, she had severe difficulty separating from her adoptive mother, who even needed to sit next to Jackie during circle time. Jackie was hesitant to share with or be near peers. Yet at the end of the session she typically resisted leaving the program and would cry.

Intervention Strategies

Jackie was allowed time over several sessions to adapt to the play environment. The environment initially was adjusted to provide less sensory stimulation and more structure for children like Jackie who were demonstrating difficulty in coping with the amount of sensory stimuli present in the form of visual, auditory, and tactile media. Gradually Jackie was encouraged to expand her play with materials into more complex actions and themes. The following example from the third session illustrates how a program volunteer coupled verbal invitations with physical assistance for support and comfort while encouraging Jackie to explore new and unfamiliar equipment placed in the gross motor room:

> Eileen holds Jackie and brings her to the top of two bolster swings suspended horizontally which compose a "double-decker bus." She says "Did you see this one?" as she appears to be guiding Jackie in exploring the equipment. Jackie reaches for the suspended ring above the bolster swing unsuccessfully. She puts both hands on the top bolster at Eileen's suggestion, then grasps the ring with both hands. Eileen swings her back and forth while supporting her at the hips and thighs. Eileen then suggests that Jackie try sitting on the top bolster as she lifts the child up. Eileen reassures Jackie that she is holding her and reminds her to hold on. Jackie holds the ring with her left hand and sits on the bolster swing.

Many opportunities were presented for fine motor exploration and skill development during free play and group play time. Activities incorporated use of a variety of sensory materials as well as tools to encourage a multitude of fine motor experiences. Songs with hand movements, puppets, craft tasks, drawing and coloring, tabletop games requiring use of precision with tools and eye–hand coordination, puzzles, and constructional activities were examples of those used. Gross motor activities that strengthened body scheme and eye–hand coordination were also provided.

Gradually the distance from her adoptive mother was increased, whereas interaction with staff and peers in proximity was encouraged. Many opportunities were also presented to develop praxis on verbal command during both free play and group activities. Songs with instructions, games reliant on auditory skills, the posing of questions for encouragement of problem solving during free play, and gradual incorporation of more multistep directions were playfully utilized to build skills in this area. In addition, suggestions for home-based activities to promote praxis on verbal command and fine motor skills were made to her mother.

Intervention during play with peers was aimed at increasing the amount of structure to encourage more purposeful play. Cooperative activities were implemented during circle time, starting with staff as a partner, then progressing to a peer partner with staff assisting, and eventually encouraging Jackie to interact with peers on her own.

Outcome

By the end of the 15-week program, Jackie was initiating, persisting with, and developing play themes more independently. She was demonstrating increased ability to attend to group activities and free play without intervention. In addition, she began to ask where certain peers were, to choose to be near them, and to engage in cooperative play. During the last week of the program, Jackie participated with two other children in an imaginative and cooperative play activity without adult support. However, the cooperative play was relatively disorganized, lacking a developed theme, role playing, and verbal interactions.

Jackie was also able to tolerate being away from her adoptive mother for most of the session if she left the room or remained in a corner of the room. Overall, Jackie was enjoying activities more independently. She began attending a preschool independently without requiring accompaniment from her mother.

reminders, physical assistance, and protection through use of such objects as mats and helmets are all techniques that are critical to the safety and perceived safety of the children. Some children need specific assistance in this area since their safety awareness is so poor.

Therapeutic Use of Objects, Materials, and Activities

Therapeutic use of objects, materials, and activities was the second general category of strategies deemed successful with the children in the pilot program (Ewald, 1993). Two main types of strategies fall under this category: reduction of number of objects in the environment and judicious use of preferred play materials.

Number of Objects in the Play Environment. In preparation for play sessions, it is tempting to set out a large variety of toys for the children to choose from and play with. This can be far too overwhelming for these children and tends to encourage wandering and fleeting play encounters. In addition, this can hinder complex play because there are too many sensory (visual, auditory, tactile) distractions in the environment. One therapeutic strategy consists of drastically reducing the number of toys and visual paraphernalia from the play environment. If possible, different segments of the program should be located in separate rooms or in clearly demarcated areas. For example, in the pilot program, the gross motor activities were moved to a separate room from the fine motor and imaginary play materials. Afterward, the children appeared much less distractible, with less wandering. This is illustrated in the following excerpt from field notes taken on the day that the children were introduced to the new arrangement:

> There are much fewer materials present in the large room—two to three activities set up on tables, a smaller imaginary play area. … overall the children are calmer, the atmosphere is *much* quieter and everything and everyone is more organized.

Preferred Play Materials and Activities. Throughout the program certain materials and toys were favored by the children more than others. These materials tended to be associated with relatively more sustained, productive play. Staff of the pilot program discovered a number of therapeutic strategies, discussed later in this subsection, that involved the judicious presentation of preferred play materials. However, it should be noted that in the pilot program it appeared that the specific toys and materials provided did not seem as important, generally, as the ways in which the staff and volunteers encouraged the children to explore and engage in play with them.

Preferred toys and activities consisted of play dough; household items or domestic toys within the imaginative play area; constructive tabletop toys; tabletop games with animal characters, which challenged visual-perceptual and fine motor skills; foam soap; books; records; the bubble ball bath

(a large container filled with plastic balls); and a climbing structure. When the videotaped sessions were reviewed, it was clear that the children chose to engage in these activities more frequently than other activities and that they stayed with them longer. Overall, the children appeared most independent and stayed longest with the play dough and household item toys.

Less popular items included toys and activities that required a sequence of actions, turn taking, or an unusual or complex procedure. The children depended on adult direction to do these activities, and perhaps this was why independent selection of these activities was noted less often than was the case with preferred activities.

Field notes indicated that "the use of tangible, visual, and kinesthetic cues to gain the children's attention," as opposed to solely auditory–language cues, was highly effective in involving them in play activities. It is recommended, therefore, that concrete objects be used to augment instruction when teaching these children a new activity. Use of tangible objects is also recommended to facilitate extended engagement in play, particularly cooperative play, which tends to be challenging for these children. Play materials that provide tactile, proprioceptive, and visual feedback are recommended because the children seemed to respond to, and seek out, these kinds of activities. Examples of these are play dough, foam soap, brushes, books, household items, and climbing and jumping activities (Fig. 12-5).

In the pilot program, the most successful activities involved an optimal level of challenge for the children and simultaneously provided tangible feedback. Ineffective activities typically were too unstructured, made demands that were too complex for the children's abilities, or were overstimulating, as when too many choices of play or craft materials were set out. Such overstimulating situations created overarousal and disorganized activity. Many of the children in the program were sensory defensive, which made it particularly difficult for them to focus attention

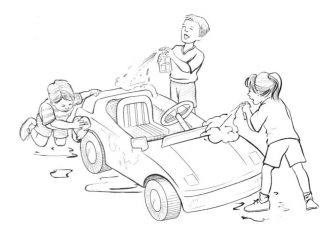

FIG. 12-5   The tactile defensive child often avoids materials such as soap foam, but once the child has become focused in a calm environment the incorporation of such tactile media into an imaginative play theme can entice him or her into productive exploration of tactile materials. (Illustration by Jeanne Robertson.)

when a great deal of noise or visual distraction was in the room.

It is recommended that activities that impart a calming and organizing influence be used before the introduction of more challenging ones. In the pilot program, calming activities usually involved heavy work (proprioceptive input from activities providing resistance, often with concomitant deep touch pressure) or gross motor activity (Fig. 12-6).

Another strategy involving presentation of preferred toys is to structure the first few sessions of a group program so

that the demand level for task success is very low. Later, as the children become more familiar with the play setting, more complex activities can be gradually introduced and encouraged.

Since the play of the children in the pilot program was primarily at a sensorimotor stage of development, it is suggested that activities and materials that primarily offer sensorimotor experiences be provided when working with similar children, especially in the early stages of the intervention program. The therapist can gradually increase the level of developmental challenge over time.

It is important that planned activities not be overly complex or demanding in areas of the children's developmental weaknesses. For example, in the pilot program, the original use of the *Movement Is Fun* curriculum (Young, 1988) was not successful because it required the children to attend closely to verbal directions and then motor plan their responses to the verbal commands, both of which were areas of weakness for most of the children in the group. This movement curriculum was successful only after the activities were modified using tangible objects to augment verbal instruction.

Materials such as dress-up clothes and other props for imaginative play are strongly recommended as facilitators of cooperative social play. An incident involving Eric provides a striking example of the potential for encouraging social play through utilization of certain play materials. This usually quiet, reclusive boy suddenly became animated and spontaneously began to interact with a peer in cooperative, imaginative, dramatic play after dress-up clothes were brought out one day (Fig. 12-7).

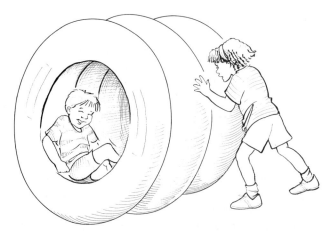

FIG. 12-6 Play activities that involve heavy work and active movement can be organizing, calming, and motivating and thus facilitate sustained cooperative play with turn taking. (Illustration by Jeanne Robertson.)

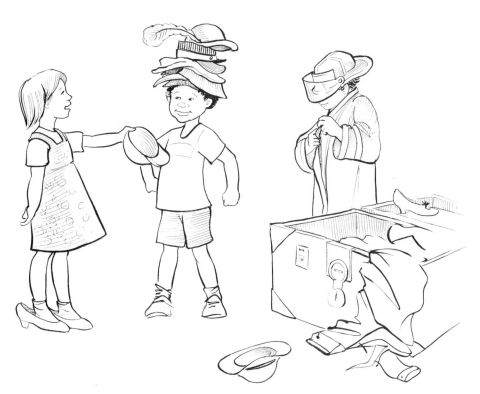

FIG. 12-7 Dressup play can be especially helpful in encouraging social interactions. (Illustration by Jeanne Robertson.)

Spatial and Temporal Organization of the Program

Spatial and temporal organization of the play setting relates to how the play environment and daily routine are structured. Spatial organization refers to the structure and arrangement of activities and persons within the play space. Temporal organization relates to the arrangement of the activities in relation to time.

Spatial Organization. Three types of strategies that relate to spatial organization are identified. First, strategies that establish spatial definition involve the designation of particular places for specific activities, belongings, and caregivers. A second grouping of spatial strategies involves consideration of the number of children within a space. The final type of spatial strategy entails the consideration of the sensory characteristics of the play space.

Spatial definition. Establishing spatial definition involves breaking a large play area into smaller sections, each of which provides environmental cues that are conducive to a particular type of activity. The effect is a less overwhelming and distracting environment for the children. For example, in the pilot program, the large playroom was sectioned into four spaces designated for imaginary play, fine motor (tabletop) activities, circle time (the movement curriculum), and a reading area. In addition, the separation of gross motor activities into another room assisted with activity focus. By creating "niches" within the program for imaginative, fine manipulative, and gross motor play areas, more structure was added to the play environment (Fig. 12-8). In addition, an area was designated for personal belongings. This contributed to the organization of the daily routine by demarcating the space devoted to entering and exiting the program from the space devoted to play.

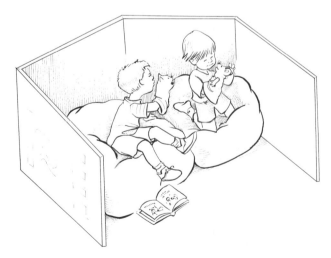

FIG. 12-8 By creating niches within the play environment, therapists can add structure, minimize extraneous sensory stimulation, and thereby increase the child's comfort level, focused attention, and potential for cooperative play. (Illustration by Jeanne Robertson.)

A related strategy involved designating a special place where parents and other caregivers could sit and talk while the children played. In the pilot program, it was reasoned that provision of this space would support the goal of shifting the social interactions of the children from parents to peers, while at the same time meeting the needs of parents. Providing a space for parents to sit and talk over coffee is recommended as it supports relationships among the parents and caregivers and gives them some respite. It is likely that this, in turn, enhances program attendance, which of course is ultimately of benefit to the children.

Number of children. Another property relating to spatial arrangement involves consideration of the number of children placed within a designated play area. During the pilot program, the children appeared to demonstrate greater complexity and longer duration of time spent in play activities when no more than three or four children were present in a particular play area. In contrast, situations in which all seven children participated in an activity simultaneously tended to be less organized. This may have been because of the amount of distracting sensory stimuli generated by larger numbers of children sharing a space. These experiences indicate that small numbers of children should be grouped within a play area whenever possible to enhance ability to focus upon play activities.

Sensory characteristics. Consideration of the sensory characteristics of the play environment is critical. In the pilot program, certain types of visual, auditory, and tactile sensory input appeared to be problematic for the children. For example, the soap foam generated a disturbing tactile sensation for some of the children. For many of them, the incidental sounds generated by toys and people were distracting or distressing. A common reaction when the environment was visually busy was to disengage from the activity at hand. In general, when the children became overwhelmed by sensory stimuli, they tended to "tune out" of the activity and withdraw or become overly excited and disorganized.

It is recommended that a calm, quiet environment with as little background noise or visual distraction as possible be used, especially when the children are being introduced to a new program, a new play activity, or a new play space. This helps the children to feel that they are in a safe, comfortable place and also helps them to attend to the activities presented. The first few sessions of a new program could focus solely on acclimation to the environment and routine. This is done by designing the environment so that extraneous sensory, social, and task demands are minimized and the routine is simple. Examples of strategies include reducing the number of people present in the setting, having fewer pictures and decorations up in the room, choosing a quiet room, and establishing a quiet area in the room such as a reading corner. A blanket of background sound using soft music, a fan, or a white noise machine may be helpful for children who demonstrate difficulties in habituating to incidental noises. Later, as the children become familiar with the setting, more environmental stimuli can be added.

Temporal Organization. "Temporal organization" refers to the time spent in play activities and the sequencing of activities in time. During the pilot program, staff developed two temporal organization strategies that appeared to be very effective in helping the children sustain productive involvement with play activities.

First, within a session, it seemed helpful to allow the children to spend time in familiar environments and activities before introducing them to less familiar, potentially threatening activities. For example, the younger children in the program were generally more successful when allowed time to play with familiar fine motor and imaginative play materials before proceeding into the gross motor room, which was equipped with novel suspended equipment and other challenging therapeutic materials. The second strategy was to structure shorter periods of free play time within smaller play spaces, using simple exploratory play materials first before proceeding to more challenging activities. These two temporal strategies, then, were integrated with spatial strategies and with carefully selected play materials to help the children make the most of their play experiences in the program. In essence, these strategies together provided the children with a "warmup time" in which they could experience feelings of comfort and competence before tackling more difficult challenges.

Over the course of a program such as the one described here, children gradually become able to handle longer periods of time in more complex kinds of play. In our pilot program, the most complex imaginative play activities and the longest durations of sustained attention were observed on the twenty-third session, nearly 3 months after the beginning of the program. Because they were very involved in imaginative play on that particular day, the children were allowed to continue to play for an extended amount of time. It appeared that more complex play was an outcome of their high level of comfort in a familiar environment with familiar materials and peers, combined with a flexible program that responded to their needs by allowing them more time to play in a given activity when this was appropriate.

CONCLUSION

Preschoolers who have been prenatally exposed to illicit drugs, although not usually developmentally delayed, may have difficulty engaging fully in age-appropriate play activities. It is not known why this is so, but it is plausible that prenatal drug exposure may interfere with the regulation of arousal, attention, and emotion. Research indicates that environmental influences are powerful in shaping the developmental outcomes of these children. This gives us reason to expect that intervention efforts, if undertaken with sensitivity, can potentially make a difference in their lives. These authors have identified several types of therapeutic strategies that appear to be successful in promoting more complex and satisfying play experiences for a small group of preschoolers with prenatal drug exposure. This discussion of therapeutic strategies is hoped to be a stimulus for therapists who are committed to helping the lives of children with prenatal drug exposure and for researchers who are interested in evaluating the effectiveness of therapeutic efforts.

REVIEW QUESTIONS

1. Differentiate between the known developmental effects and the suspected developmental effects of prenatal drug exposure for each of the following age groups: neonate, infant, toddler, and preschooler.
2. Discuss why developmental outcomes for these children are still being questioned by researchers. Why are so many research results inconclusive?
3. What are some behavioral manifestations of self-regulatory problems? How might these kinds of problems affect the mother–infant relationship? How might they influence the child's risk for later difficulties with learning and behavior?
4. What is the evidence that childrearing environments make a difference in the developmental outcomes for children with prenatal drug exposure? What are the implications for intervention?

5. Describe what is meant by pejorative labeling. Why should this be avoided? What are the implications for professionals working with children who have been prenatally drug exposed?
6. What is meant by "therapeutic use of self"? What are the eight types of strategies identified by the authors that fall into this category? Give an example of a specific strategy for each of these.
7. What is meant by "therapeutic use of objects, materials, and activities"? Name the two types of strategies that fall into this category and provide examples of each.
8. What is meant by "spatial organization" of the program? Name the three types of strategies that relate to this and give examples of each.
9. What is meant by "temporal organization" of the program? Give examples of specific strategies related to this.

REFERENCES

Adintori, L. (1995). *Fine motor skills of two- to three-year-old drug-exposed children.* Unpublished Master's thesis, University of Southern California, Los Angeles.

Ayres, A. J. (1989). *Sensory Integration and Praxis Tests.* Los Angeles: Western Psychological Services.

Azuma, S. D. & Chasnoff, I. J. (1993). Outcome of children prenatally exposed to cocaine and other drugs: A path analysis of three-year data. *Pediatrics, 92,* 396-402.

Bauman, P. S., & Dougherty, F. E. (1983). Drug-addicted mother's parenting and their children's development. *International Journal of the Addictions, 18,* 291-302.

Bauman, P. S., & Levine, S. A. (1986). The development of children of drug addicts. *International Journal of the Addictions, 21,* 849-863.

Bayley, N. (1993). *Bayley Scales of Infant Development.* New York: Psychological Corporation.

Bingol, N., Fuchs, M., Diaz, V., Stone, R. K. (1987) Teratogenicity of cocaine in humans. *Journal of Pediatrics, 110,* 93-96.

Chasnoff, I. J. (1988). Drug use in pregnancy: Parameters of risk. *Pediatric Clinics of North America, 35,* 1403-1412.

Chasnoff, I. J., Burns, K. A., Burns, W. J., & Schnoll, S. H. (1986). Prenatal drug exposure: Effects on neonatal and infant growth and development. *Neurobehavioral Toxicology and Teratology, 8,* 357-362.

Chasnoff, I. J., Burns, K. A., Schnoll, S. H., & Burns, S. J. (1985). Cocaine use in pregnancy. *New England Journal of Medicine, 313,* 666-669.

Chasnoff, I. J., Chisum, G. M., & Kaplan, W. E. (1988). Maternal cocaine use and genitourinary tract malformations. *Teratology, 37,* 201-204.

Chasnoff, I. J., Hunt, C. E., Kletter, R., & Kaplan, D. (1989). Prenatal cocaine exposure is associated with respiratory pattern abnormalities. *American Journal of Diseases of Children, 143,* 583-587.

Chouteau, M, Namerow, P. B., & Leppert, P. (1988). The effect of cocaine abuse on birth weight and gestational age. *Obstetrics and Gynecology, 72,* 351-354.

DeGangi, G. A., & Greenspan, S. I. (1989). *Test of Sensory Functions in Infants.* Los Angeles: Western Psychological Services.

Edmondson, R., & Smith, T. M. (1994). Temperament and behavior of infants prenatally exposed to drugs: Clinical implications for the mother-infant dyad. *Infant Mental Health Journal, 15,* 368-379.

Ewald, J. L. (1993). *A qualitative study of play in three children, three to four years of age, with prenatal exposure to drugs.* Unpublished Master's thesis, University of Southern California, Los Angeles.

Folio, M. R., & Fewell, R. R. (1983). *Peabody Developmental Motor Scales and Activity Cards.* Allen, TX: DLM Teaching Resources.

Fulroth, R., Phillips, B., & Durand, D. J. (1989). Perinatal outcome of infants exposed to cocaine and/or heroin in utero. *American Journal of Diseases of Children, 143,* 905-910.

Griffith, D. R. (1988). The effects of perinatal cocaine exposure on infant neurobehavior and early maternal-infant interactions. In I. R. Chasnoff (Ed.). *Drugs, alcohol, pregnancy, and parenting.* Lancaster, UK: Kluwer Academic.

Griffith, D. R., Azuma, S. D., & Chasnoff, I. J. (1994). Three-year outcome of children exposed prenatally to drugs. *Journal of the American Academy of Child and Adolescent Psychiatry, 33,* 20-27.

Hans, S. L. (1989). Developmental consequences of prenatal exposure to methadone. *Annals of the New York Academy of Sciences, 562,* 195-207.

Hawley, T. L. (1994). The development of cocaine-exposed children. *Current Problems in Pediatrics, 24,* 259-266.

Householder, J., Hatcher, R., Burns, W., & Chasnoff, I. (1982). Infants born to narcotic-addicted mothers. *Psychological Bulletin, 91,* 453-468.

Howard, B. J., & O'Donnell, K. J. (1995). What is important about a study of within-group differences of "cocaine babies"? *Archives of Pediatric and Adolescent Medicine, 149,* 663-664.

Hurt, H., Brodsky, N. L., Betancourt, L., Braitman, L. E., (1995). Cocaine-exposed children: Follow-up through 30 months. *Developmental and Behavioral Pediatrics, 16,* 29-35.

Hyde, A., & Trautman, S. (1989). Drug exposed infants and sensory integration: Is there a connection? *Sensory Integration Special Interest Section Newsletter, 12*(4), 1, 2, 6.

Johnson, H. L., Diano, A., & Rosen, T. S. (1984). 24-month neurobehavioral follow-up of children of methadone-maintained mothers. *Infant Behavior and Development, 7,* 115-123.

Johnson, H. L., Glassman, M. B., Fiks, K. B., & Rosen, T. S. (1991). Resilient children: Individual differences in developmental outcome of children born to drug abusers. *Journal of Genetic Psychology, 151,* 523-539.

Kaltenbach, K., & Finnegan, L. P. (1989). Children exposed to methadone in utero: Assessment of developmental and cognitive ability. *Annals of the New York Academy of Sciences, 562,* 360-362.

Kaltenbach, K., Graziani, L. J., & Finnegan, L. P. (1979). Methadone exposure in utero: Developmental status at one and two years of age. *Pharmacology Biochemistry & Behavior, 11,* Suppl. pp. 15-17.

Lane, S. J. (1992). Assessment of infants born after prenatal cocaine exposure. *Developmental Disabilities Special Interest Section Newsletter, 15*(3), 2.

Lifschitz, M. H., Wilson, G. S., Smith, E. O., & Desmond, M. M. (1985). Factors affecting head growth and intellectual function in children of drug addicts. *Pediatrics, 75,* 269-274.

Little, B. B., Snell, L. M., Klein, V. R., & Gilstrap, L. C. (1989). Cocaine abuse during pregnancy: Maternal and fetal complications. *Obstetrics and Gynecology, 2,* 157-160.

Lodge, A. (1976). Developmental findings with infants born to mothers on methadone maintenance: A preliminary report. G. Beschner & R. Brotman (Eds.) *National Institute on Drug Abuse Symposium on Comprehensive Health Care for Addicted Families and Their Children* (pp. 79-83). Rockville, MD: National Institue on Drug Abuse.

Los Angeles Unified School District. (1989). Today's challenge: Teaching strategies for working with young children prenatally exposed to drugs/alcohol. Unpublished manuscript.

Mayes, L. C., Bornstein, M. H., Chawarska, K., & Granger, R. H. (1995). Information processing and developmental assessments in 3-month-old infants exposed prenatally to cocaine. *Pediatrics, 95,* 539-545.

Miller, L. J. (1988). *Miller Assessment for Preschoolers (Revised).* San Antonio, TX: Psychological Corporation.

Neuspiel, D. R. (1993). On pejorative labeling of cocaine exposed children. *Journal of Substance Abuse Treatment, 10,* 407.

Oro, A. S., & Dixon, S. D. (1987). Perinatal cocaine and methamphetamine exposure: Maternal and neonatal correlates. *Journal of Pediatrics, 111,* 571-578.

Persic, A. (1995). *Comparison of Preschoolers With and Without Prenatal Drug Exposure on the Miller Assessment for Preschoolers.* Unpublished Master's thesis, University of Southern California, Los Angeles.

Ritchie, J. M. & Greene, N. M. (1980). Local anesthesia. In A. G. Gilman, L. S. Goodman, & A. Gilman (Eds.). *The pharmacologic basis of therapeutics* (6th ed., pp. 300-320). New York: Macmillan Publishing Co.

Robert, M. (1992). *A Pilot Study on the Relationship between Prenatal Exposure to Drugs and Sensory Dysfunction in Minority Infants 10 to 12 Months of Age.* Unpublished Master's thesis, University of Southern California, Los Angeles.

Rodning, C., Beckwith, L., & Howard, J. (1989). Characteristics of attachment organization and play organization in prenatally drug-exposed toddlers. *Development and Psychopathology, 1,* 277-289.

Rosen, T. S., & Johnson, H. L. (1982). Children of methadone-maintained mothers: Follow-up to 18 months of age. *Journal of Pediatrics, 101,* 192-196.

Ryan, L., Ehrlich, S., & Finnegan, L. (1987). Cocaine abuse in pregnancy: Effects on the fetus and newborn. *Neurotoxicology and Teratology, 9,* 295-299.

Schneider, J. W., Griffith, D. R., & Chasnoff, I. J. (1989). Infants exposed to cocaine in utero: Implications for developmental assessment and intervention. *Infants and Young Children, 2,* 25-36.

Strauss, M. E., Lessen-Firestone, J. K., Chavez, C. J., (1979). Children of methadone-treated women at five years of age. *Pharmacology Biochemistry and Behavior, 11,* 3-6.

Strauss, M. E., Starr, R. H., Ostrea, E. M., Chavez, C. J., & Stryker, J. C., (1976). Behavioral concomitants of prenatal addiction to narcotics. *Behavioral Pediatrics, 89,* 842-846.

van Baar, A., & de Graaff, B. M. T. (1994). Cognitive development at preschool-age of infants of drug-dependent mothers. *Developmental Medicine and Child Neurology, 36,* 1063-1075.

Wachsman, L., Schuetz, S., Chan, L. S., & Wingert, W. A. (1989). What happens to babies exposed to phencyclidine (PCP) in utero? *American Journal of Drug and Alcohol Abuse, 15*(1), 31-39.

Wilson, G. S. (1989). Clinical studies of infants and children exposed prenatally to heroin. *Annals of the New York Academy of Sciences, 562,* 183-194.

Wilson, G. S., Desmond, M. M., & Verniand, W. M. (1973). Early development of infants of heroin-addicted mothers. *American Journal of Diseases of Children, 126,* 457-462.

Wilson, G. S., Desmond, M. M., & Wait, R. B. (1981). Follow-up of methadone-treated and untreated narcotic-dependent women and their infants: Health, developmental, and social implications. *Journal of Pediatrics, 98,* 716-722.

Wilson, G. S., McCreary, R., Kean, J., & Baxter, J. C. (1979). The development of preschool children of heroin-addicted mothers: A controlled study. *Pediatrics, 63,* 135-141.

Young, S. (1988). *Movement is fun.* Torrance, CA: Sensory Integration International.

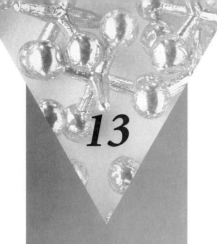

13

DOING WITH—NOT DOING TO: PLAY AND THE CHILD WITH CEREBRAL PALSY

Erna I. Blanche

Several years ago a therapist treated a 3-year-old girl, Sandra, who had been diagnosed with hypotonic cerebral palsy. She was barely able to maintain her head against gravity, she was unable to coordinate reach and grasp, and she did not communicate her needs other than by blinking her eyes and making sounds. Sandra liked to participate in baking cookies, she liked Barbie dolls, and she enjoyed the interaction with other children; however, she did not enjoy puzzles or any motor activity that she was asked to perform during the course of treatment. Sandra demonstrated her dislike by closing her eyes or pretending to be unable to hold her head up.

Treating Sandra was a challenge. Her nontestable cognitive abilities appeared to be significantly higher than her motor skills, and so she was somewhat able to control her environment by opening and closing her eyes to express interest. When motivated, she participated in the treatment session by being alert. When the activity was not appealing to her, she closed her eyes or leaned her head against the table. It took the therapist a long time to figure out that physical fatigue was not the main reason for lack of participation. At that point the therapist decided that to have a successful session would require careful observation of the activities during which Sandra appeared alert and attending.

During one of these treatment sessions the therapist noticed that Sandra appeared very interested in a little girl her own age, the sibling of another child who was receiving treatment at the same time. In her hope to actively involve Sandra, the therapist incorporated this little girl in the treatment session. The sibling carried her Barbie dolls into the treatment room and the therapist, following Sandra's sudden interest, decided to incorporate the dolls and the other little girl into a tea party. The session went well. The children later played simple board games, made a picture, and played with cars. The therapist attended to Sandra's tendency to withdraw from an activity as an indicator of her intrinsic motivation. She also looked for other activities that could be enjoyable, not necessarily activities chosen to address the child's multiple limitations.

When the therapist left that facility, the mother expressed her gratitude to the therapist and added that during her treatment sessions she "did with" rather than "did to" her daughter, and that difference made the experience meaningful for the child. The therapist thought about her words and wondered whether, in reality, she "did with" all the children she treated or whether the desperation of not being able to have Sandra participate in the treatment prompted her to move in that direction. She decided that entering into play with children regardless of their diagnoses was the key and that "doing with" was what she needed to do with all her clients.

The general interest in the value of play in an individual's life has prompted occupational therapists during the last decade to become increasingly concerned about the role of play in the life of the child with cerebral palsy (Anderson et al., 1987; Missiuna & Pollock, 1991; Rast, 1986).

Cerebral palsy (CP) is described primarily as a permanent impairment affecting automatic postural control and movement as a result of a nonprogressive brain disorder (Bobath & Bobath, 1975; Moore, 1984). However, CP is better understood as a multiple disorder that may have impacts on several areas of development, including sensory processing, perception, cognition, and social–emotional relationships (Cruickshank, 1976; Erhardt, 1993; Moore, 1984). Cerebral palsy is most often classified according to the topographical distribution of tone and presence of abnormal movements. Categories of CP include spastic, which is further subdivided into quadriplegia, diplegia, and hemiplegia; athetoid, which can be further subdivided into nontension, dystonic, choreoathetoid, and tension athetoid; ataxia; flaccid hypotonia; and mixed type (Moore, 1984; Wilson, 1991). Children with CP are also classified according to the severity of the movement disorder and the presence of cognitive limitations. Therefore children diagnosed with CP constitute a heterogeneous group whose limitations in entering play diverge from one to another.

The current view of CP portrays the deficit as a sensorimotor disorder that affects the child's interactions with the environment, including exploration and function (Fetters, 1991). The nature of the disorder restricts play and overall development in two ways, reduced interactions affect the use of play as a context for learning and for practicing adaptive behaviors, and limited ability to enter into play restricts the experience of play as a spontaneous, intrinsically motivated, joyous activity.

This chapter emphasizes the need to incorporate play into the treatment and into the life of the child with CP. It stresses the importance of play as a context for learning as much as an intrinsically rewarding experience. The first part of the chapter addresses the limitations of CP and its impact on play; the second part addresses how to incorporate play into the treatment session and the life of the child. Sections of treatment sessions are utilized to depict each concept. Because play is a spontaneous, intrinsically motivated activity, most successful events described in this chapter were not planned and occurred "accidentally" during a treatment session. However, the successful resolution of the event depended on the therapist's ability first to recognize the potential of that activity; next, to follow the child's lead; and last to trust her skills to handle the process while suspending the

consequences of not following her plans for the time being. In other words, it required the therapist to enter into play "with" the child.

CHARACTERISTICS OF PLAY

Play is described in different ways. The most frequently cited views of play describe it as an activity which is intrinsically motivated and flexible (Bruner, 1972), enjoyable (Piaget, 1962), arousing (Ellis, 1973), active, spontaneous, and during which reality might be temporarily suspended (Singer & Singer, 1977). During the performance of daily occupations, elements of play are intertwined with functional tasks. For an activity to be considered play, it needs to have some of the characteristics just mentioned. The literature on play often attempts to make a distinction between play and work or play and drudgery. Drudgery, defined as "the enforced engagement in distasteful physical or mental effort to obtain the means of survival" (Pugmire-Stoy, 1992, p. 4), is considered the opposite of play. An activity is experienced as approaching play if it contains a greater share of play characteristics and less of drudgery.

With the child with CP, play and therapy are sometimes mutually exclusive activities. Rast (1986) states: "In the therapeutic setting, play often becomes a tool used to work toward a goal, despite the fact that the goal-oriented, externally controlled aspects of the therapy situation conflict with the essence of play itself" (p. 30). Pugmire-Stoy (1992) reinforces this point by writing that some of the "so-called 'play'" (p. 4) presented to handicapped children is closer to drudgery. Therefore, including the essence of play into the session can be a challenge. As clinicians, therapists tend to utilize play as a motivator or a context for learning adaptive skills; however, it is important to understand the value of play as a context for fun as much as a context for learning. Only by understanding this context for fun will therapists be able to promote intrinsic motivation, spontaneity, and the feeling of being able to actively direct one's own actions and have mastery over the environment. Thus a whole new dimension and potential can be added to the therapeutic process and the life of the child with CP.

In reference to the child with physical and/or cognitive impairment, play can be summarized as having three roles. The first role of play is as an important childhood occupation that provides context for learning and adaptation (Bruner, 1972; Bundy, 1992; Munoz, 1986; Reilly, 1974; Robinson, 1977). The literature that uses this view of play often emphasizes the assessment of developmental levels of play as valuable because it provides a "window" to the child's level of skill development (Casby, 1992; D'Eugenio, 1986; Fewell & Glick, 1993). This role of play views it as important because it serves a function of preparation for adult performance.

The second role of play described in the OT literature is as a reward or motivation instigating the child to interact with the environment and, thus, reach treatment objectives. This view of play often describes the use of appropriate toys, activities, and games to encourage active participation when using an neurodevelopmental treatment (NDT) approach in the treatment of CP (Boehme, 1987; Rast, 1986). Both the first and second views of play regard it as a means to an end or as an experience that serves a purpose: the first view of play regards it as serving the purpose of preparing the child for adult work performance; the second view of play regards it as having the immediate purpose of motivating the child to interact within the treatment session. Positioning during play (Diamant, 1992; Finnie, 1975) and adaptation of toys for the child (Batty, 1989; Langley, 1990) can be considered part of these traditions. In general these traditional approaches to play in the child with CP fail to explore fully the inherent worth of play itself and, instead, reinforce its role in the acquisition of functional skills.

Recent literature challenges this initial emphasis placed on play as a vehicle for learning skills for future performance (Caldwell, 1986) and explores another aspect of play by emphasizing the basic characteristics that define the quality of the experience as an end in itself (Bundy, 1993). Bundy (1993) describes a play–nonplay continuum based on the individual's perception of control, source of motivation, and suspension of reality and urges therapists utilizing a sensory integration (SI) approach to evaluate each activity in reference to this continuum. The need to assess each activity as providing the potential for play should also be used with other approaches (such as NDT) in the treatment of the child with CP. Being aware of these basic characteristics assures a better utilization of play as a context for the acquisition of treatment goals. However, fostering these characteristics in the child with CP is a challenge and, hence, is seldom observed in treatment. This chapter proposes that the purpose of incorporating play into treatment lies not only in its role in fostering the acquisition of functional skills but also in its role as an enriching experience in its own right. The role of play in the individual's development of a sense of mastery over the environment has been identified in the nonhandicapped child as well as in the child with CP (Bruner, 1972; Rast, 1986); however, play may also involve experiencing pleasure, learning to be flexible and spontaneous, and developing intrinsic motivation to participate in the decision making process, eventually leading to an increased perception of the self as capable of mastering the environment. This view of play incorporates play in the treatment session in the context of for fun as well as in a context for learning, within which all treatment activities are included.

Fostering play in the child with CP involves many factors. First, it requires understanding the child's limitations in movement, sensation–perception, and cognition. Second, it requires awareness of the limitations imposed on the child by the physical environment and the adult's predisposition to play. Third, it requires understanding the fundamental characteristics of the experience and the use of activities that may lead to it. The impact of these areas on play are described in the following section. As they read the following sections

therapists need to be aware that, regardless of the nature and extent of their limitations, children with CP often spontaneously rise above these to seek ways to engage in play.

LIMITATIONS IN THE CHILD WITH CEREBRAL PALSY

The multiple disabilities that accompany cerebral palsy interfere differentially with the child's participation in everyday tasks such as self-care, schoolwork, and play. Play as a context for learning and as a joyful activity is limited in children with CP. As a context for learning, play is limited primarily by the child's own physical challenges. Yet, as an enjoyable, spontaneous, intrinsically motivated activity, play is further limited not only by the disability itself but also by the limitations imposed by those surrounding the child. These limitations imposed by people and the environment are often more restrictive than the child's own physical handicaps. The child is often able to engage in spontaneous playful interaction that doesn't require the use of the less developed skills; however, people in the child's environment often unconsciously interfere with the expressions of these behaviors. The limitations both inherent and environmental are described fully in the following subsections.

Limitations in Movement

The movement limitations in the child with CP have been extensively described (Bly, 1983; Bobath & Bobath, 1975). The severity of these movement deficits have impacts on play in two ways. First, they affect the child's ability to access actively and thus explore the environment; second, once the child finds something that interests him or her, the movement deficits limit the potential to enter spontaneously into active play. These two factors affect the child's sense of mastery over the world. Children with severe movement disabilities have great difficulty engaging in activities for their sensorimotor pleasure. As this is the first expression of play observed in the child (Piaget, 1962), reduced exposure to this form of play may, in turn, further restrict the child's development of motor coordination in addition to affecting perceptual and cognitive development. Since play is also an arena that leads to mastery (Bruner, 1972; White, 1959), the inability to enter fully into play early in life may also affect the child's own perception of control over the environment and hence his or her development of intrinsic motivation. Simply stated, these children are used to "being done to" rather than "doing with" and may tend to perceive themselves as spectators rather than actors.

Older children who have movement deficits but no severe limitations in cognitive development are often able to enter into other forms of play through social interactions, fantasy play, and humor. Hence they may utilize their communication skills to initiate contact with others and feel that they have an impact on the environment. Play in those children with less severe movement deficits may also be significantly affected. Even when they may be able to ambulate and, hence, increase their accessibility to play materials, these children may exhibit various degrees of perceptual and cognitive limitations that confine their engagement in play. The play of children with mild movement disorders is often affected more by perceptual and cognitive deficits than by the movement deficit per se. Thus it is important when evaluating the play of these children to identify each limitation's impact on the experience of play.

Sensory Processing Limitations

Sensory and motor deficits presented by the child with CP have been often viewed as interrelated (Fetters, 1991; Moore, 1984). These sensory and perceptual deficits may occur secondarily to the movement limitations or may result from primary neurological damage (Moore, 1984). Sensory processing deficits presented by the child with CP affect play in different ways: first, they have impacts on the child's preference for certain play materials and activities; second, sensory processing deficits affect modulation and hence sustained attention. For instance, tactile discrimination and tactile modulation deficits have impacts on children's ability to obtain information about an object and hence influence their toy preference (Curry & Exner, 1988; Danella, 1973). This preference may mask motor as much as sensory–perceptual restrictions. Research studies as well as clinical observations indicate that multiply handicapped children exhibit a strong preference for vibratory toys (Danella, 1973) and for hard over soft toys (Curry & Exner, 1988). This preference for toys that provide distinct somatosensory inputs may indicate a sensory modulation problem that needs to be addressed during treatment.

Children who are able to move in space but exhibit vestibular modulation deficits may avoid moving equipment because of a hypersensitivity to movement and/or a gravitational insecurity. These sensory modulation deficits added to the postural limitations affect the child's active participation in treatment and on the playground.

Deficient visual perception may also affect the child's choice of play activity. Children with CP may not choose to play with toys that require refined perception of visual figure ground, spatial relations, or visual discrimination, such as puzzles, nesting toys, and construction materials. Although these areas may need to be addressed in treatment, they are not good choices for recreation or to foster autonomous play, at least not initially.

Sensory modulation deficits affect the child's ability to maintain an optimal level of arousal so attention and learning of new concepts can occur. Children with modulation deficits have difficulty engaging in play either because their arousal level is too low and interferes with active movement and motivation to participate or because it is extremely high and thus interferes with the child's ability to maintain attention on the play activity.

Limitations in Cognitive Abilities

Cognitive impairments are often described as accompanying cerebral palsy and may be more handicapping than the restrictions in movement. In children with severe spastic quadriplegia, intellectual level has been found to have a greater impact on the acquisition of early cognitive milestones than severity of physical limitations (Eagle, 1985). Consequently, in the child with both severe movement and severe cognitive deficits the cognitive limitations affect the development of play to a greater degree than do motor abilities.

Cognitive limitations may also affect the ability to enter into make-believe and fantasy play. During fantasy play the child replays the past and anticipates the future. Therefore fantasy play has impacts on the development of the capacity to anticipate practical consequences of actions (Singer & Singer, 1977). Children with CP may spontaneously enter in this form of play, whereas therapists and parents tend to focus on play with objects and may neglect to consider the value of make-believe or pretend play. This is an area that needs to be valued by the adult working with children.

Limitations in Environmental Interactions

In addition to the limitations that are inherent in a diagnosis of CP, the outside environment imposes physical and social restrictions that may be as confining as, or even more confining than, the disorder itself. The physical limitations include several factors of decreased accessibility: to materials, such as appropriate toys; to environments, such as recreational facilities; and to extracurricular activities that promote play, such as sports, drama, and art. Social barriers occur as a result of the imposition of others' values and beliefs, which limit social interactions. Physical limitations to recreational and leisure facilities in the environment are widely recognized. This section focuses on the limitations that occur in social interactions.

Limitations in Social Interactions. Social constraints on play are evidenced in the child's interactions with adults and peers. The influence of teachers, caregivers, and other adults in the development of play and other activities has been widely documented (Caldwell, 1986; Hanzlik, 1989, 1990; Kogan et al., 1974; Missiuna & Pollock, 1991; Shevin, 1987). Several external factors contribute to different patterns of activity and diminished play in children with CP.

First, because of the nature of the physical limitations, the child with CP needs more adult intervention to perform simple activities and spends more time interacting with adults than his or her nondisabled counterpart does. Caregivers often tend to overprotect the child and this adult interaction typically contains little play (Missiuna & Pollock, 1991). Furthermore, the amount of free time available is reduced because of the need for therapy (Missiuna and Pollock, 1991). These children usually participate in "tightly defined sequencing of objectives" and "tightly defined in-structural approaches" that do not allow much flexibility or spontaneity (Shevin, 1987, p. 237). This happens in the classroom and in other settings.

Finally, contributing to these factors, children with CP are exposed to attitudes toward play in which play is infrequent and not connected to the development of autonomy and self-direction (Shevin, 1987). Children with CP often demonstrate the intrinsic motivation and potential to enter into play, but they experience physical and environmentally imposed obstacles that result in different daily activity patterns compared to their nonhandicapped peers. When activity patterns of children with CP and spina bifida were compared to those of nondisabled children, the former exhibited specific differences from the latter. Children with CP and spina bifida spent more time in quiet recreation, dependent activities, and activities of personal care; and they spent less time in active recreation, activities away from home, and household tasks than the nondisabled children. Their activities were less varied and were often accompanied by social interaction (Brown & Gordon, 1987).

In summary, physically challenged children spend larger amounts of time in structured activities that may further constrict the sense of freedom necessary to explore the environment and engage in play. Additionally, they have decreased opportunity to make decisions about what to do, where to go, whom to be with, and how to do something. Hence this often results in a decreased belief that one may be able to act on the environment.

The impact of adult intervention on the experience of play in the child with CP may start early in life. Mother–infant verbal and nonverbal interaction may be the primary component of play. In this interaction with the caregiver, children learn to respond with cognitive, motor, and social adaptations (Hanzlik, 1990). In turn, the caregiver adjusts to and reinforces the child's responses, and hence infants and caregivers mutually contribute to the interaction (Hanzlik, 1990). If the child is unable to respond to these interactions adaptively, there is a risk for deviations to develop. These anomalies in the interactive process may affect the social, cognitive, and physical development of the infant (Hanzlik, 1990).

In addition, a professional's emphasis on the child's physical limitations indirectly affects the parent–child interaction in that the caregiver may overfocus on physical development and tend to neglect other facets of development (Kogan et al., 1974), including play. Professionals often teach parents about the importance of therapeutic intervention during the daily routine. This further constrains the parents' time and disposition to engage in spontaneous play (Hanzlik, 1989, 1990). The degree of physical limitations affects the interaction in such a way that it has been noticed that, over the years, parents tend gradually to decrease their affection during play and therapy sessions, particularly in those cases where children make less physical progress (Kogan et al., 1974).

Furthermore, the difficulties and frustrations experienced by the child with CP may cultivate apathy and withdrawal (Mogford, 1977) and thereby negatively affect interaction with other children (Missiuna & Pollock, 1991). Children

with CP have limited access to playing with nonhandicapped children unless it is carefully planned. This occurs because, first of all, there is still stigma attached to these children; second, their responses are slower and therefore affect the playful interaction. In addition, when these children have the opportunity to play with nonhandicapped peers, such as when they are placed in mainstream programs, interaction between these groups is seldom encouraged (Shevin, 1987).

It is a paradox that adults who know little about play teach children how to play (Caldwell, 1986). This certainly applies to children with CP. Caregivers, teachers, and therapists need to become more aware of not only the importance of play as a means to an end, but also of how to foster the child's intrinsic motivation to seek opportunities to experience play as a pleasurable activity in itself. Playful interaction among children with similar physical difficulties is limited by the presence of multiple disabilities and may need adult facilitation. The following example illustrates this point:

CASE EXAMPLE 1

Three parents carry their children, Sam, Jenny, and Rick, into the treatment room and place them on the mat. Sam and Jenny have a diagnosis of spastic quadriparesis, and Rick is diagnosed with spastic athetosis. They are unable to sit independently but can roll and creep. Soon after Sam is placed on the floor, he recognizes Rick and Jenny, smiles, and creeps toward them. His spasticity becomes more evident as he pulls his weight on his arms. When he reaches Jenny he says, "Hi" and looks around searching for Sarah, his therapist. Jenny, prone, hyperextends her head, smiles in response, but is unable to change her position. Rick attempts to catch Sam's attention by vocalizing but his sounds do not make clear words. Sam stays near them, smiling while he continues to wait for his therapist.

This description illustrates spontaneous interaction among children with CP. Sam approached the other children and initiated a potentially playful interaction. However, Jenny's and Rick's responses were limited to smiles and vocalizations and did not further evolve into a playful interaction, probably because the required movement adaptations were beyond their capabilities. Children with CP may initiate a playful interaction by reaching, smiling, or bringing a toy over to another individual; however, they tend to rely on the other person's expansion on this initial interaction. Therefore a group of children with similar deficits may have difficulty entering into a playful interaction together.

In summary, the play of a child with CP is restricted by the inherent limitations of the diagnosis and by sociocultural constraints imposed by others in the environment; however, these children possess the intrinsic motivation to enter into alternate forms of playful interaction. When serving these children, it is important to be aware of the nature of the disorders presented by the child and how these disorders interfere with the capacity to play. More importantly, therapists need to be aware of the adult's responsibility in either facilitating or inhibiting play.

THE ROLE OF PLAY IN TREATMENT AND EVERYDAY LIFE

As previously discussed, fostering play in the child with CP requires understanding the role of play in everyday life and how it is constrained by factors in both the child and the environment, including the adult's values and predisposition to play. Fostering play requires having appropriate play materials, play space, play time, and playmates (Pugmire-Stoy, 1992). However, since these elements are not enough to spark play in the child with CP, the adult needs to view him- or herself as a primary tool in facilitating play in treatment and everyday life.

Play in the Treatment Session

In the United States the preferred approach to treating movement disorder of the child with CP is NDT. Neurodevelopmental treatment's goals include increasing the child's functional ability through the facilitation of normal postural control and movement patterns. The purpose of NDT is to enhance functional performance by addressing the movement component of that performance. Although some authors believe play and NDT can be easily combined (Anderson et al., 1987; Erhardt, 1993), NDT's focus on postural adjustments during function requires much creativity so that the possibilities of entering into spontaneous play are not inhibited. The most often described relationships between NDT and play are depicted in Box 13-1. Play can be utilized during the treatment session to motivate the child to move by providing a meaningful context and distracting him or her from the therapeutic objectives; Anderson et al., 1987; Rast, 1986). Improved movement abilities gained during the NDT session in turn affect the child's potential to engage in exploration and free play outside the treatment session.

Traditionally, the use of NDT techniques did not provide room for a serious consideration of play in the treatment session. It is interesting to note, however, that although play was considered an important topic in occupational therapy treatment of the child with CP from early on (Craig & Hendin, 1951; Robinault, 1953), the introduction of NDT principles into the occupational therapy (OT) literature did not address the context of play (Fiorentino, 1966; Myzak & Fiorentino, 1961). Interest in play increased later after the NDT approach was firmly established among occupational therapists, and probably as

a result of the increased interest in play in the OT literature (Reilly, 1974). The view of play that evolved during the 1970s and 1980s has been described at the beginning of this chapter. It is this view that is expanded on now, in the 1990s. From this perspective, play has the following purposes in the treatment of the child with CP:

- As a motivator or reinforcer (often through the use of a toy or as promised time at the end of the session)
- As an arena or meaningful context where skills are acquired for future performance
- As an enjoyable, intrinsically motivated, spontaneous, process-oriented activity.

Caldwell (1986) proposes that "we have so overweighed our research toward play as a means to an end that we have lost the essence of what play means in the life of the young child" (p. 307). This section addresses all three uses of play but emphasizes the importance of the often neglected third use as the one that restores the essence of play into the life of the child with CP. To embrace this view in treatment therapists need to be able to distinguish among play as a motivator, play as context for acquisition of adaptive skills, and play as an intrinsically motivated, process-oriented activity.

Play as Motivator or Reinforcement. When play is utilized to serve the purpose of motivating the child to interact and participate in treatment, it is important to consider all the possibilities that it can offer. First, therapists need to make a differentiation between play and play materials and how to utilize the materials and space to their maximum potentials. Second, therapists need to be aware that if they are to use play as motivation, they need to allow play time during the session. Third, therapists need to consider that there are other forms of play that may be more productive than forms of play requiring the child to use fine motor manipulation. Finally, therapists need to discourage some common practices during treatment.

Play materials. In reference to the first point, play materials refer generally to toys. The sensorimotor toys used in therapy are often not conducive to play but have been chosen by therapists to affect motor coordination and other deficit areas. Hence, they are seldom regarded as play by the child. (Fig. 13-1 *A* and *B*). When asked whether he wanted to play with some coordination toys while waiting for his mom, Sam, a 5-year-old child with spastic diplegia, emphasized this point by saying: "No. That is not fun; that is work!" If therapists want to encourage play rather than solely functional motor performance through the use of an educational "toy," then they need to pay attention to the way they utilize space and toys. Even when they utilize colorful and attractive spaces and materials, the most difficult challenges for clinicians are finding a toy that addresses both the therapist's goals and the child's motivation and interests and treating the child without having total control over the space in which he or she plays. In the therapeutic setting, clinicians often sacrifice motivation for therapeutic value and transform play into a vehicle for meeting motor goals. For exam-

<table>
<tr><td>Box
13-1</td><td>THE RELATIONSHIP BETWEEN PLAY
AND NDT</td></tr>
</table>

Play as motivation → NDT treatment → impacts on movement → ability to play

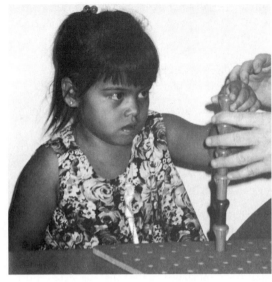
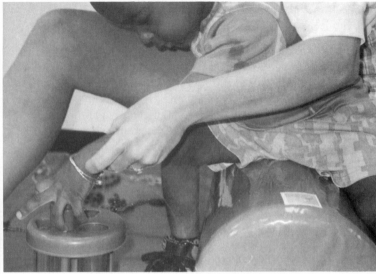

FIG. 13-1 A and **B,** The use of coordination toys to facilitate reach, grasp, release and trunk control. The use of these activities may or may not be considered play by the child.

ple, therapists control the toys the child uses and the space that the child can explore. Exploration often leads to play; however, in the child with CP, the need to use positioning equipment in the home and classroom often restricts that possibility (Graham & Bryant, 1993). In treatment, handling of the child should take place during free exploration and should not be limited to a confined space (Fig. 13-2 A, B & C). The following case example illustrates that point.

CASE EXAMPLE 2

The treatment room is large and inviting. There are colorful balls, rolls, and toys on the blue mats. A therapist, Marcie, treats Mark, an attractive 3-year-old boy with spastic diplegia. His mother sits nearby with the younger sibling. Mark lies prone on the mat, his head rests on his arms. Upon a request from the therapist, he raises his head and begins to move slowly toward her. He stops and rests. His muscle tone is low but increases when he attempts to move in space. His movements are slow and ponderous. All of a sudden his younger sibling runs by him to get a toy. Mark raises his head eagerly, follows her movements with his head and chases her by pulling on his arms and creeping in her direction. As he moves, his muscle tone increases and flexion is observed in his body. The therapist calls him and asks him to stop and instead come to her. Mark stops, yet ignores the request to creep back. Marcie approaches him and helps him sit on a red bolster. Mark has little control over his movements. His balance is poor and he tends to use his arms for support.

Marcie places a ring stack in front of him and asks the youngster to reach. He attempts to reach slowly and with difficulty, his trunk is slouched, his head is laterally tilted and he leans on his hands against the bolster. The therapist wonders whether the activity is too demanding and changes the child's position. He now side-sits against the bolster. Marcie then shows him a book; she plans to maintain his attention and work on his sitting balance by pointing to the pictures in the book. At first Mark appears interested in the book, but he soon slouches against the bolster and leans his head on his upper extremities as he looks around the room.

In this example Mark indicated little intrinsic motivation to engage in the sensorimotor activities presented to him. However, he did appear interested in the other child moving around him. The therapist's goals included the development of postural control to participate in functional activities. At this point in treatment, it might have been more beneficial to use the other child as a playmate to motivate Mark to maintain an erect position. In this case the use of sensorimotor play materials was too demanding and not motivating enough for the child.

If therapists want to encourage genuine play rather than motor performance with an educational "toy," then they need to pay attention to the toys they provide. The choice of appropriate toys to encourage active participation during treatment has been extensively documented (Ayrault, 1977; Musselwhite, 1986). The choice of toy depends on the purpose of play. Toys are chosen for their educational and therapeutic value or for their recreational value (Tebo, 1986). Therapeutic toys are chosen based on the needs of the child, yet recreational toys are chosen to facilitate independent play and are based on the child's acquired skills and motivation. When choosing a toy, it is necessary to consider the features inherent in the toy (safety, durability, degree of structure offered by the toy, responsiveness of the toy, and the motivational value of the toy), the age appropriateness of the toy, and the therapeutic value of the toy (Musselwhite, 1986).

The toys for children with severe movement deficits need to be carefully chosen. Sometimes commercially available toys can be adapted so that their responsive nature is enhanced and can be easily triggered by the child's limited movements. The more severely involved child often chooses to play if the toy is colorful and produces dramatic rewards for simple movements (Mogford, 1977). In reference to the therapeutic value of toys, children with fluctuating muscle tone benefit from toys that are heavier and offer resistance

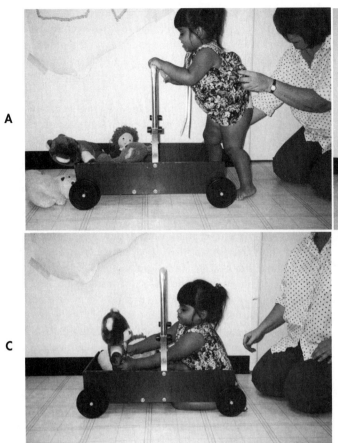

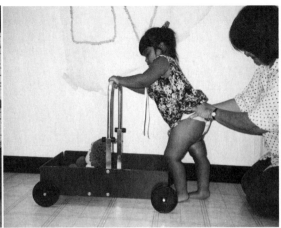

FIG. 13-2   A, A carriage with dolls can motivate the child to move. **B,** In some cases (see right knee) adequate body alignment is lost in the enthusiasm of performing the activity. **C,** In other cases the child's motivation to play may take momentary priority over the treatment goal.

because they facilitate proximal stability and increase sensory feedback (Boehme, 1987). Children with hypertonicity need toys that are lighter and offer some unpredictability because they facilitate greater ranges of movement and decrease the tendency to fixing (Boehme, 1987). Toys that require less precise manipulative skills, such as textured play dough, action toys, stickers, magnetic toys, rice, brushes, and shaving cream or foam may also prove to be appropriate choices for most children (Fig. 13-3). Toys that do not have rigid, preset rules and that allow flexibility may increase motivation to participate and enhance the child's feeling of mastery over the material.

Play time. In reference to the use of play time as a reinforcer, therapists need to be careful not to banish it consistently until the end of the session. If play is used to reinforce a specific action, then it needs to be consistently allowed at some point during the session, not necessarily at the end. In the classroom setting, the timing of the free-play activity at the end of the day, before lunch, or after a class period makes it particularly vulnerable to interruption and postponement (Shevin, 1987). The same occurs in the therapeutic session. Play time allowed only at the end of the session may carry the message of decreased importance and lack of regard for what the child deems important.

Different forms of play. Different forms of play include fantasy play, social interactions, and sensation seeking. These are sometimes more powerful sources of motivation than manipulation of toys. The incorporation as playmates of other children, who may or may not have a disability, into the treatment session with the purpose of motivating movement, active participation, and social interaction can often prove to be enriching (Fig. 13-4).

Practices to be discouraged. A habit that needs to be discouraged is the use of toys as lures to prompt the child to participate. For example, therapists often display a toy to instigate a specific movement such as reach or ambulation; however, when the child is close to the promised toy, therapists automatically move it further away so that a more perfect movement or a longer sequence of movement is forthcoming. These practices lead to decreased motivation and decreased active participation on the part of the child.

A further practice that needs to be discouraged is the introduction of a toy that requires manipulation while facilitating a gross motor skill such as balance. Although it is important to facilitate movement within a meaningful context, in everyday life people seldom perform activities that require simultaneously gross motor and fine motor–perceptual and cognitive effort. It may be more beneficial to encourage fantasy play, as in pretending and storytelling, rather than forms of play that require fine motor manipulation when working on the development of gross motor skills. Later, once the new gross motor skill is developed, therapists can incorporate it into forms of play that require reach, grasp, release, and fine motor manipulation.

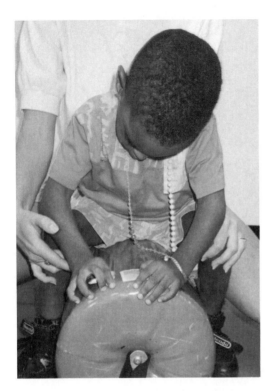

FIG. 13-3 This 4 year old expressed interest in playing with stickers. The therapist accommodated her treatment goals (weight bearing) to include this activity in the treatment session.

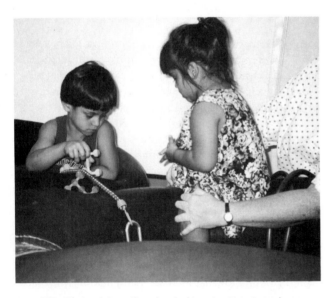

FIG. 13-4 Interactive play during a treatment session.

An additional practice that needs to be discouraged is that of repeating the same activity several times consecutively. For example, when utilizing toys such as construction toys, puzzles, blocks, or action figures, therapists sometimes ask the child to place pieces into a container or put a puzzle together. Once the child performs the activity successfully, the therapist dumps the pieces out and asks the child to repeat the activity. This habit may be effective in facilitating a

desired movement; however, it takes perceived control away from the child and reinforces the child's perception of lack of mastery over the environment. If play, rather than toys, is used to motivate the child, then it is necessary to consider alternate forms of play and the use of playmates to enhance the experience.

In summary, when utilizing play as a motivator therapists need to consider several aspects, such as the treatment goal, the child's motivation and interest in play, and the role of play and toys in the session. Once these points are clarified, the therapist can move on to incorporate play by manipulating the materials, the space, the use of peers, and the timing of the interactions with people and objects.

Play as Context. Play has been described as an activity that provides context to the development of adaptive skills (Munoz, 1986; Rast, 1986; Robinson, 1971; Sparling et al., 1984). In one way, this view of play considers it to be useful in the service of the development of motor, cognitive, and social skills for future use, rather than as a purely enjoyable experience. The playful activity is still chosen for its educational and/or therapeutic value. However, this view also recognizes play as a valuable activity with distinct characteristics and not just as a reward or motivation for some other goal.

When thinking about play as a context (for developing functional skills), the therapist needs to understand that the child's and therapist's purpose, and therefore how the activity is viewed by both parties, may differ. Activities that appear to be enjoyable to the adult may not be considered play by the child. All functions performed by children are not play; however, many activities can be spontaneously transformed into play. A treatment session may be transformed into play by allowing the child to choose an activity, be spontaneous, and have fun. Activities can be transformed into play by the child's willingness to enter an enjoyable world in which reality is momentarily suspended and the goal of the activity is the performance of it. Hence, even when the therapist's motivation is to incorporate play for the acquisition of specific developmental skills, taking into consideration the child's perception of play increases the probability of the child's full participation. This point is elaborated further in the next section.

The use of play as context for NDT techniques can now be discussed in reference to the impact of recent findings in motor control theories. These findings are based on an ecological approach that views the actor and environment as inseparable in the acquisition of skills (Gliner, 1985). They emphasize the need for a treatment environment that is "critical in eliciting the type of action (movement if you will) that is adaptive" (Fetters, 1991; p. 222). Hence the goal of the therapist is to create an environment with "opportunities for normal, or at least preferred movement patterns" (Fetters, 1991, p. 222). The recent findings in motor control theories advocate teaching motor problem solving skills using a less "hands on" approach. This line of reasoning suggests that the therapist should elicit child self-initiated movement and active exploratory experiences while considering environmental restrictions and musculoskeletal constraints, the child's motivation, opportunities to practice abilities, and opportunities to develop effective compensations when necessary (Fetters, 1991; Gliner, 1985). This chapter proposes that, in such a model, play provides a relevant context for the acquisition of skills. Play proves to be pivotal as a motivating, freely chosen activity during which the therapist can elicit active movement and exploration, the child can develop problem-solving skills and strategies in a task-oriented context, and the child can practice newly acquired skills.

Principles of motivation and environmentally relevant activities are central to theories of occupational therapy and were long ago incorporated in sensory integrative treatment (Ayres, 1972; Gliner, 1985). However, they are only recently being emphasized as part of the treatment of motor skill for the child with CP. The findings in motor control theories emphasize the importance of context-relevant, self-initiated movement, not only as a concern for the occupational therapist but as a concern for other professionals working with the child as well. Box 13-2 summarizes the considerations for using play in treatment for the child with CP. These considerations are discussed in detail in the following sections.

Play as an End in Itself. Incorporating play into the treatment session and the life of the child with CP requires understanding the characteristics and essence of play. The basic components of play that can be incorporated into treatment are:

1. Spontaneity in starting, changing, or ending an activity. For the child, spontaneity may lead to increased variability of behavioral responses and may have an impact on creativity (Singer & Singer, 1977).
2. Intrinsic motivation to initiate, create, or be part of an activity. Fostering intrinsic motivation may enhance the child's sense of control.
3. Ability to suspend reality, which may affect the child's motivation to participate in treatment activities.
4. Enjoyment of the process rather than focusing on the end product. This may increase active participation.
5. Active participation either physically, cognitively, or socially. This will affect learning and overall performance.
6. Increased arousal. Play can be used to increase arousal level and, hence, can be incorporated into treatment. Level of arousal has an impact on the child's attention and active interaction with the environment.

These concepts are next described in relationship to the use of play as motivator, as context, and as enjoyable activity.

Spontaneity. Freedom to be spontaneous is often inhibited by physical limitations. When therapists evaluate play, children are often placed in an inviting environment in which they are encouraged to play spontaneously. Sheridan (1975) refers to the importance of systematic observations of spontaneous play in handicapped children. These observations often yield valuable information about the child's ability to self-organize to interact with the environment.

Levitt (1975) describes the interactions of cerebral palsied children with an adventure playground designed to

---

Box 13-2	CONSIDERATIONS: PLAY IN TREATMENT

CONSIDERATIONS—PLAY TO MOTIVATE PARTICIPATION
Use of materials and space
- Features of the toys: safety, motivational
- Structure provided, responsiveness
- Age appropriateness
- Therapeutic value: treatment goals

Use of play time
Use of playmates
Use of multiple forms of play
- Social interaction
- Sensory input
- Fantasy (suspension of reality)

CONSIDERATIONS—PLAY AS A CONTEXT FOR THE DEVELOPMENT OF ADAPTIVE SKILLS
- Therapist's treatment goal
- Child's motivation to participate

CONSIDERATIONS—PLAY AS AN END IN ITSELF
- Intrinsic motivation
- Spontaneity
- Enjoyment
- Suspension of reality
- Active engagement—sense of control
- Increased arousal

---

stimulate motor and sensory experiences. In this situation children demonstrated two types of behaviors. On the one hand, the opportunity for the child to move spontaneously allowed an opportunity to practice movements that were already established in therapy. Some of these behaviors included movement skills that were rarely possible in the school, clinic, or hospital setting. On the other hand, children regressed to lower levels of motor ability if the play activity was overly demanding yet highly interesting (Levitt, 1975). These are important considerations in treatment as the child who engages in spontaneous play may need additional support so he or she progresses to the next level of motor development rather than regressing to previous ones.

The role of the adult in encouraging spontaneity is pivotal. Spontaneity can be incorporated during the treatment session by being less directive and providing activities that are flexible, with rules that can be bent or that allow modifications. Puzzles and coordination toys do not allow for a great deal of spontaneous behavior. On the contrary, they follow preestablished patterns and discourage the child from spontaneously choosing to end or prolong activity as she or he sees fit.

Intrinsic motivation. Being intrinsically motivated requires having basic ideas of how to interact with objects and space. Because of motor and other limitations, children with CP do not have much freedom to choose and carry out a task. In addition, adults seldom provide these children with the opportunity to express their opinion and/or select among several alternatives. Their very structured daily routines greatly reduce the possibility to express intrinsically motivated behavior. When children with CP are asked to choose between several alternatives, they often respond, "I don't know." Intrinsic motivation may be hindered by several factors: cognitive limitations that affect the development of new ideas, physical limitations that may limit the choices, and finally, externally produced limitations set by caregivers and other adults for the child at home, school, and in therapy.

Recent findings in motor control research emphasize the importance of motivation in task performance and in the treatment of CP (Giuliani, 1993). The use of sensory integration principles in conjunction with NDT provides a useful frame of reference to facilitate intrinsic motivation. Intrinsic motivation can be fostered during the treatment session by providing choices of activities and encouraging decision making. Hence, the environment and the therapist need to be flexible to allow for it.

CASE EXAMPLE 3

Erika, a 4-year-old girl diagnosed with spastic diplegia, received occupational therapy once a week in a setting that served multiple diagnoses and utilized several treatment approaches. The treatment goals included facilitation of sitting balance, shoulder flexion against gravity, and bilateral activities. Erika was inquisitive; she often asked what the other children were doing and tended to prefer to observe the other children instead of playing with the play dough, puzzles, blocks, and stickers that the therapist presented to increase her perceptual–motor skills.

On one occasion Erika appeared particularly uninterested in the activities she was asked to choose from, and she looked up at the glider and asked the therapist whether they could do that. Although this had not been one of the choices given to Erika, she appeared to have her heart set on doing that activity. The therapist realized that hanging from the glider could trigger increased spasticity in the lower extremities; plus, Erika's hands were not strong enough to hold the weight of her entire hanging body. At that point, the occupational therapist decided that as long as one of her goals was to facilitate upper extremity movement above her head in conjunction with active trunk extension against gravity, she could try to do just that by holding Erika up in her arms so she could reach for the glider. When the child reached, the therapist, still problem solving, lowered her hands to Erika's lower extremities and maintained these in abduction to avoid an abnormal extensor pattern. Erika laughed as she moved in space holding onto the glider, and she then "fell" into a pillow. After that she sat on the bolster and continued happily with the perceptual–motor activities provided by the therapist.

This vignette illustrates how the child's intrinsic motivation to perform an activity was respected and encouraged by the therapist. Making this a successful activity required physical and mental effort from the therapist. The activity itself lasted at most a minute; however, the memory of the experience stayed with Erika. On subsequent sessions Erika continued to choose some of the activities that she wanted to perform. Some of these activities worked well with the treatment goals; other were cut short by the therapist because they facilitated increased tone and abnormal posturing and

therefore conflicted with some of the treatment goals. Erika did not mind having some activities eliminated as long as she could choose others.

It is important to emphasize that during the treatment session both functional tasks and playful experiences are important. Both work and play are part of the lives of people and both need to be incorporated into the treatment without always considering one at the expense of the other. The vignette about Erika illustrates how therapist and child negotiated an agreement that allowed for both work and play.

Suspension of reality in fantasy play. Fantasy play requires the individual to be able temporarily to suspend reality and its consequences. The ability to suspend reality and enter a makebelieve world has an important role in the child's development and it may contribute to creativity (Singer & Singer, 1977). Fantasy can be used throughout a treatment session to motivate a child or to encourage him or her actively to use creative thought processes. Clinicians are sometimes not aware of the value of social interaction and fantasy play as assisting treatment sessions. The following case example illustrates that point:

CASE EXAMPLE 4

A summer storm starts as Luisa, a physical therapist, is ready to begin the treatment session with Johnny. She is aware that Johnny is extremely sensitive to noise and therefore very afraid of the storm that is coming. At first Luisa hopes that the child will not notice that it is getting darker and that the rain is coming harder. When the child expresses his discomfort, she knows that the session may be over unless she figures out how to distract him from the whole situation. Luisa decides to enter into fantasy with the child as she tells him a story that she makes up as the thunder and rain are coming down. She explains that this is just a party happening somewhere in the sky. The angels are having fun, and they are getting mighty rowdy. The noise of thunder is interpreted as barrels of soda that they are rolling down to be refilled, and the lightning occurs because the angels are quite mischievous and play with the lights. The entire storm is translated into the angels having a merry good old time!

Johnny enters into the story by asking about each sound that he hears: "Is that a barrel rolling down?" or "Are they dancing?" The session continued successfully and Johnny had a good time. Both therapist and child viewed the time as meaningful: for the child the meaning was provided by the story telling; and for the therapist the meaning was derived from the success of the treatment activity.

In this vignette fantasy play was used to shift attention and motivate the child to stay with the activity while the therapist continued to facilitate postural control. Luisa entered into fantasy play as a way to distract the child; however, she unconsciously incorporated all the elements that make play an end in itself: she was spontaneous, she respected the child's intrinsic motivation to participate in the making of the story and thus did not control the outcome. The storyline suspended reality, and they had fun while doing it. Fantasy play could also have been utilized to encourage a creative thought process by having the child create the story himself. In that case play would have been used as motivator, as context, and as an intrinsically motivated joyous activity in its own right.

Closely related to fantasy and creativity is the use of educational drama and educational art to foster development in physically challenged children. Sparling et al. (1984) report the use of controlled experience of drama and art with 14 physically challenged children. Their findings suggested that art and drama had a significant effect on cognitive, social–emotional, motor, language, and activities of daily living (ADL) performance, with drama having a greater effect on the first three areas and art having a greater effect in the last three areas.

Fantasy play can be used to encourage the child to suspend reality and use creative thought processes. Some games that can be used during the session and that encourage active participation by the child include alternate storytelling. In this situation the child and the therapist take turns making up a story. Each of them needs to adapt to the changes made by the previous person and is required to continue the story. Other less demanding incorporation of fantasy play is the use of hats, jewelry, and social games that incorporate the ability to pretend (Fig. 13-5 and 13-6). Children with CP often enjoy treating a doll on a ball. One might view this behavior as an illustration of the major emphasis in their lives.

Fun and enjoyment. To increase the child's enjoyment of a task, it is important to include activities that are process oriented rather than end product or goal oriented. The consideration of an activity as process oriented or as end product oriented is ultimately determined by the person performing the task: the child. For example, for some children the process of making a picture is fun, for others the same pleasure is derived from the completed task, and for others it may simply be drudgery. If the process is a chore, the pleasure of the completed picture may not be enough to make the activity fun. It is difficult to find sensory motor activities that are fun for the child with CP. As previously mentioned,

nonstructured materials such as play dough, water, and bubbles allow the child to have fun while manipulating the material. Social play and action toys such as dolls, cups, and cars also allow some freedom and enjoyment (Fig. 13-6). Activities that provide enhanced sensory input such as playing in the sand or water, swinging, and pounding play dough are often enjoyable and process oriented (Fig. 13-7, *A* and *B*).

In the treatment of children with CP therapists tend to provide play activities that address their movement limitations. Hence these are seldom considered fun and are seldom chosen by the child. But the child may choose to repeat an activity because it is fun, and this activity may prove to bea useful context for practicing specific skills. Practicing newly acquired skills increases the child's motor ability and provides a sense of mastery that may increase pleasure derived from the activity.

Increased arousal. The incorporation of play as an activity that increases arousal can be accomplished through the use of sensory input. This input can be utilized to modify the child's arousal level and hence facilitate attention. Play is often described as an activity that is sought because of its arousing qualities (Ellis, 1973), as when children twirl and swing. The child with CP may be limited in his or her search for an arousing experience. In treatment, a session can be started with some arousing play experience that has been transformed to meet the treatment goals.

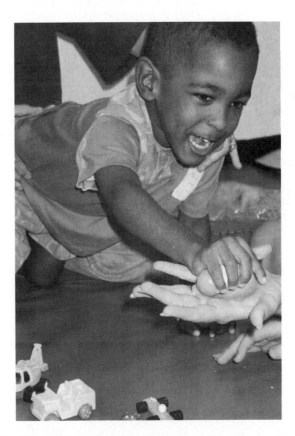

FIG. 13-6 Little people, cars, and other social toys are sometimes less demanding and more motivating for the child. Most functions that can be facilitated with a coordination toy can be performed with action toys.

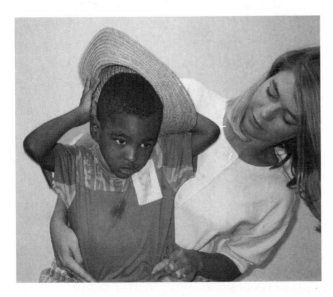

FIG. 13-5 Hats can be used during fantasy play to facilitate head control and upper extremity reach.

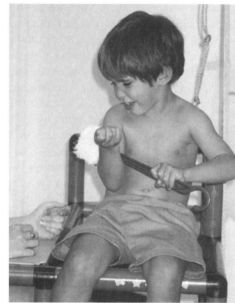

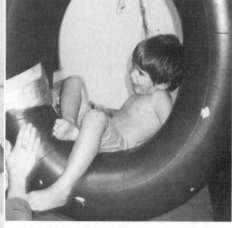

FIG. 13-7 The integration of equipment that provides sensory input such as brushes (**A**) and swings (**B**) assists in preparing the child's arousal level and motivation to actively engage in an activity.

CASE EXAMPLE 5

Brian, a 5-year-old child with spastic hemiplegia, had been treated for most of his life. The treatment goals included improving postural control, hand skills, and visual–motor coordination. On one occasion, the treating clinician noticed that he became more cooperative after he entered an arousing play activity that involved tactile input. They called it "Ninjas." In this game Brian was the Ninja Turtle and the therapist was "Shredder" or the "bad guy." Each carried a long handle brush that could be used to brush the other's feet. The big treatment balls and bolsters lying around the treatment room became the obstacles that needed to be sorted out while running away. Both therapist and child can chase each other. During this activity, Brian, who was usually inattentive and tripped often, was able to maneuver through most obstacles in space, go up and down ramps, and maintain his balance while climbing onto equipment (Fig. 13-8, *A, B,* and *C*). This activity was performed for a short time; however, the increased arousal that occurred during that time affected Brian's ability to attend and he was able to participate more actively in the subsequent tabletop activities.

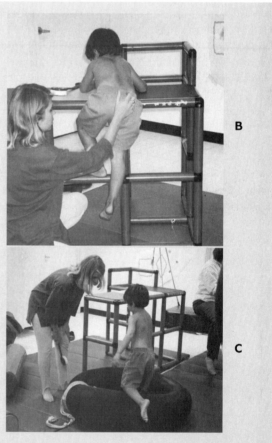

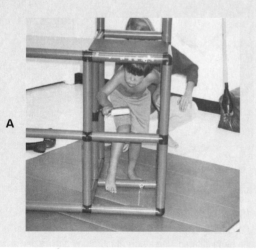

FIG. 13-8 **A** and **B,** Children are often motivated to participate in active games (role playing Ninja Turtles, Power Rangers, etc.), which can be used to facilitate movements in space while negotiating obstacles. **C,** The use of tires and large equipment can encourage balance, upper extremity weight bearing, and active movements in space.

Encouraging Independent Play and Recreational Activities

The ultimate goal of encouraging play during school and treatment sessions is to enhance the child's motivation to engage independently in play. Yet external factors such as the daily routine and the physical environment may need to be modified for play to occur outside the controlled environment. Fostering play outside the structured environment requires offering the child the opportunity to have appropriate play materials, play space, play time, and playmates (Pugmire-Stoy, 1992). Box 13-3 summarizes the areas to consider when fostering play outside the treatment area.

In reference to play materials when fostering independent play, it is important to have a selection of novel material and/or toys available for the child. Toy lending libraries offer the opportunity to have a large selection of toys and games from which the child can choose (Munoz, 1986). Sometimes the materials must be adapted to meet the needs of the child. When independent play is to be facilitated the selection of play materials needs to relate to the everyday environment, such as playing in the snow, piling and jumping into leaves, and splashing water (Musselwhite, 1986). Toys for independent play may also

> ### Box 13-3 FOSTERING PLAY OUTSIDE THE TREATMENT AREA
>
> **PLAY MATERIALS**
> - Type of toys
> - Toy variety (construction, sociodramatic, etc.)
> - Need for adaptive toys
> - Toy lending libraries
>
> **PLAY SPACE**
> - Consideration of distractions
> - Seating and positioning
> - Adapted playgrounds
> - Backyard activities
>
> **PLAY TIME**
> Individual and with others
> - At home
> - Play dates
>
> In the community and with others
> - Art classes
> - Theater productions
>
> **PLAYMATES**
> Non–physically challenged children
> - Siblings and neighbors
> - Classmates (in mainstreamed program)
>
> Children with similar difficulties

need to be more responsive and easier to handle than those that are used with adult guidance. In summary, the choice of materials should allow the child to explore, master, and control.

Play space includes having a specific space for the child to play. The space and the materials should allow for novelty and surprise. In some cases the child needs to be offered novel environments and allowed to explore space freely. In other instances he or she may need positioning equipment to engage in play. Play space includes adapted playgrounds, adapted backyards, and adapted ways to explore the community as an alternative for the child. Children with physical disabilities can enjoy outdoor activities such as gardening, nature walks, picnics, and animal husbandry if a few adaptations are made (Greenstein et al., 1993). Occupational therapists need to assume an active role not only in adapting the child's playground but in planning community playgrounds (Stout, 1988).

Even when children with CP have busy routines that do not allow for free time to engage in spontaneous play, play time needs to be scheduled during the day. It may be free time before dinner, scheduled time with a friend, or time for a recreational activity such as an art class. Some schools plan a theater production in which parents and children participate. Such a program provides an opportunity for the parents, teachers, and children to engage in potential play.

When considering playmates the possibility of playing with nonhandicapped siblings, neighbors, and friends can prove to be an enriching experience for the child with CP and the playmates. Socially inclined children may enter more easily into play when other children are present. Other children may prefer to observe peers rather than enter into play with them. Nonhandicapped children offer better role models of spontaneous play behavior than adults. Yet, when the child with CP participates in a mainstream special education program, this interaction is seldom encouraged by teachers and other adults (Shevin, 1987).

The Role of the Adult in Facilitating Play

Adults play a pivotal role in enhancing or inhibiting the child's capacity to play (Jones & Reynolds, 1992; Musselwhite, 1986; Newson & Head, 1979). In the case of the child with CP, adults may have to take a more active directive role in encouraging the child to interact actively with the environment (Newson & Head, 1979). However, the adult may also sometimes need to just have an inviting role in encouraging play. Therefore, when fostering play therapists need to take into consideration their own readiness to allow play to occur, the role in it they take, and the tactics they utilize to facilitate play (Musselwhite, 1986). Musselwhite (1986) and Jones and Reynolds (1992) identify several roles taken by the adult during play with the child. These roles can be summarized as follows:

- *The stage manager.* The adult takes the responsibility to provide the time and arrange the physical environment so it invites play (Jones & Reynolds, 1992). This is the role often taken by preschool teachers and therapists utilizing an SI approach.
- *The mediator.* The adult assists in child-to-child and child-to-physical world interaction by modeling problem-solving skills during play (Jones & Reynolds, 1992). This approach is often utilized by occupational therapists when taking into account the context of play to problem solve a situation.
- *The director.* The adult takes a very active role in getting and maintaining the child's attention and interest in play, demonstrates specific skills and behaviors, and controls the playful interaction between two children or between the adult and the child (Jones & Reynolds, 1992; Musselwhite, 1986). This role may be taken by therapists when working with children who are severely limited and when utilizing play as a context for learning adaptive skills.
- *The observer.* The adult does not enter into play but sits back, takes notes, and analyzes the situation (Jones and Reynolds, 1992; Musselwhite, 1986). This role is utilized by the therapist during the assessment of play skills.
- *The player.* The adult enters into play with the child. Deciding to assume this role depends on the adult's preferred style of interaction, the child's need for challenge, and the child's ability to sustain play (Jones & Reynolds, 1992). Both adult and child may act as equal partners, taking turns in the interaction. The adult may have to initiate an interaction but then encourages the child actively to participate and respond (Musselwhite, 1986). The biggest risk of adopting this role is the risk of taking over the interaction, especially if this role is adopted from the beginning and the child is not given a chance to develop his or her own play. Adopting this role may enhance the content of play and enrich the relationship between adult and child (Jones & Reynolds, 1992). We need to strive for this last role when inviting the child to enter into play as a spontaneous, intrinsically motivated behavior.

Adults in the environment of children with CP may be inhibiting play for several reasons: because they do not believe it is important; because they do not know what to do to enter into play with the child; or because they are overeager to facilitate it. In a study of children's participation in the adventure playground, Levitt (1975) described the adult's behavior as overeager to have the child enjoy the visit. When adults are overeager to foster a successful experience they may act too fast and not allow the child to explore a given situation fully.

When Nothing Works

The treatment sessions described in this chapter illustrate how difficult it can be to have genuine play during treatment. When the activity is unsuccessful the following questions can guide the clinical reasoning process:

1. In reference to the therapists' views of play:
   a. How do they value play? What are their biases about the child's play?
   b. Are they cueing into the child's verbal and nonverbal messages about interest and motivation? Even when these motivations are weakly expressed, or their expression is severely limited?
   c. Once they have cued into the child's motivations, are they willing to be flexible enough to change the process (not the goals) of the therapeutic interaction?
   d. Are they willing to work with someone else's idea? Are they open to surprise?
   e. Are they accepting of multiple outcomes—which may not be what was initially planned?
2. What roles are they taking when facilitating play (i.e., stage manager, director, observer, or facilitator)?
3. Is the activity at the child's motor and cognitive developmental level?
4. Is the appropriate amount of sensory input being provided to the child? Is low arousal level affecting muscle tone and drive to explore the environment?
5. Is the activity structured in such a way that the meaning is eliminated, for example, in repetition of manipulative tasks?

SUMMARY

Play in the child with CP can be used as motivation, as context to promote competence, and as spontaneous, enjoyable activity. This chapter emphasizes the importance of understanding the characteristics of play and the role of the adult in promoting play in the child with CP. For that to occur, play must be considered not only a means to an end but also an end in itself.

REVIEW QUESTIONS

1. The author discusses the roles of play in normal development. Consider how these roles are relevant to the child with cerebral palsy.
2. Consider how limitations in movement, sensory processing, cognition, and environment may have an impact on the play of the child with cerebral palsy. How may treatment address each of these types of limitations?
3. Contrast the ways in which play is used in treatment as a motivator, as a context for skill acquisition, and as a process-oriented activity.

4. Describe considerations that need to be made when selecting toys for children with severe movement deficits.
5. How may the therapist encourage spontaneity and enjoyment in the play of the child with cerebral palsy?
6. What are the roles that adults may take on when facilitating play? Under what circumstances are the roles typically assumed?

REFERENCES

Anderson, J., Hinojosa, J., & Strauch, C. (1987). Integrating play in neuro-developmental treatment. *American Journal of Occupational Therapy. 41*(7) 421-426.

Ayrault, E. W. (1977). *Growing up handicapped—A guide for parents and professionals to helping the exceptional child* (pp. 97-107). New York: A Continuum Book/The Seabury Press.

Ayres, A. J. (1972). Sensory integration and learning disorders. Los Angeles, CA: Western Psychological Services.

Batty, J. (1989). Making disabled children smile is as easy as flipping a switch. *OT Week*, Feb. 23, 1989.

Blair, E., & Stanley, F. (1985) Interobserver agreement in the classification of cerebral palsy. *Developmental Medicine and Child Neurology, 27,* 615-622.

Bly, L. (1983). The components of normal movement during the first year of life and abnormal motor development (monograph). Chicago, IL: Neurodevelopmental Treatment Association.

Bobath, K., & Bobath, B. (1975). *Motor development in the different types of cerebral palsy.* London: William Heineman Medical Books.

Boehme, R. (1987). *Developing mid range control and function in children with fluctuating muscle tone.* Milwaukee, WI: Boehme Workshops.

Brown, M., & Gordon, W. A. (1987). Impact of impairments on activity patterns of children. *Archives of Physical Medicine and Rehabilitation, 68,* 828-832.

Bruner, J. S. (1972). The nature and uses of immaturity. *American Psychologist, 27,* 687-708.

Bundy, A. C. (1992). Play: The most important occupation in children. *Sensory Integration Special Interest Section Newsletter, 15,* 1-2.

Bundy, A. C. (1993). Assessment of play and leisure: Delineation of the problem. *American Journal of Occupational Therapy, 47,* 217-222.

Caldwell, B. (1986) The significance of parent-child interaction in children's development. In A. W. Gottfried & C. Caldwell Brown (Eds.). *Play Interactions—The contributions of play materials and parental involvement to children's development.* Proceedings from the eleventh Johnson and Johnson Pediatric Round Table (pp. 305-310). Lexington, Mass.:Lexington Books.

Casby, M. W. (1992). Symbolic play: Development and assessment considerations. *Infants and Young Children, 4*(3), 43-48.

Craig, H. L., & Hendin, J. (1951). Toys for children with cerebral palsy. *American Journal of Occupational Therapy, 5*(2), 50-51.

Cruickshank, W. M. (1976). The problem and its scope. In W. M. Cruickshank (Ed.). *Cerebral palsy—A developmental disability* (3rd ed.). Syracuse, NY: Syracuse University Press.

Curry, J., & Exner, C. (1988). Comparison of tactile preferences in children with and without cerebral palsy. *American Journal of Occupational Therapy, 27,* 457-463.

Danella, E. A. (1973). A study of tactile preference in multiply-handicapped children. *American Journal of Occupational Therapy, 27*(8), 457-463.

D'Eugenio, D. (1986). Infant play: a reflection of cognitive and motor development. In *Play a skill for life* (pp. 55-66). Rockville, MD: The American Occupational Therapy Association, Inc.

Diamant, R. (1992). *Positioning for play—Home activities for parents of young children.* Tucson, AZ: Therapy Skill Builders.

Eagle, R. S. (1985). Deprivation of early sensorimotor experience and cognition in the severely involved cerebral-palsied child. *Journal of Autism and Developmental Disorders, 15*(3), 269-283.

Ellis, M. J. (1973). *Why people play.* Englewood Cliffs, NJ: Prentice Hall.

Erhardt, R. (1993). Cerebral palsy. In H. Hopkins & H. Smith (Eds.). *Willard and Spackmans's occupational therapy* (8th ed., pp. 430-458). Philadelphia: J.B. Lippincott.

Fetters, L. (1991). Cerebral palsy: Contemporary treatment concepts. In M. Lister (Ed.), *Contemporary management of motor control problems—Proceedings of the II STEP Conference.* (pp. 219-224). Fredericksburg, VA: Bookcrafters.

Fewell, R. R., & Glick, M. (1993). Observing play: An appropriate process for learning and assessment. *Infant and Young Children, 5*(4), 35-43.

Finnie, N. (1975). *Handling the young cerebral palsied child at home.* New York: E.P. Dutton and Company.

Fiorentino, M. R. (1966). The changing dimension of occupational therapy. *American Journal of Occupational Therapy, 20*(5), 251-252.

Gliner, J. (1985). Purposeful activity in motor learning theory: An event approach to motor skill acquisition. *American Journal of Occupational Therapy, 39*(1), 28-34.

Graham, M., & Bryant, D. (1993). Developmentally appropriate environments for children with special needs. *Infants and Young Children 5*(3), 31-42.

Greenstein, D., Miner, N., Kudela, E. & Bloom, S. (1993). *Backyards and butterflies—Ways to include children with disabilities in outdoor activities.* Ithaca, NY: New York State Rural Health and Safety Council.

Giuliani, C. A. (1991). Theories of motor control: New concepts for physical therapy. In M. Lister (Ed.) *Contemporary management of motor control problems* (pp. 29-35). Proceedings of the II Step Conference. Fredericksburg, VA: Bookcrafters.

Hanzlik, J. R. (1989). The effect of intervention on the free-play experience for mothers and their infants with developmental delay and cerebral palsy. *Physical and Occupational Therapy in Pediatrics, 9*(2), 33-51.

Hanzlik, J. R. (1990). Interaction between mothers and their infants with developmental disabilities: Analysis and review. *Physical and Occupational Therapy in Pediatrics, 9*(4), 33-47.

Heriza, C. (1991). Motor development: Traditional and contemporary theories. In M. Lister (Ed.) *Contemporary management of motor control problems—Proceedings of the II STEP Conference* (pp. 29-35). Fredericksburg, VA: Bookcrafters.

Jones, E., & Reynolds, G. (1992). *The play's the thing . . . Teachers roles in children's play.* New York: Teachers College Press.

Kogan, K. L., Tyler, N., & Turner, P. (1974). The process of interpersonal adaptation between mothers and their cerebral palsied children. *Developmental Medicine and Child Neurology, 16,* 518-527.

Langley, M. B. (1990). A developmental approach to the use of toys for facilitation of environmental control. *Physical and Occupational Therapy in Pediatrics, 12*(4), 69-91. (Special issue on rehabilitation technology.)

Levitt, S. (1975) A study of gross motor skills of cerebral palsied children in an adventure playground for handicapped children. *Child: Care, Health and Development, 1,* 29-43.

Missiuna, C., & Pollock, N. (1991). Play deprivation in children with physical disabilities: The role of the occupational therapist in preventing secondary disability. *American Journal of Occupational Therapy, 45*(10), 882-888.

Mogford, K. (1977). The play of handicapped children. In B. Tizard & D. Harvery (Eds.). *Biology of play* (pp. 170-184). London:Spastics International.

Moore, J. (1984, May). The neuroanatomy and pathology of cerebral palsy. Selected proceedings from Barbro Salek Memorial Symposium. *Neurodevelopmental Treatment Association Newsletter,* pp. 3-58.

Munoz, J. P. (1986) The significance of fostering play development in handicapped children. *Play a skill for life—A monograph project of the Developmental Disabilities Special Interest Section of the American Occupational Therapy Association* (pp. 1-11). Rockville, MD: The American Occupational Therapy Association.

Musselwhite, C. R. (1986). *Adaptive play for special needs children.* San Diego, CA: College-Hill Press.

Mysak, E., & Fiorentino, M. R. (1961). Neurophysiological considerations in occupational therapy for the cerebral palsied. *American Journal of Occupational Therapy, 15*(3), 112-117.

Newson, E., & Head, J. (1979). Play and playthings for the handicapped child. In J. & E. Newson (Eds.). *Toys and playthings* (pp. 140-158). New York: Pantheon Books

Piaget, J. (1962). *Play, dreams and imitation in childhood.* (C. Gattegno & F. M. Hodgson, Trans.). New York: W. W. Norton. (Original work published in 1951).

Pugmire-Stoy, M. C. (1992). *Spontaneous play in early childhood.* Albany, NY: Delmar Publishers.

Rast, M. (1986). Play and therapy, play or therapy. In *Play a skill for life—A monograph project of the Developmental Disabilities Special Interest Section of the American Occupational Therapy Association* (pp. 29-41) Rockville, MD: The American Occupational Therapy Association.

Reilly, M. (1974). Defining a cobweb. In M. Reilly (Ed.), *Play as exploratory learning—studies of curiosity behavior* (pp. 57-116). Beverly Hills, CA: Sage Publications.

Robinault, I. P. (1953). Occupational therapy technics for the pre-school hemiplegic—toys and training. *American Journal of Occupational Therapy, 7*(5), 205-207.

Robinson, A. (1977). Play: the arena for acquisition of rules for competent behavior. *American Journal of Occupational Therapy, 25,* 281-284.

Sheridan, M. D. (1975). The importance of spontaneous play in the fundamental learning of handicapped children. *Child: Care, Health and Development, 1,* 3-17.

Shevin, M. (1987). Play in special education settings. In J. H. Block & N. R. King (Eds.). *School play—A source book* (pp. 219-251) New York: Teachers College Press.

Singer, D., & Singer, J. (1977). *Partners in play—A step by step guide to imaginative play in children.* New York: Harper and Row.

Sparling, J. W., Walker, D. F., & Singdahlsen, J. (1984) Play techniques with neurologically impaired preschoolers. *American Journal of Occupational Therapy, 38*(9), 603-612

Stout, J. (1988). Planning playgrounds for children with disabilities. *American Journal of Occupational Therapy, 42*(10), 653-657

Tebo, S. E. (1986). Evaluating play selection and its possible effects on play behaviors of children with severe mental impairment. In *Play a skill for life* (pp. 13-25). Rockville, MD: The American Occupational Therapy Association, Inc.

White, R. W. (1959). Motivation reconsidered: The concept of competence. *Psychological Review, 66,* 297-333.

Wilson, J. (1991). Cerebral palsy. In S. K. Cambell (Ed.). *Pediatric Neurologic Physical Therapy* (2nd ed.) (pp. 301-360). New York: Churchill Livingstone.

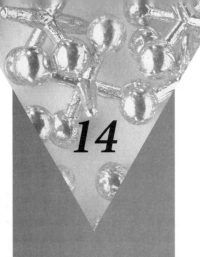

14

ACCESSING PLAY THROUGH ASSISTIVE TECHNOLOGY

Jean Crosetto Deitz and Yvonne Swinth

Adrienne, a 3 year old with spinal muscular atrophy, whips across her preschool playground in a shiny yellow car with black roll bars. She's chasing Jason, who rides a red tricycle. Her teacher holds a remote control, a safety feature designed so that she can stop the car with a flick of a switch and, if necessary, redirect the car.

Thomas, a toddler with cerebral palsy, hits a big red switch to activate a tape player. He smiles and attempts to sing as his favorite song plays.

Jennifer, a high school student with juvenile arthritis, plays a video adventure game with a friend. They are taking a break during an annual staff meeting. Jennifer is an expert at using her computer to design graphics for the high school yearbook.

All of these children lack most of the motor skills of their typically developing peers. However, technology helps to equalize the environment, allowing them to play both alone and with others. It provides them with opportunities to participate in play or leisure activities and socialize in the same settings as their peers without disabilities.

Although there are many definitions of play, most include the concept that play is "an activity voluntarily engaged in for pleasure" (Simon & Daub, 1993, p. 118). Play is one of the primary occupations of childhood, and Simon and Daub (1993) contend that through play "the child learns to explore, develop, and master physical and social skills" (p. 118) and to adapt within his or her environment and culture. According to Piaget (1952), play and cognitive development are interdependent, with play fostering the child's competence in his or her world; however, for some children, because of a disability the ability to play is compromised. The result may be frustration, unsuccessful experiences, and ultimately learned helplessness.

Brinker and Lewis (1982) maintain that an important competence of young infants is the "ability to detect and utilize cooccurrences" (p. 1). Since infants with impairments—"Loss or abnormality of cognitive, emotional, physiological, or anatomical structure or function…" (U.S. Department of Health and Human Services, 1993, p. 33)—have difficulties in utilizing these cooccurrences, further impairments may result. This in turn may lead to disability, or the "inability or limitation in performing tasks, activities, and roles to levels expected within physical and social contexts" (U.S. Department of Health and Human Services, 1993, p. 33).

219

According to Cotton (1984), play helps a child learn to cope with frustration, anxiety, and failure. Consider the difference between repeated failure when there is no chance of success, for instance, an 8-year-old boy with severe motor impairments trying to move the pieces in a chess game. No matter how hard he tries, success is never achieved. By contrast, consider the same child equipped with a computer, software for playing chess, and an alternative access system he can use successfully. This enables him to compete as an equal with able-bodied peers, experiencing and learning to cope with anxiety when questioning the advisability of a given move, and the frustration of thinking a move is ideal and then experiencing failure when an opponent announces checkmate. Although some efforts bring realistic frustration and failure for the child, every effort doesn't bring failure. Practice has the potential of leading to favorable moves and experiences of success. These experiences can help the child learn the joy and benefit of involvement and acquire skills in coping effectively with realistic frustration (Fig. 14-1).

Missiuna and Pollock (1991) distinguish between primary and secondary forms of play deprivation experienced by children with physical disabilities. According to these authors, primary forms of play deprivation refer to those play experiences the child is deprived of because of impairments. For example, consider the child with a visual impairment who will not have the opportunity to play with mixing colors when painting. Regardless of the intervention, this primary form of play deprivation will remain unchanged. By contrast, secondary forms of play deprivation occur when no analogous forms of play are substituted for play experiences the child is deprived of because of impairment. In the previous example, a toy or device that allows the child to mix sounds instead of colors could allow the child to control the play and participate in a creative process. The failure to provide such alternative forms of play is believed to be related to learned helplessness and dependence. According to Missiuna and Pollock, children who are unable to experience normal childhood play because of impairments "may encounter secondary social, emotional, and psychological disabilities" (1991, p. 883), many of which could be avoided through the use of alternative play experiences. Often, in such cases, assistive technology can enable children with disabilities to engage, either independently or with their peers, in alternative forms of play.

ASSISTIVE TECHNOLOGY

An assistive technology device is "any item, piece of equipment, or product system, whether acquired commercially off the shelf, modified, or customized, that is used to increase, maintain, or improve functional capabilities of individuals with disabilities" (H.R. Rep. No. 100-819, 1988). These devices are available on a continuum ranging from low to high technology. Although there is no clear distinction between low and high technology, generally, as assistive technology becomes more complex it is considered high technology. This typically includes computers, some alternative or augmentative communication systems, environmental control systems, and power mobility devices. By contrast, low technology solutions tend to be less complex (e.g., simple devices to stabilize toys, large fasteners on doll clothes, or nonelectronic communication aids). If selected with care, technology, whether low or high, can empower children with disabilities so they can maximize their potential to engage in play activities and other developmentally appropriate occupations.

The specific toy adaptations and devices described in the following sections are used as examples. The clinician should be reminded that numerous other options exist; new technologies are being developed daily, and when considering the use of assistive technology, responsibility for being knowledgeable about current devices lies with the clinician.

Enhancement of Play Through Simple Toy and Environmental Adaptations

Occupational therapists often use simple toy and environmental adaptations to enable children with disabilities to play. Typically these solutions are low cost, low maintenance, readily available, and limited only by the imaginations of the therapist and those working with the child with a disability. In many cases, some of the best low-technology solutions have been envisioned by children with disabilities and their families. Examples of low-technology solutions are Velcro fastenings on doll clothes so that the child can engage in symbolic play (make-believe); jigs and other stabilizers (i.e., using Dual-Lock™ [Ablenet, Inc.]) on wheelchair lap tray surfaces and on the backs of toys to stabilize play materials; and handles on pieces of puzzles and board games. Also, for children with fine motor difficulties, some play materials can be enlarged and, for others, handles on play materials with special grips can be designed. Adaptations and/or careful

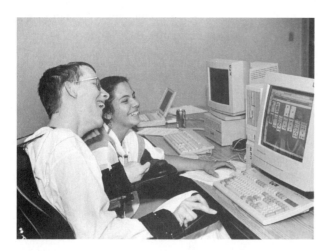

FIG. 14-1 Teens use a computer to play cards. (Courtesy Mary Levin, DO-IT Project, University of Washington, Seattle, WA.)

selection of riding toys also can enable a child with a disability to participate in play with his or her peers that would not be possible using many of the traditional toys (e.g., tricycles, scooters, bicycles). For example, for a child with lower extremity limitations, riding toys propelled by arm movements rather than leg movements could be considered; for a child with poor trunk stability, a tricycle seat could be adapted to provide additional support; and for a child experiencing difficulty with keeping his or her feet on the pedals of a tricycle, straps could be added.

For creative ideas on simple adaptations specific to outdoor activities for children with disabilities, refer to *Backyards and Butterflies* (Greenstein, 1993). According to the author, most of the ideas in her book were developed by rural parents to enable their children to enjoy and participate in outdoor activities. The solutions presented apply predominately to the home environment and are relatively inexpensive, homemade assistive technology solutions. Included are creative designs for a wheelchair-accessible plant table; adapted handles for gardening supplies (hoses, trowels, etc.); special carriers for garden tools; adapted fishing poles; accessible bird feeders; spillproof containers for holding wildflowers; easily accessible insect houses; custom-made horseback riding aids; adaptations for large toys with wheels (i.e., tricycles, bicycles, wagons); and safe and accessible swings and slides. In addition, Greenstein (1993) deals with accessibility in the berry patch; caring for animals; and backyard design including factors such as porches, ramps, fences, and picnic tables. Though these solutions were contributed predominately by parents in rural environments, many are equally applicable to children living in cities.

Other simple technology solutions involve the use of toys with switches. Typically, these toys run on batteries and when activated they produce action, sound, visual effects, and/or tactile sensations (e.g., vibrations). Examples of toys with switches are monkeys who clang their cymbals; dogs that bark, wag their tails, and roll over; trains that travel around tracks chugging and periodically whistling; and a variety of busyboxes. Some switch-activated toys can be purchased in toy stores and no adaptations are required; others can be purchased with switches designed for children with disabilities (e.g., Ablenet, Inc.; Toys for Special Children); and still others must be adapted. An example of the former is "Shout 'N' Shoot" (Cap Toys), a voice-activated, head-mounted water gun. Jean Isaacs describes use of this toy by her 10-year-old son, Forrest, who uses a wheelchair for mobility and has limited motor control (Isaacs, 1994). Once the gun was strapped to Forrest's head and the microphone was positioned he was able to participate independently in a water-gun party, soaking peers by looking at them and making a sound.

Numerous resources are available to assist therapists and parents with the process of using and making switches (Glennen & Church, 1992; Parette et al., 1986; Williams & Matesi, 1988; Wright & Nomura, 1991). Also, most battery-operated toys can be easily adapted for switch use via a Battery Device Adapter™ (Ablenet, Inc.). This device is cost effective and can be used with multiple battery-operated toys and games. A listing of addresses of the manufacturers of products and other resources mentioned in this chapter can be found in Appendix 14-A.

Appropriate application of toys with switches has several strengths. First, compared to higher technology solutions, they are relatively simple and in many cases make it possible for the child to access developmentally appropriate toys. Most important, involvement with this type of toy is useful for the chronologically or developmentally young child because it enables the experience of cooccurrence between the child and the environment. Drawing on Piaget's work, Brinker and Lewis postulate that cooccurrences act on the child in four ways:

> First, cooccurrences orient the organism to attend to the environment. Second, they arouse the organism and help to modulate its state. Third, the detection of cooccurrences leads to a positive affective tone. Fourth, through the operation of memory, they become the aliments for subsequent intentional actions and ultimately for the development of mental structure. (1982, p. 3)

Therefore these toys are highly appropriate for children starting in substage 3 (4 to 8 months) of the sensorimotor period, during which time children repeat acts involving objects outside of themselves. In the early stages, toys and switches can be carefully selected and designed so that gross, random movements produce a result. For example, a large switch, sensitive to lower extremity movement, could be placed under the feet of a child with a severe motor impairment. When the child moves the lower extremities, the switch would activate a music box. As the child matures and develops a beginning understanding of cause and effect, more complex toys can be employed that are activated by more complex access systems such as multiple switch arrays or joysticks. Also, as the child develops, toys need to be changed often and should be selected for providing variety. Examples are a tape recorder that plays favorite songs or stories and a remote control car that can be driven at a variety of speeds and in a variety of directions. Through playing with switch-operated toys, children may develop basic skills in such areas as object permanence, cause–effect relationships, and directionality. In addition, they begin to learn that the surrounding environment can be controlled. Since many children with limited motor control are unable to manipulate toys independently at the appropriate stage in development, switch toys can provide a viable alternative, allowing them to play and explore similarly to their peers who are not disabled (Swinth & Case-Smith, 1993).

Use of toys with switches has limitations, and therapists are cautioned to avoid misuse. First, for most children developmentally beyond 18 months to 2 years, many of the toys that can be activated with switches are repetitive and become boring after the first few times of use. Second, many of these toys typically provide limited opportunities for creativity. Third, use of a variety of switch toys can become costly.

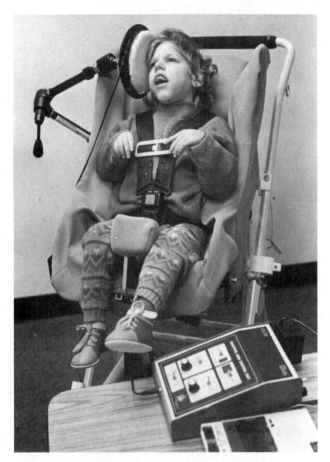

FIG. 14-2 A child uses a switch to activate a tape recording of her favorite music. (Courtesy Bruce Terami.)

Therefore, switch toys are most appropriate for use with very young children or as transitional toys leading to play facilitated through higher technology solutions involving computers, communication augmentation systems, environmental control systems, and power mobility (Fig. 14-2).

Enhancement of Play Through Computers

Computer use for play or leisure is becoming increasingly common in most school and some home environments. Children who are typically developing as well as those with disabilities are being introduced to computers at younger ages. The computer, combined with thoughtfully selected access systems and software, can enhance play or leisure experiences in three ways. First, it can provide simulations of experiences that would be difficult, if not impossible, for the child to engage in without the computer. For example, a child with severe motor impairments may never be able to experience the excitement of a game of chase and capture on the playground or in the neighborhood. However, the chasing and capturing can be simulated through computer games, with resultant excitement and intense involvement. Second, the computer and related software provide a variety of play or leisure opportunities unique to the modality

(e.g., interactive stories with audiovisual flexibility, adventure challenges or mysteries involving problem solving). Provided the child with the disability can access the computer, the child can engage in these play or leisure activities as an equal with peers and adults. Third, the computer and related software can be used to facilitate play between children with and without disabilities. This was demonstrated by Spiegel-McGill et al. (1989). These researchers used a single-subject alternating treatments design to study the effect of three play conditions (microcomputer play, remote-controlled robot play, play without technology) on the amount of time each of four preschoolers with disabilities interacted with a peer who was socially competent and without disabilities. All of the children were in an integrated preschool. Findings from this study suggested that microcomputers facilitated social interaction for the two children with significant social and language deficits and physical disabilities. However, for the two children with only mild social interaction deficits, the microcomputer did not appear to enhance social interaction with peers without disabilities.

One of the primary benefits of the computer as an assistive device to enhance play is that it is highly adaptable in terms of both methods of access and types of play activities available through software. With children with disabilities, computer access systems often need to be selected and modified to meet individual needs. Some children cannot use the computer via the standard keyboard or the mouse and as a result require an alternative access system such as the Adaptive Firmware Card for Apple computers or the Ke:nx™ for Macintosh computers (both available from Don Johnston Developmental Equipment, Inc.). These types of devices allow for alternate input methods to meet a wide range of physical access needs. Categories of computer access include (1) physical keyboard adaptations, such as changes to the standard keyboard and expanded or minikeyboards; (2) virtual keyboards such as Morse Code input, voice input, and on-screen keyboards; and (3) mouse emulators such as the Headmaster (Prentke Romich Company), the Headmouse (Madenta Communications Inc.), and the Touch Window (Edmark Corporation). It is important to remember that these alternative access systems are not necessarily compatible with all software selected to enhance play. Some access systems, such as the Muppet Learning Keys (Sunburst Communications), work only with specially designed programs, whereas others are compatible with most standard programs. This latter group, known collectively as keyboard and mouse emulators, allows for input from a source other than the standard keyboard or mouse to be interpreted as input from either of these sources. Therefore, before an access system is purchased compatibility with software the child is likely to use needs to be evaluated (Fig. 14-3).

In addition to being adaptable in terms of access, the computer is ideal because of its adaptability to the types of play activities available through software. These programs range from being extremely simple and appropriate for use with very young children to being highly complex and challenging

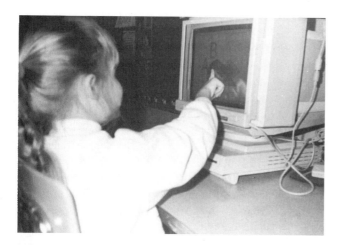

FIG. 14-3   A child uses a computer with a Touch Window (Edmark Corporation) to play a simple game.

for precocious teens. Examples of the former are *Baby Smash* and *Switches, Pictures and Music,* both of which are public domain, cause–effect software operated by a single switch. When using *Baby Smash* via a switch a child adds graphics (e.g., lightning bolts, circles) to the computer screen while the computer concurrently plays music or makes a sound. Switches, Pictures and Music, plays a series of common children's songs such as "BINGO" and "I'm a Little Teapot," while simultaneously displaying a face that alternately winks and smiles at the child. In all, 60 percent of the 20 typically developing 6- through 8-month-old infants in a study by Swinth et al. (1993) demonstrated ability to access the computer to play successfully an adapted version of the latter cause–effect program. Adaptations involved shortening the time the music played following switch activation so that infants had to reactivate the switch to continue playing.

Examples of highly complex programs are SimCity Classic (Maxis) and Myst CD (Broderbund). SimCity Classic allows participants to create and run their own city including houses, roads, people, etc. Myst involves the participant in exploring, solving riddles, and looking for treasures in a three-dimensional world. Because these games require deductive reasoning, involve dealing with abstract and hypothetical situations, and necessitate organizing and systematizing, they are appropriate for preteens and teens at Piaget's formal operations stage of development.

Between these extremes are a variety of programs for children with a diversity of interests and at various developmental levels. There are programs such as *KidPix* (Broderbund) that allow a child to use the computer as a crayon or paint brush to "color" or "paint" a picture; CD ROM programs such as *Grandma and Me* and *Arthur's Teacher Trouble* (Broderbund) that encourage a child to interact with the program as a story is being told; and public domain programs such as checkers and solitaire that allow a child to play board and card games, either alone or with a peer. This flexibility is important as the child develops and his or her interests and capabilities change.

Another benefit of the computer is that via the internet a school age child or teen can access more of the world. This capability is particularly beneficial for individuals with severe motor or sensory (e.g., blind, deaf) impairments. Randy Hammer, a teen who is blind, exemplifies effective use of the internet for educational and recreational purposes (Hammer, 1994). Relative to the latter, Randy described using the internet with a screen reader to browse through the newspaper, selecting articles to read for enjoyment. In addition, he described telneting to chat systems to "talk to people in California about the earthquakes there" or to "ask people in Kansas City about the Chiefs' chances in the Superbowl" (Hammer, 1994, p. 25). He further stated that chat systems provide a way to "make new friends" (Hammer, 1994, p. 25).

Enhancement of Play Through Augmentative and Alternative Communication Systems

Communication, both verbal and nonverbal (e.g., gestures, signs), is an important part of play for children. If communication is compromised by impairments, this can limit children's opportunities to engage in play and other relevant occupations. When this occurs, the use of augmentative or alternative communication systems should be considered and the final selection should reflect the child's communication needs. Carefully selected augmentative or alternative communication systems can make it possible for children with communication impairments to engage in a variety of play and leisure activities such as participating in a game of Simon Says with neighborhood children, engaging in the necessary interactions required for playing a board game with a friend and sharing stories with peers at lunch.

Augmentative and alternative communication are modes of communication such as gestures, sign language, and aids that do not require oral language skills (Church, 1992; Glennen, 1992). The distinction between augmentative and alternative communication is that the former supplements, enhances, or supports oral communication, whereas the latter replaces it (Lewis, 1993). The possibilities for alternative or augmentative communication are numerous. Many children start with simple communication boards or picture exchange systems (PECS). The former typically are boards displaying pictures, letters, words, or word symbols and the child communicates by pointing or looking at the desired picture or symbol. Picture exchange systems allow a child to initiate "a communicative act for a concrete outcome within a social context" (Frost & Bondy, 1994). For example, a child using the PECS might give a picture of a desired item or activity to another child or adult in exchange for that item or the opportunity to engage in the activity. These simple types of communication systems can facilitate play.

More complex, high-technology solutions involve computerized systems that are operated through special software (Lewis, 1993). Some high-technology solutions, referred to as dedicated systems, involve microcomputers that can only be operated as communication aids (Lewis, 1993). Examples of these are the Liberator (Prentke Romich Co.) and the Dynavox (Sentient Systems Technology, Inc.). In other cases, portable microcomputers are adapted for use as augmentative or alternative communication aids. In either situation, choices exist in terms of access and output methods. For access, both direct selection (e.g., pointing directly to the desired symbol) and scanning may be considered. For some children, direct selection is facilitated with special aids such as mouthsticks or light beam pointers. Scanning, by contrast, is an indirect selection process whereby the user is presented with communication aid symbols (i.e., letters, pictures) until the user indicates that the selected symbol is his or her desired choice (Glennen, 1992). Output methods for high-technology systems vary and can be spoken (i.e., taped speech, synthesized speech), printed, or a combination of both spoken and printed.

Use of communication systems can be frustrating for both the receiver and the speaker for three primary reasons. First, these systems can be difficult to learn to use; second, synthesized speech can be hard to understand; and third, communication using any type of system takes longer than speaking. As a result, selection of an alternative or augmentative communication system for a child or teen should take into consideration both the needs of the user and the anticipated communication partners. For example, if communication partners are likely to be very young children or individuals with poor reading skills or vision, then a system with spoken output should be considered as opposed to one that exclusively provides printed output. By contrast, if the primary communication partner has a hearing impairment, printed output may be preferred. It also is important to teach communication partners (even very young children) strategies to facilitate interaction with the individual employing a communication system. With children this can be incorporated with play in such a way that communication via the system augments play, and play using the system ultimately enhances communication skills.

Enhancement of Play Through Environmental Control Systems

As previously noted, one of the ways children play is by interacting within their environments. For children with disabilities, such opportunities can be severely limited. However, with the use of environmental controls, possibilities for an increased variety of play and leisure activities become available. Environmental control systems can be simple, involving minor adaptations to one appliance in the home, or they can be complex, involving elaborate control systems and multiple appliances. Whether simple or complex, such systems can make it possible for children to engage in activities such as turning lights on and off, activating a stereo or television, talking on the telephone, and helping to cook in the kitchen. When considering environmental controls it is first necessary to determine what parts of the environment it is appropriate and possible for the child to control and what parts of the

environment the child desires to control. This requires evaluating the child's environment and daily routine as well as the functional capabilities and motivation of the child. For instance, it is important to know whether the child enjoys music, stories on tape, cookie baking, or television programs. Typically, young children start with single-switch systems that allow them to participate in such activities as "helping mom" mix cookies by being in charge of turning the mixer on and off. As the child progresses developmentally, more complex environmental control systems, many of which are microprocessor controlled, can be employed to allow the child or teen to operate multiple appliances (i.e., television, computer, stereo, lights) using a single system. Use of such systems, whether simple or complex, can help children increase their functional independence and their ability to participate in a broader range of play and leisure activities than would be possible without environmental controls.

Enhancement of Play Through Mobility Devices

Movement is integrally tied to play at all stages of development. Children in the sensorimotor stage of development move (crawl, creep, walk, and run) for the pure pleasure of the experience and as a means of exploring their environments. As the children grow older, movement continues to be an important component in their play. On playgrounds, preschoolers can be observed chasing each other, negotiating playground equipment, and riding toys with wheels. As children reach school age, games requiring movement become more complex in terms of skills required and rules for participating. At all stages of development, if a child's movement is compromised by impairments, there is a need to explore alternative methods of mobility for engagement in play and leisure activities.

The literature supports the introduction of power mobility to young children (20 months and above) with motor impairments for two reasons (Butler, 1986; Butler et al., 1983, 1984; Douglas & Ryan, 1987; Wright & Kohn, 1993). First, it is an attainable skill for young children that can partially compensate for gross motor movement limitations. Second, it appears to be associated with an increase in self-initiated behaviors, especially those related to spatial exploration. Butler (1986) observed that onset of a passive, dependent pattern "coincided with failure of the normal development of locomotion about 12 months of age, and was increasingly manifested as inhibited locomotion progressively interfered with normal childhood activities" (p. 325). Therefore, it seems desirable to explore alternative mobility options as soon as a child's impairment impedes his or her mobility. Some options involve low technology (see Case Example 1: Infant), whereas others require high technology. The Transitional Power Mobility Aid, the Maddak Inc. award winner at the 1994 American Occupational Therapy Association (AOTA) National Conference, is an example of the latter. This device is designed for children 1 through 6 years (up to a maximum of 45 pounds or 42 inches in height). Created as a transitional device for power mobility, it was designed for indoor use in home and school settings and has a power base and an adjustable frame allowing for growth and for positioning in sitting, semistanding, and standing (Javernick, 1994). Using up to four switches or a joystick, a child can experience self-initiated exploratory mobility and can physically interact with the environment. Advantages of this mobility device are its small size and design features that facilitate access to preschool tabletops and positioning on a level with peers. Wright and Kohn (1993) described use of this device in a mainstreamed preschool classroom by a 3-year-old child with a diagnosis of spinal muscular atrophy, type II. This child had a power wheelchair but would not use it in the classroom because "it positioned her above the level of her peers, and she could not access table top activities" (Wright & Kohn, 1993, p. 29). By contrast, after the first day the Transitional Power Mobility Aid was introduced into the child's classroom, the child moved independently from one tabletop activity to another and her teachers reported an increase in her interactions with peers. This suggests that an important consideration in choice of a mobility device is positioning of the child, both in relationship to aspects of the environment that the child wants to access and in relationship to peers (Fig. 14-4).

A variety of power mobility devices designed for children and teens are currently available and new options are being developed regularly. To facilitate play and leisure involvement, when a power mobility device is selected, activities in which the child or teen currently wants to engage and potential future activities should be considered in relationship to design features. For example, an early school age child whose primary concern is vertical positioning might prefer a mobility device such as the Chairman Robo™ (Permobil). The Chairman Robo™ resembles a small forklift with the child independently being able to control the vertical position of the seat from an on-floor position to 28 inches from the seat to the floor. This requires the addition of a seat elevator. This ability to control the vertical position of the seat enables the child to play on the floor with peers; to be positioned appropriately at school desks, dining tables, etc.; and to access play materials on shelves of varying heights. However, this strength needs to be balanced against potential limitations. Its predecessor, the Turbo, was noted as having a relatively large turning radius and a slow maximum speed (Deitz et al., 1991). In making a final selection, the child, family, and interdisciplinary team should weigh these and other variables and often are required to establish priorities since one device typically does not meet all needs.

Other options that have been employed successfully for young children, as either transitional mobility devices or as toys, are electric cars available in toy stores. These have the advantages of being relatively low in cost (typically under $200 for the car without adaptations), being easy to trans-

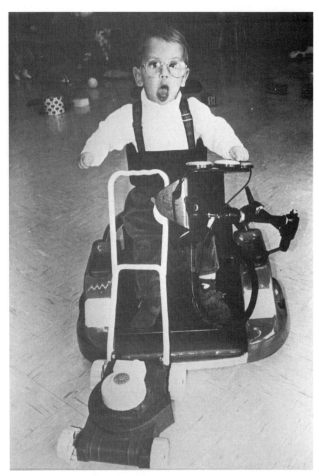

FIG. 14-4   A toddler in the Transitional Power Mobility Aid (TPMA) pushes a toy lawnmower. (The TPMA was designed and developed at Lucile Salter Packard Children's Hospital through a grant from the U.S. Department of Educations, OSERS.)

port in a station wagon or trunk of a large car, being adaptable in terms of positioning and controls, and looking like a toy. The use of a toy as a transitional mobility device not only facilitates play but also may help the child and family progress to the use of another type of mobility aid. Disadvantages of electric cars are that they tend to be noisy and are less durable than power wheelchairs. However, as mobility toys for use in large spaces (e.g., playgrounds, gyms), electric toy cars allow children with disabilities to join peers in typical childhood games involving moving, bumping, turning, and chasing (Fig. 14-5) (also see Case Example 3: 5 years).

As the child gets older, the types of play and leisure activities in which he or she wants to engage should be taken into consideration when selecting manual or power wheelchairs. Some manual and power chair users, especially in the teen years, choose to participate in wheelchair competitive sports such as tennis, basketball, and racing. For manual chair users, participation in these activities can be enhanced by use of lightweight and ultralightweight sport wheelchairs weighing from approximately 40 pounds to less than 25 pounds. Many of the newer designs allow for adjustable

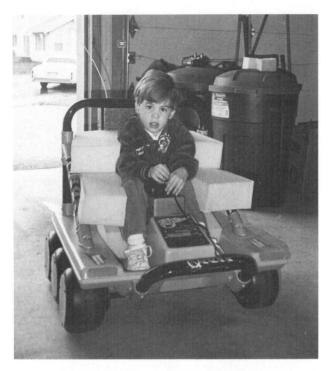

FIG. 14-5 A child drives a toy car in the family garage.

wheel positions and seat heights, making it possible to optimize biomechanical efficiency (Masse et al., 1992). An added advantage of these chairs is that they are highly portable, in most cases fitting easily in trunks of cars. This makes it possible for a teen with a disability to travel to recreational events (e.g., football games, movies, parties) with peers without requiring special accommodations for transportation.

Enhancement of Play and Leisure Through Adaptive Sports Equipment

Often it is important for children and teens with disabilities to be able to participate in outdoor leisure activities with their families and peers. This can be facilitated through the use of adaptive sports equipment combined with special instruction. Recreational programs for people with disabilities are typically manned by volunteers and provide equipment, instruction, and transportation for children and teens. As a result of these programs and specialized equipment, children and teens with disabilities can bicycle, water ski, snow ski (both Alpine and Nordic), and sail. For biking, there are three major classes of adaptations: (1) hand-powered three wheelers for individuals with lower extremity impairments; (2) foot-powered three wheelers for individuals with balance difficulties; and (3) tandems (either regular tandems or tandems with recumbent seats that provide additional trunk stability and that allow for either foot or hand pedaling) for people with sensory or motor impairments or developmental disabilities. Tandems have the advantage that another person can travel on the same bicycle as the individual with the disability, thus allowing participation in the leisure activity while compensating for the individual's impairment (e.g., eyes to see the road, additional strength and endurance to pedal, judgment about traffic).

Adaptive equipment is available for both downhill and cross country skiers with disabilities. Examples are sit-skis, bi-skis, and mono-skis for people with lower extremity impairments, and a variety of adapted poles suited to individual needs. For example, an individual with a lower extremity amputation often can use one ski aided by adapted poles that circle the forearm like lofstrand crutches and have small skis on the tips. Similarly, adaptive equipment such as the Kan-Ski (Quickie Designs, Inc.), a wide single ski on which the participant sits, makes it possible for a person with mobility and balance impairments to water ski. The Shake-A-Leg Foundation, operating out of several locations in the United States, has been instrumental in adapting sailboats and related facilities to accommodate the needs of people with disabilities, especially those who are normally wheelchair bound. In addition, they provide instruction and support for those interested in participating in recreational or competitive sailing and other leisure activities such as archery, scuba diving, rowing, kayaking, horseback riding, bowling, volleyball, basketball, tennis, swimming, and quad rugby.

Assistive devices such as those described make it possible for children and teens to participate in a wide range of sports activities. To assist children and teens and their families in exploring options, occupational therapists should be familiar with recreational programs in their communities that provide equipment, evaluation, training, and outings for people with disabilities. In addition, they must be sensitive and responsive to family interests and needs. For example, if a family has a history of downhill skiing and a child is born with spina bifida, it is important to make sure the family is aware of adaptive ski equipment and specialized instruction for people with lower extremity limitations. Thus, instead of either giving up a favorite leisure activity or leaving the child at home, the child can participate with the family on their winter outings by using adapted equipment (Fig. 14-6).

Adapted Cars and Specialized Drivers' Education

Most teenagers look forward to obtaining a driver's license, one of the activities within our society that signals passage to maturity (Dacey & Travers, 1994). Driving enlarges the world teens can access independently. For many this skill is perceived as increasing competence and independence and becomes a gateway to a variety of developmentally appropriate leisure activities. Therefore, it is important for the sensitive therapist to consider the value of driving for an older teen with a disability. This may require adaptations for vehicles such as ramp and lift systems, reduced-effort steering, and hand controls for accelerating and braking. In addition, drivers' education that is modified to meet individual needs

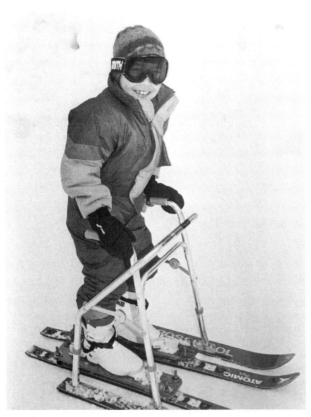

FIG. 14-6 A child uses adapted equipment for skiing. (Courtesy SKIFORALL Foundation.)

should be considered. If the resources are available and the teenager is able to drive with appropriate adaptations, independent driving may allow the teen to pursue such activities as attending sports events, meeting with peers at community restaurants, and participating in school or church functions. Given the need of teens to establish their independence, the value of driving as opposed to being transported by a parent should not be minimized.

CASE EXAMPLES

Throughout the following sections of this chapter, case examples are presented involving the use of assistive technology to enhance play experiences for children with disabilities. These vignettes are intended as realistic examples, rather than model solutions, of the application of assistive technology to enhance play and leisure involvement for children and teens at a variety of developmental levels. Many of these vignettes also reflect consideration of multiple factors in the selection and design of assistive technology solutions that are sensitive to the needs of the child or teen and the characteristics of his or her environment. Both low-technology and high-technology solutions are presented.

CASE EXAMPLE 1: 3½ TO 7½ MONTHS

Lynn was born with a congenitally dislocated hip and as a result was in a spica cast (extending from waist to ankles) from age 3 to 7 months. As she began to reach for toys, she was frustrated when her attempts resulted in pushing the toys out of her range. Two solutions were effective. First, when prone, Lynn was positioned facing the corner of her crib, within reach of the bumper guard. Toys were positioned between Lynn and the bumper guard. Thus, when Lynn's early attempts to reach a toy resulted in pushing the toy away, the toy was stopped by the bumper guard and as a result stayed within the radius of her reach. The second solution involved rigging a sturdy line from one end of Lynn's crib to the other and then tying a toy to the line in such a way that when Lynn was supine, she could reach the toy but not the ribbon attaching the toy to the line. This was important to avoid injury caused by the ribbon's wrapping around a body part. Typically 10 or more toys were attached to the line at the foot of Lynn's crib. One toy was slid into position for play, and when Lynn tired of that toy, "mom," in the course of doing her housework, slid the present toy to the head of the crib, and moved the next toy within reach. This allowed Lynn to play independently for short periods of time and met her needs until she was 6 months old. At that time, when in a prone position, Lynn would try futilely to move forward using her arms. The spica cast was like an anchor. Lynn's unsuccessful attempts resulted in temper tantrums and inconsolable crying. In an attempt to allow Lynn to move independently, she was strapped to a scooter board, positioned so that her shoulders and arms were free. Using this device she happily and independently explored her home environment. These low-technology, low-cost solutions facilitated involvement in developmentally appropriate activities and assisted with state regulation while Lynn was immobilized by her cast. When the spica cast was removed, no further intervention was required and Lynn quickly learned to crawl like other infants her age.

CASE EXAMPLE 2: 10 MONTHS

Susie, a child with cerebral palsy resulting in quadriplegia, appeared to be cognitively normal. At 10 months of age, she was demonstrating an awareness of and interest in her surroundings. However, when she tried to use her upper extremities to manipulate toys, she appeared to be frustrated by her lack of control.

As a result, Susie's parents and therapists decided it was time to introduce Susie to simple cause–effect computer games to provide her with (1) play opportunities she could control; and (2) a modality for developing prerequisite computer skills for later use in school. When positioned properly, Susie had adequate upper extremity control to use a touch window as long as refined or accurate motor movements were not required. At the developmental center, Susie appeared to enjoy computer play and did not exhibit the frustration she displayed when attempting to manipulate toys. Through a grant, her parents were able to purchase a computer system for home. Susie's parents reported that playing computer games with Susie became a favorite family activity. Susie appeared to enjoy the mutual interaction, and her siblings reported that they liked being able to play "with" her, rather than doing something "to" her.

The early introduction of assistive technology provided Susie with some control over her environment during play and opportunities to interact with family members and peers during this process. In addition, computer play helped Susie develop some of the prerequisite skills for using the computer for later school work since it was anticipated that Susie would be more functional at word processing as opposed to writing with a pencil.

CASE EXAMPLE 3: 5 YEARS

Julia, a 5-year-old child with spinal muscular atrophy, had limited motor control of her upper extremities and no voluntary control of her lower extremities. She attended a regular preschool, where she was the only child with a disability. Julia enjoyed interacting with her peers but became frustrated when her highly mobile classmates moved away from her and she could not follow independently. She had a travel wheelchair and, although her parents and therapists were working on obtaining funding for a power wheelchair, it was anticipated that it would be an additional 9 months before Julia would receive her new chair.

While waiting for funding and for processing of paperwork for Julia's new wheelchair, Julia's therapists and her parents began to look for a transitional method for mobility that would allow her to participate in active play both in the classroom and on the playground. One therapist recommended obtaining and adapting a battery operated ride-on toy car because it was an age-appropriate toy that Julia could control independently. After being provided with information by the therapist, the family obtained the car and materials necessary for adapting it to meet Julia's needs. These adaptations included the addition of a remote control device with an emergency shutoff button that could be used by the adult supervising Julia while she played in the car, adjustable speed settings for different environments (e.g., slow for in the classroom, fast for on the playground), a large ball on top of the joystick for Julia to grasp, a foam insert to provide additional trunk control and stability, and a seat belt for safety and support.

Julia quickly adjusted to her car. Since it was low to the ground and she had some control of her upper extremities, she was able to transfer in and out of it independently. Her therapist added a bar on one side of the car that Julia could hang on to for stabilization during transfers. Julia appeared to enjoy the car most at recess when she joined her peers who were "driving trikes." The group members would ride in circles, bump into each other, and play chase. Before getting her car, Julia could only observe these activities. It was noted that during car play, Julia began to initiate more interactions with her peers and her peers tended to interact more with her. Nine months later, Julia received her power wheelchair and made the transition to a public school kindergarten class. In that setting Julia used her power wheelchair for mobility during playground games.

CASE EXAMPLE 4: 8 YEARS

It was late summer and Jeff was recovering from a left upper extremity amputation above the elbow. Because of the severity of his injury, plans for fitting and training with a prosthesis were not scheduled for another month. Jeff, an active 8 year old, was frustrated and bored during this phase and identified that he would like to join his siblings and peers when picking blackberries, playing with Legos, and riding bicycles. He was experiencing difficulty with the former because he couldn't hold a container for berries and pick at the same time. The therapist cut a large hole in the top of a small plastic bleach bottle, leaving the handle intact; thoroughly cleaned the bottle; and then showed Jeff how he could strap the bottle to his waist using his belt. This freed his hand for picking berries.

Jeff had given up playing with interlocking blocks, his favorite quiet activity, because he couldn't stabilize the vehicle or building he was constructing when he attempted to add additional pieces. Jeff's father, working with the therapist, constructed a solid, flat work surface for Jeff and his friends that was covered with base plates so that the object Jeff was building could be attached to the surface and wouldn't slide around each time a new block was added. Last, Jeff's parents had Jeff's bicycle braking system adapted for right-hand control of both the front and back wheels. These assistive technology solutions helped Jeff engage in play and leisure activities both alone and with his peers during a transitional period. It was anticipated that he would continue to use the interlocking block building surface and bicycle adaptations even after fitting with the prosthesis.

CASE EXAMPLE 5: 12 YEARS

Sam, a 12-year-old boy with cerebral palsy and severe quadriparesis, used a power wheelchair for mobility and a light talker for communication. Sam was fully included in all classes at his school and interfaced his light talker with a computer to complete his academic assignments. Sam, like his sixth grade peers, began to notice girls and soon had a "girl friend" who often called him at home. To Sam's dismay someone always had to hold the phone for him and he could only listen and provide occasional verbalizations. Sam complained to his parents and therapists that he wanted to talk on the phone "like his friends." As a result, Sam's family and therapists worked together to develop a system for phone talking. This involved adapting a telephone headset so that it didn't interfere with the placement of Sam's optic light and so that the phone mouthpiece extended toward his light talker. Sam and his family also put the phone numbers he used most frequently on automatic dial and adapted the latter so Sam could activate it independently. Sam still had to be set up on the system, but once set up he was free to make private phone calls and join in the common preteen leisure activity of "talking on the phone."

CASE EXAMPLE 6: 14 YEARS

Karl, a freshman in high school who had sustained a head injury during elementary school, valued participating in intramural sports on Tuesdays. Though reminded before leaving for school, by Tuesday afternoons Karl would forget the day of the week and take the bus home immediately after school. As a result, he regularly missed out on a favorite activity. To help Karl remember this variation in his schedule, Karl was supplied with a watch with an alarm feature. Before school on Tuesdays, Karl's mother would remind Karl about intramural sports. Karl would set his alarm for a preprogrammed time (2 minutes after the dismissal bell at the end of the day). The alarm served as a sufficient reminder that the schedule was different on Tuesdays. This method was chosen rather than having the teacher assume responsibility for reminding Karl because it gave Karl more responsibility for his leisure time activities.

CASE EXAMPLE 7: 17 YEARS

Teenage students with physical disabilities frequently voice frustration that emphasis is placed on therapy and assistive technology to aid in movement about school and participation in academic classes, but little attention is given to extracurricular activities. Dawn, a sophomore in high school with cerebral palsy with triplegia, voiced this concern. When questioned about her desires, Dawn indicated that she was interested in basketball even though she could not play. She decided that the next best thing would be to take statistics for the boys' basketball games. Working with her parents and her therapist, she developed a plan. First, she talked to the basketball coach and found out what would be required to assume the role of "official stats person." The coach was supportive and willing to work with Dawn and her therapist. Because Dawn required use of either a manual chair or an electric scooter for mobility, transportation to and from away games as well as accessibility of all gyms was addressed. Next, Dawn and her therapist worked together to develop a "statistics sheet" on the laptop computer that Dawn used with a word prediction program for all written work. During her sophomore year, Dawn kept statistics for the junior varsity team; during her junior year she advanced to the varsity team. She reported that she enjoyed her new circle of friends from basketball and that she wanted to explore other possible ways to get involved in extracurricular activities.

THE RESULT AND THE IMPORTANCE OF WORKING AS A TEAM

Most children requiring technology to enable or enhance play experiences also need technology to maximize their participation in other daily occupations (i.e., work and self-care). As a result, these children benefit from integrated technology solutions assessed, developed, and implemented through a team process. According to Carney and Dix (1992), using the interdisciplinary team model fosters a "whole child" approach, taking into consideration intellectual, physical, sensory, and psychosocial factors. In complex situations teams should be composed of a variety of individuals, including but not limited to occupational therapists, rehabilitation engineers, teachers, speech–language pathologists, physical therapists, psychologists, vision specialists, physiatrists, and aides. Last, and most important, the family or care providers and, if possible, the child should be active members of the team. Burnett and Dutton (1994) stated, "Parents can bring a broad knowledge of what has and has not worked for their child in the past, a wealth of experience, a set of family goals and values, and an understanding of how the child communicates" (p. 4). They further contend that parents must be fully involved in the team and the decision making process and that this involvement increases the likelihood of technology strategies' being carried out at home. For children within the school system, this same level of involvement is important for teachers who are directly involved with these children (Swinth, 1994).

Often, because of the challenges of daily demands related to self-care and school, play and leisure are forgotten. It is important to communicate directly with the child or the teen regarding his or her desires related to play and leisure. With the chronologically or developmentally young child, this may involve presenting two alternatives and allowing a choice. By contrast, a child who is older and cognitively able can be involved directly in selecting types of play and leisure activities, describing or demonstrating challenges encountered in attempting to engage in those activities, and arriving at possible solutions. Solutions should be sensitive and responsive to preferences of the child and family concerning comfort for the child and the caregiver, energy conservation for the child or teen, the environments in which the child lives including cultural and ethnic factors, and the flexibility of the device. The latter must be considered in relationship to use in multiple settings such as home, school, playground, and community and in relationship to compatibility with technology devices likely to be selected for future use or for use in other occupations. For example, consider a preschool child who has been using a variety of switch-activated toys. The team might decide that computer games would provide developmentally appropriate and varied play experiences. Because of the cost of computers, when making a selection, the team would need to consider not only the child's immediate play needs but also potential future uses of the computer (e.g., word processing, drawing).

In addition, attention should be focused on cost and funding issues; the durability of the selected technology in relationship to anticipated frequency and length of use; and the availability of repair options and ease of repair. Last, provisions should be made (1) for training the child, caregivers, and teachers to use the technology; (2) for monitoring progress; and (3) for providing thorough, periodic reevaluation. The latter is necessary because children change developmentally, their needs may change because of disease processes, and they may develop new ideas about what they want to do.

Equally important is the need for therapists to remain current about new technology options and the function, capability, and durability of these options. Resources in this process are continuing education programs (Deterding et al., 1991), venders, colleagues, individuals who use technology, and ABLEDATA (Landers, 1994). The latter is a database of information on assistive technology distributed in the United States. Products may be from domestic or foreign companies. In addition, the database includes " 'Do-It-Yourself' designs and prototype descriptions" (Landers, 1994, p. 56). Each entry in this database includes a description of product features and specifications, pricing data, and manufacturer and distributor information. Regardless of the resources used, therapists are responsible for maintaining current knowledge of technology options and regularly sharing this information with children, their families, and other team members.

DIRECTIONS FOR THE FUTURE

The development and use of technology for helping children with disabilities access play is in the early stages. New computer programs and technology options merit exploration and development. Consider the possibilities for computer games involving less repetition and more creativity. For example, imagine a 5-year-old child lacking the motor capability to engage in imaginative play with a doll house equipped with a family, a dog, and furniture. If a program existed for creative doll house play, this child could engage in similar imaginative play using the computer. An elaborate doll house could be depicted on the screen and surrounded by a variety of options such as a family (including individuals with disabilities), furniture for the living room, furniture for the bedroom, etc. By clicking on specific options, the child could move desired objects to rooms of his or her choice and then arrange the furniture or people. By clicking on a specific section of the doll house, a room could be enlarged to allow for more detailed play within that room. A paint palate also could be included so that the child could reupholster the couch, dye mom's hair, or refinish the woodwork. Clicking on kitchen cupboards would open doors to reveal dishes and food. With additional clicks these could be removed from the cupboards and arranged for a dinner party. Clothes for the family could be found in drawers and closets. Switching to another program, the child could build a spaceship with Legos. The possibilities are endless and the final advantage is that after minutes or hours of play with tiny pieces (e.g., blocks, doll house furniture) putting away the toys is like magic, involving only a click.

Virtual reality, " a looking-glass technology that transports the user into an imaginary, three-dimensional universe created with software" (*The New York Times,* April 13, 1994, p. B6), is a new technology whose potential for use

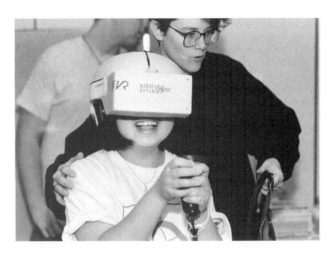

FIG. 14-7 A teen uses a virtual reality system to "chase sharks." (Courtesy Mary Levin, DO-IT Project, University of Washington, Seattle, WA.)

with children with disabilities is just beginning to be explored. This technology originally was developed for training pilots and astronauts. Recently, in pediatric rehabilitation, virtual reality is being used to help children learn to operate power mobility devices. For example, at the Oregon Research Institute, Christopher, a 5-year-old child with cerebral palsy, is taking wheelchair driver's education in a virtual world. Securely strapped into a power mobility device and wearing a special headset, he uses the joystick to " negotiate challenging terrain: grassy fields, pools of mud, long panes of ice" (*The New York Times,* April 13, 1994, p. B6). Could this same technology be used to allow children with disabilities to explore and roam freely in a variety of environments (e.g., the woods, the mountains, an ocean beach, the streets of a city)? The extent to which this technology will open doors to more play and leisure options for children and teens with disabilities is limited only by funding constraints and the creativity and motivation of software developers (Fig. 14-7).

REVIEW QUESTIONS

1. Define assistive technology. Provide implications for encouraging the play of the child with a disability.
2. Discuss how simple toy and environmental adaptations may be made to enhance the play of children with a variety of types of disabilities.
3. Describe several ways that computer use can enhance the play of children with disabilities.
4. Differentiate between augmentative and alternate communication, and describe how each can contribute to

the play and leisure experiences of children with disabilities.
5. What are the kinds of activities that environmental control systems and mobility devices can enable children with disabilities to do? Provide specific examples of each.
6. Define modes of adaptation that can enhance the potential of children and teens to engage in sports.
7. What resources are available to an older teen who wants to drive?

REFERENCES

Brinker, R. P., & Lewis, M. (1982). Discovering the competent handicapped infant: A process approach to assessment and intervention. *Topics in Early Childhood Special Education, 2,* 1-15.

Burnett, S., & Dutton, D. (1994). Responsiveness to consumers. *Technology Special Interest Section Newsletter, 4*(2), 3-4.

Butler, C. (1986). Effects of powered mobility on self-initiated behaviors of very young children with locomotor disability. *Developmental Medicine and Child Neurology, 28,* 325-332.

Butler, C., Okamoto, G., & McKay, T. (1983). Powered mobility for very young disabled children. *Developmental Medicine and Child Neurology, 25,* 472-474.

Butler, C., Okamoto, G., & McKay, T. (1984). Motorized wheelchair driving by disabled children. *Archives of Physical and Medical Rehabilitation, 65,* 95-97.

Carney, J., & Dix, C. (1992). Integrating assistive technology in the classroom and community. In G. Church & S. Glennen (Eds.). *The handbook of assistive technology* (pp. 207-240). San Diego, CA: Singular Publishing Group.

Cotton, N. (1984). Childhood play as an analog to adult capacity to work. *Child Psychiatry and Human Development, 14,* 135-144.

Church, G. (1992). Glossary of Assistive Technology. In G. Church & S. Glennen (Eds.), *The handbook of assistive technology* (pp. 343-359). San Diego, CA: Singular Publishing Group.

Dacey, J., & Travers, J. (1994). *Human development across the lifespan.* Madison, WI: WCB Brown & Benchmark Publishers.

Deitz, J., Jaffe, K., Wolf, L., Massagli, T., & Anson, D. (1991). Pediatric power wheelchairs: Evaluation of function in the home and school environments. *Assistive Technology, 3,* 24-31.

Deterding, C., Youngstrom, M. J., & Dunn, W. (1991). Position paper: Occupational therapy and assistive technology. *The American Journal of Occupational Therapy, 45,* 1076.

Douglas, J., & Ryan, M. (1987). A preschool severely disabled boy and his powered wheelchair: A case study. *Child: Care, Health and Development, 13,* 303-309.

Frost, L. A., & Bondy, A. S. (1994). *PECS: The picture exchange communication system training manual.* Cherry Hill, NJ: Pyramid Educational Consultants, Inc.

Glennen, S. (1992). Augmentative and Alternative Communication. In G. Church & S. Glennen (Eds.). *The handbook of assistive technology* (pp. 93-122). San Diego, CA: Singular Publishing Group.

Glennen, S., & Church, G. (1992). Adaptive Toys and Environmental Controls. In G. Church & S. Glennen (Eds.). *The handbook of assistive technology* (pp. 173-205). San Diego, CA: Singular Publishing Group.

Greenstein, D. (1993). *Backyards and butterflies.* Ithaca, NY: New York State Rural Health and Safety Council.

Hammer, R. (1994). Overcoming challenges via the Internet. *Windows on Computing, 15,* 25-26.

H.R. Rep. No. 100-819, 100th Congress, 2d Session (1988).

In virtual reality, tools for the disabled. (1994, April 13). *The New York Times,* p. B6.

Isaacs, J. (1994). Forrest pumps: A sound-activated water gun works without adaptations. *Exceptional Parent, 24,* 40-41.

Javernick, J. (1994). Maddak Inc. Awards OT Practitioners' Creativity. *O.T. Week, 8,* September 1, 62.

Landers, A. (1994). The ABLEDATA database of assistive technology. *Exceptional Parent, 24,* 56.

Lewis, R. B. (1993). *Special Education Technology.* Pacific Grove, CA: Brooks Cole Publishing Company.

Masse, L. C., Lamontagne, M., & O'Rianin, M. D. (1992). Biomechanical analysis of wheelchair propulsion for various seating positions. *Journal of Rehabilitation Research and Development, 29,* 12-28.

Missiuna, C., & Pollock, N. (1991). Play deprivation in children with physical disabilities: The role of the occupational therapist preventing secondary disability. *The American Journal of Occupational Therapy, 45,* 882-888.

Parette, H., Strother, P., & Hourcade, J. (1986). Microswitches and adaptive equipment for severely impaired students. *Teaching Exceptional Children, 19,* Fall, 15-18.

Piaget, J. (1952). *The origins of intelligence in children.* New York: International Universities Press.

Simon, C. J., & Daub, M. M. (1993). Knowledge bases of occupational therapy, Section 2A: Human development across the life span. In H. L. Hopkins & H. D. Smith (Eds.). *Occupational therapy* (pp. 95-130). Philadelphia: J. B. Lippincott.

Spiegel-McGill, P., Zippiroli, S. M., & Mistrett, S. G. (1989). Microcomputers as social facilitators in integrated preschools. *Journal of Early Intervention, 13,* 249-260.

Swinth, Y. (1994, September). The role of the special education team in selecting and implementing assistive technology. *School System Special Interest Section Newsletter, 1,* 1-3.

Swinth, Y., & Case-Smith, J. (1993). Assistive technology in early intervention: Theory and practice. In J. Case-Smith (Ed.). *Pediatric occupational therapy and early intervention* (pp. 342-368). Boston: Andover Medical Publishers.

Swinth, Y., Anson, D., & Deitz, J. (1993). Single-switch computer access for infants and toddlers. *The American Journal of Occupational Therapy, 47,* 1031-1038.

U.S. Department of Health and Human Services. (1993). *Research plan for the National Center for Medical Rehabilitation Research* (NIH Publication No. 93-3509). Rockville, MD: Author.

Williams, S., & Matesi, D. (1988). Therapeutic intervention with an adapted toy. *The American Journal of Occupational Therapy, 42,* 673-676.

Wright, C., & Kohn, J. G. (1993). A transitional powered mobility aid for a toddler with quadrimembral limb deficiency and a preschooler with spinal muscular atrophy. *Journal of the Association of Children's Prosthetic-Orthotic Clinics, 28,* 28-29.

Wright, C., & Nomura, M. (1991). *From toys to computers: Access for the physically disabled child.* Available from C. Wright, P. O. Box 700242, San Jose, CA 95170.

APPENDIX 14-A

Addresses of Manufacturers of Products and Resources Referred to in this Chapter

- Ablenet, Inc.
  1081 Tenth Ave. S.E.
  Minneapolis, MN 55414-1312
- Broderbund
  P.O. Box 6130
  Novato, CA, 94948-6130
  Phone: 415-382-4700
- Cap Toys
  26201 Richmond Road
  Bedford Heights, OH 44146-4139
- Don Johnston Developmental
  Equipment, Inc.
  PO Box 639
  1000 N. Rand Rd, Bldg 115
  Wauconda, IL 60084-0639
- Edmark Corporation
  6727 185th Ave. NE
  P.O. Box 3218
  Redmond, WA, 98073-3218
- Madenta Communications Inc.
  #216 Advanced Technology Center 965020
  Ave.
  Edmonton, Alberta T6N 1G1 Canada

- Maxis
  2 Theatre Square
  Orinda, CA 94563-3346
- Permobil
  6 B Gill Street
  Woburn MA. 01801
- Prentke Romich Company
  1022 Heyl Road
  Wooster, OH 44691
- Quickie Designs Inc.
  2842 Business Park Ave.
  Fresno, CA 93727
- Sentient Systems Technology, Inc.,
  2100 Wharton St.
  Pittsburgh, PA, 15203
- Shake-A-Leg Foundation Headquarters
  University of Rhode Island
  25 West Independence Way Ste. H.
  Kingston, RI 02881
- Sunburst Communications
  101 Castleton St.
  Pleasantville, NY 93727
- Toys for Special Children,
  385 Warburton Ave.
  Hastings-on-Hudson, NY 10706

Note: This list is provided to assist therapists in locating available resources. It is not exhaustive, nor does it represent an endorsement of companies or products.

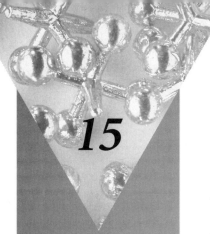

STORYTELLING, STORYMAKING, AND FANTASY PLAY

Linda S. Fazio

Practitioners, regardless of discipline, have long used play in therapeutic exchanges with children. Therapeutic play is generally thought to be goal directed and purposive. According to Knox (1993), "for play to be used successfully in treatment, the child should feel responsible for choosing or directing the play episode" (p. 265); this is of particular importance when "the goal is to increase competence in play development" (p. 265). Theoretical and interpretative motivation for the use of play in therapy has varied among disciplines. Historically, occupational therapists have been accustomed to the use of play concepts and modalities in their work with children. It was not at all uncommon for the pediatric occupational therapist to be introduced to a child as the "play lady." That therapist and child engaged in a positive therapeutic play experience may, in fact, be the essence of pediatric occupational therapy.

Occupational therapy practice in pediatric psychiatry, historically, has been much less common than in other areas of pediatrics, as it continues to be today; however, programs that exist both clinically and in private practice are rich in their eclectic use of developmental, social-transitional, sensory-integrative, and behavioral approaches to treatment. Much of the work with pediatric psychosocial intervention before the 1980s was strongly influenced by Freudian psychoanalytic interpretation in all the disciplines, and it still is today in those disciplines allied with more traditional psychiatry.

The occupational therapist is accustomed to examining the "occupations" of the patient and to looking at these "occupations" not only as the mode to determine progress, or lack of it, but also as the actual determinent of therapeutic milieu. For the child, of course, play and the accoutrements of play are central. Perhaps another attribute of many occupational therapists that has caused some identity problems for the profession, although a strong plus for the patient, has been their insatiable need and ability to see the potential for the attainment of therapeutic goals in virtually every activity they encounter. This ability to create rich and exciting therapeutic environments with few restraints and, at times, without consideration of other disciplines' boundaries may cause laypeople not to distinguish the occupational therapist from the teacher, the counselor, the social worker, the recreation therapist, or the "play-lady volunteer"! Over the course of time other disciplines have recognized the value of occupational therapy's rich tool box and have likewise borrowed selected media and modalities for their therapeutic purposes. Whatever the circumstance initiating the choice of therapeutic environment and modality, it is to the child's best interest that therapists are dedicated; and in today's world of print and visual media, interactive computer software, and a beautiful array of games and toys, therapists must be even more alert to the myriad of choices for therapy. Oftentimes, though, it is the traditional modalities that are the most novel and for that reason offer the most appeal for the child.

It is to one of these traditional modalities that this chapter is devoted, that of the *story*.

THE STORY AS A PLAY TECHNIQUE FOR THERAPEUTIC INTERVENTION

Stories and storytelling are familiar to every child and every adult regardless of culture, socioeconomic circumstances, or tradition. Jay O'Callahan, a professional storyteller quoted in Baldwin (1995), notes that the tradition of storytelling by parents has suffered in the competition with television. He encourages parents to read stories and then tell them. "Parents make wonderful storytellers because they have strong bonds with the listener and they know their child's needs better than anyone else" (p. 32). Parents do, of course, frequently tell stories to their children; often these take the form of short, on the spot vignettes told to teach a moral lesson with regard to "what might happen, if" or "when I was a little girl, grandma used to …"; these are ways to pass on family values and traditions and are perhaps more effective than any other teaching tool a parent may use.

A therapeutic story is, in fact, not much different. It serves to assist in the resolution of a problem or issue and is sometimes done through a moral lesson, although it is perhaps less spontaneous than a parental story and is selected as a modality to bring about a therapeutic goal or goals. Baldwin recounts a story told by a therapist who worked with terminally ill children. Her patient, an 11-year-old boy named Jonathan, had leukemia. After his death his wishes were to have his ashes scattered over Lake Michigan. When the child died, his parents and younger brother, Charlie, age 5, went out on the lake to scatter the ashes. "A monarch butterfly flew down and Jonathan's mother said, 'Look! That's Jonathan!' The next day they were out on their boat and again a monarch butterfly flew down to them, and this time Charlie said, 'Look! That's Jonathan.' Later, they were sitting on the beach and a gray moth flew up from the sand. Charlie shouted, 'Look! That's Jonathan…but he's wearing a different shirt.'" (p. 34). This story, told for the benefit of the younger brother, had healing benefit for the family unit as well as for each individual family member.

Stories may involve parents and families in other ways. Kral (1986) provides discussion of the use of stories to assist in widening the range of options available to a parent, or perhaps a teacher, in dealing with a child. Parents of children with problems often generate "solutional" stories spontaneously when together in a group. Shared stories of how they deal with a child's difficult behaviors prompt other stories and therefore offer potential solutions. Therapists are all familiar with the stories they tell each other regarding their patients, and they have all benefited from these exchanges. Most often the benefit gained has been in the creation of scenarios that they can then try with their own patients; but perhaps more importantly, therapists are able to encourage a sense of security and professional empowerment in their abilities to utilize their therapeutic skills.

Kral goes on to discuss social–emotional therapy for children in the school setting. Whereas direct skill–based approaches are often used to treat behavioral problems related to school, indirect methods can be particularly effective in that they make use of the child's existing strengths and abilities, rather than perhaps assuming that none exist. The telling of stories is such an indirect method.

Frequently, in storytelling and storymaking, the therapist functions as a translator or guide in what may be considered a potentially confusing sea of communication, where the child's interpretation may be inaccurate or skewed. The telling of stories can be utilized to elicit the child's interpretation of an event or series of events that may have been disturbing, to share the meaning the child attaches to such events, to determine how the child incorporates this meaning into his or her emotional action plan, and further, in shared group storytelling, to provide a nonthreatening sounding panel of how this "action plan" is perceived to be culturally and socially appropriate. The latter is what Bruner (1990) describes as "felicity conditions…a method of negotiating and renegotiating meanings by the mediation of narrative techniques" (p. 67).

Children learn a language as a tool with which to mediate interactions within their environment. Whether this language is verbal or nonverbal it is, as John Austin describes, learning "how to do things with words" (1962, Preface). This communicative environment includes spoken and nonspoken language and the child is expected to learn how to negotiate and operate within it. Hassibi and Breuer (1980) note that "behavioral or psychological normalcy is a value-laden concept, varying broadly in its application from community to community and subject to changes in interpretation in different times" (p. 1). All of the elements of a communicative environment may not be present, or their appropriate combinations and sequential orderings may not be such that the child receives the kinds of experiences suited to his or her needs (Robertson & Barford, 1976). This is an even more complicated task for children who receive and encode communications in alternate or obscure ways, such as those experienced by cognitively, visually, or hearing impaired children.

Bruner (1990) makes a claim that very early in a child's development, before language actually develops, there is an ability to grasp "folk psychology." This is an initial understanding of how the group of which the child is a part interprets events; in the child's development it is a "feature of praxis before the child is able to express or comprehend the same matters by language" (p. 74). It appears that very young children, perhaps before age 4 years, have some understanding of the way their particular social–cultural group ascribes meaning to the actions of those around them and particularly to the circumstances in which actions occur because someone has held a false belief. Children younger than 4 years seem to be capable of witholding information and giving false information, as in, for example, the often heard explanation "I didn't do it! She did it" to cover an accident or some occurence that the child wishes not to share with the parent or caregiver. The point here is that a child learns a complicated series of communicative gymnastics necessary to give and to acquire the social and emotional necessities he or she needs as a member of a functioning sociocultural group. For whatever reasons it appears that the cognitively or emotionally disabled child may not develop those protolinguistic competencies necessary to attend to all the meaning variables required for successful adult interactions within a folk group.

Praxis begins with ideation or forming an idea of what to do; this bears a direct relationship to the process of knowing how to do it. A. Jean Ayres (1985) described ideation as a cognitive process that involved understanding that possibilities might take place in relation to actions of self, objects, or people. Ideation allows the child to begin to plan what to do. Guided imaging, in the form of a therapist–child created story, allows the child to sample and create "just-right" challenges without risk. This is a particularly important experience when there is a gap between forming the idea and knowing how to translate the idea into action, as is often true for the cognitively and emotionally disabled child.

One of the functions of play, according to Florey (1981), is the organizing effect on behavior realized through the conceptualization of possibilities. This process of conceptualizing can be guided for the disabled child through therapeutic storytelling and storymaking. There is little risk if the possibilities, ideas, or actions generated by a child in a story format are proven ineffective or unrealistic. Through this process the therapist can assist the child in developing more appropriate possibilities, ideas, and actions.

The therapist can also function as a translator or guide to the child's interpretation of how actual events transpired and to the meanings attached to them. The therapist or other children in a mutual storytelling group can also function as interpreters of social and cultural appropriateness of actions. The process of hearing the child's story can provide a window for the therapist to view the child's world and his or her perceived impact on it.

Children often perceive the world in strongly structured categories or dichotomies; furthermore, they are persistent in their attachment to these dichotomies of good and bad, lie or truth, for or against. Russo and Jaques (1976) describe the case of a child who relied so heavily on the stubborn use of categories that when they became frustrating or painful, "he could not realistically reconsider the situation, but resorted to sulking, crying, and temper tantrums...not reacting to the realistic environment but to the world created by his own faulty and pervasive generalizations" (p. 395). Stories were used to assist the child in developing insights regarding his

inability to deal with the gray areas of his experiences as he approached the developmental phases of adolescence. Through mutual stories practice was gained in the general classification of the child's experiences and the abstraction of different scenarios with resultant repercussions and potential outcomes.

According to Gardner (1976), children have no great interest in developing insights into their own or others' behavior. In Gardner's interpretation, conscious awareness of unconscious processes is a form of therapy best reserved for adults, although it can also be useful for adolescents. The development of the therapist's insights into the child's frustrations and resulting behaviors is, of course, critical to the advancement of therapy.

Dorothy Singer's work in play therapy and the use of stories has relied heavily on the interpretation of the symbolic play of children (1986, 1988, 1990). "A major component, then, of pretend play is the capacity of young children actually to experience symbolic or imagery-laden thought" (1990, p. 189). The child's capacity to use imagery or fantasy as a coping skill can be encouraged through storytelling therapies. Use of fantasy can help a child explore feelings and ideas, assist a child in the resolution of conflicts, and bring about cognitive change.

For the young child, life probably is a "story." Young children have an ability to humanize objects in their environment and to endow them with human feeling and emotion. The following illustration is a brief excerpt from a group storytelling transcription where a snow dome was used to initiate the stories (Fig. 15-1, *A* and *B*):

Jean: I think that little deer is shaking; it must be very cold in that snow.
Kent: That's not real snow; it's fake; plastic probably. It's probably really warm in that ball.
Nancy: Yeah; I'd like it in there; it's so cozy and nobody could bother you unless you wanted to let them in...I wouldn't let any of you in!
Kent: So, who cares; if you let someone in, the dome would have to be broken and you wouldn't be safe anymore would you?
Jean: Soooo; that's why she's not going to let you in, dummy.

When therapists attempt to understand how stories affect therapeutic outcomes they must consider them in what Bandler and Grinder (1975) describe as surface and deep meaning. "Surface meaning" refers to the more obvious storyline or literal interpretation. For the previous illustration the "surface story" involved the small deer in the dome. Deep meaning exists at the core of the story, its implicit meaning. Deep meaning can be interpreted differently by each individual. For Nancy the dome may have offered safety and security. For Kent, the aggressive realist, it was a barrier to be broken. And for Jean, the creative philosopher, it was an opportunity to defend her friend. Fairytales such as *Sleeping*

FIG. 15-1 **A,** This photograph depicts mutual storymaking that spontaneously occurred during a videotaped treatment session. The therapist is using a snow dome to facilitate the storymaking process. **B,** "I think that little deer is cold."

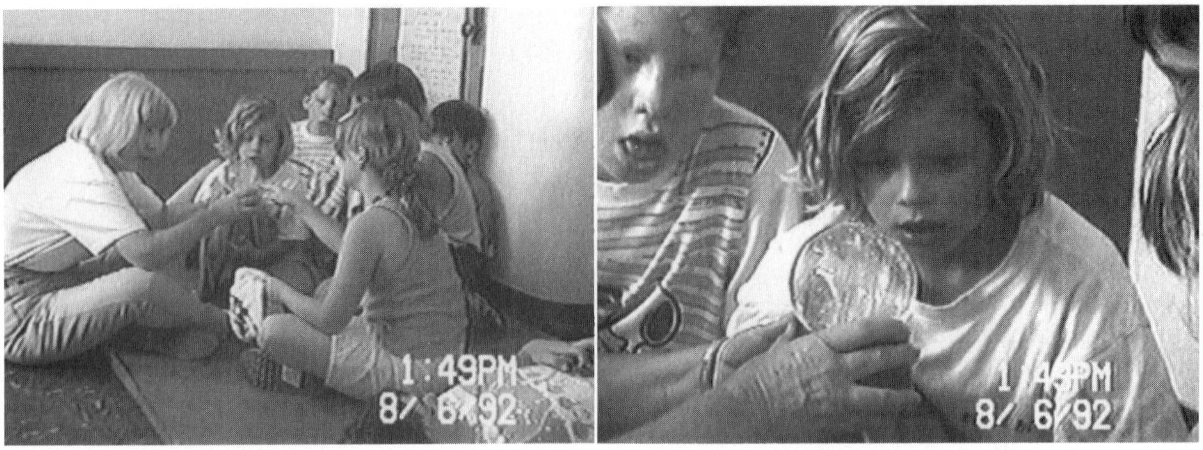

Beauty, Cinderella, and *The Ugly Duckling* are skillfully crafted stories of charming people, parties, and kindnesses, but also of evil and harmful people. These observations represent the surface structure of the stories. The deep structure exhibits intricacies of courage, love, sacrifice, and trust. It is often through this deep structure that the therapist works. However, therapy using surface structure can be equally effective. This is particularly the case within the dimensions of much of occupational therapy pediatric practice that involves the goals of improved social interactions, verbal expressions of feelings, encouragement of developmentally appropriate fantasy, and creativity. Such behaviors as taking turns, being kind to others, listening, using words to describe feelings, using self-control, being a group member, cooperating with others, empathizing with others, and understanding the impact of one's own actions and words on others are all sensitive to surface story construction. In general these stories fall into the categories of "What?" "What if?" and "How?"

The remainder of this chapter presents descriptions of frequently used storytelling and storymaking techniques.

MUTUAL AND SERIAL STORYTELLING

The mutual storytelling technique was originally proposed by Richard Gardner (1971) as a way to use children's stories for therapeutic purposes. The process of mutual storytelling is one in which the child begins a story as the therapist listens. The intent, as proposed by Gardner, is that the therapist look for unspoken psychodynamic meaning in the story. The therapist then responds to the story by telling one of his or her own. In the original use of this method the therapist's story contains the same characters and occurs in a similar setting, but the therapist introduces healthier, more adaptive solutions to whatever problems or conflicts the child may have introduced. The psychodynamic supposition is that the child's unconscious receives the potential

solutions and incorporates them in the conscious. In this technique the potential solutions are subtle; the child is not told how to handle a problem(s) and therefore does not actively resist the solution. The novelty of this technique also stimulates the child's interest and perhaps contributes to receptivity.

In this author's experience children are very much interested in this process and some equate it with video and computer games in which the central figure in a story, with the assistance of the child, may select from several adventure scenarios. Verbally telling a story that is in fact based upon the child's own experience allows the child to fit this selection of scenarios to his or her own circumstances and ferret out potential solutions.

The following is a partial transcription from one of the author's therapy sessions with Jeff, a 9-year-old boy who was identified by teachers as having a behavior problem, with possible attention-deficit disorder. The therapy was after school in a practice office set up for work with children and adolescents (comfortable sofa, table lamps, carpet, computer with selected game software, and relaxation monitoring software; cabinets with board games, dolls, and toys; dollhouse; music tapes and tape player; VCR and monitor and video tapes).

Therapist: Hello, sir (hug); . . . how are you?

Jeff: Okay, I guess (moves around room; looks out of window) . . . my mom's not waiting today, she has to take Karen to the dentist . . . anyway she's mad at me.

Therapist: (sitting on sofa) I'm tired today, how about entertaining me?

Jeff: (joining therapist on sofa) Okay, I'll tell you a joke. What did the cow say when he jumped over the moon?

Therapist: I don't know.

Jeff: Uh . . . I don't know either . . . (laughing) that's the joke, get it?

Therapist: (laughing), You're too smart today; how about telling me a story?

Jeff: I don't know any stories.

Therapist: Oh, it doesn't have to be fancy . . . tell me about your day. (therapist puts feet up and closes eyes)

Jeff: Okay, but I'll just tell you some of it.

Therapist: Okay, I'm listening.

Jeff: Keep your eyes closed, but don't go to sleep; I'll know. I'm going to tell it like I'm another boy, okay?

Therapist: Okay.

Jeff: I went to get in line for the lunchroom but the teacher says "No, you stay at your desk, Jason" (that's my name) and I sit down but I'm mad and I let her know, I look as mad as I can. Like this . . . open your eyes. Keep your eyes open because you need to see what happens next (moves from sofa to small chair near center of room) . . . this is my desk . . . I get even more mad because the kids are going to the lunch room and I can't go . . . so I get up to go anyway and my desk falls over . . . like this (knocks over the chair) . . . okay, that's it, that's the end.

Therapist: Okay, my turn now?

Jeff: Okay, I'm tired, I'm going to sleep during yours (relaxes on sofa with eyes closed).

Therapist: Okay, I'll tell mine very quietly so I don't wake you. There was a boy named Jeff . . .

Jeff: No, the boy's name is Jason.

Therapist: I forgot, go back to sleep. There was a boy named Jason and he went to Mrs.—'s third grade; he was a pretty nice boy; he took care of his rabbit, Oreo; and he tried to be nice to his sister most of the time.

Jeff: (giggles) I don't think so!

Therapist: Shhhh, you're asleep. Sometimes at school, though, Jason had some problems. Seems he had some trouble listening to what the teacher said . . . and when she got upset with him . . . he got very mad! Jason's therapist knew how to solve the problem . . . This boy needs bigger ears, or maybe just more smaller ones . . . what do you think, is this a good story, or what?

Jeff: (giggles) Bigger ears, so big they look like balloons over his head.

Therapist: . . . very big ears; and when the teacher talked to Jason the ears turned toward her just like radar! But, you know what?

Jeff: Everybody laughed?

Therapist: Well, that too; but even more interesting, Jason still didn't listen to the teacher . . . so the therapist said, big ears just won't do it . . . we have to think of something else. What about better eyes? Maybe that will do the trick. So the next time the teacher asked Jason a question he looked straight at her with his really sharp eyes and watched very carefully as quietly as he could so his eyes could do their work…and what do you know, it was easier to hear her . . . isn't that funny?

Jeff: Yeah, hearing with your eyes; that is too very weird . . . I like it! Bionic eyes.

Therapist: And something else that's weird . . . when Jason looked at the teacher and let his eyes really listen . . . he didn't mind doing what she said . . . and he didn't feel so bad anymore . . . he was even smiling a lot! End of story! Well, what do you think?

Jeff: Not too bad, not too bad . . . for you, anyway (laughs).

Therapist: (hugs his shoulders and falls back against pillows) A compliment, from you . . . I can't stand it! Think the eye thing will help Jason smile more?

Jeff: I don't know . . . I have to think about it.

Therapist: Try it out for him . . . would you? Let me know what you think next week?

This was one of a number of individual sessions with Jeff. In addition, he was a member of a small group of children (boys and girls) who were seen weekly. Activities were most often board games, arts and crafts, and community outings. Individual therapy would not have been as effective without this peer-based reinforcement of individual goals.

On occasion serial storytelling was used with the group. Oaklander (1978) refers to this kind of mutual storytelling as a "story collage" (p. 94). This version of storytelling consisted of each member having the opportunity to initiate a story of their choice; each member then takes turns to continue the story. Rules were agreed on regarding the courtesy extended to each group member (e.g., no interruptions, no derogatory comments). The therapist did not usually enter into the storytelling but, instead, offered a summary of her interpretation of the "moral" of the story (it was mutually decided that each story was to have a beginning, a middle, an end, and a moral). Over time Jeff did manage his negative behaviors more effectively (as reported by his teacher and his mother); he remained emotionally and socially engaged in the therapy sessions and was more relaxed and spontaneous. Continuing, shared treatment goals were negotiated between Jeff, his mother, his teacher, and the therapist. The addition of storytelling to the therapeutic milieu offered a novel and creative avenue of play for Jeff and for the therapist.

Storytelling is not always easy for the child, or for the therapist. It is useful to work with the child's real situations, often in a "Tell me about your day," "How was the soccer game?" approach. Gardner has suggested using a tape recorder and a microphone. The child has a personal tape labeled with his or her own name and no one else is permitted to hear it. A "guest of honor" or "television program" format is used and rules are established by the therapist (no stories that you've heard, read, or seen on television). Sometimes if the child is intimidated by the idea of telling a story the therapist may begin and then suggest that the child continue with little bits of the story. For example, the therapist may offer, "Once upon a time…in a distant land…there lived a…" as the child fills in the gaps.

Focusing on a moral, or "What can we learn from this story," offers a therapeutic potential. Use of this moral to help the child change behaviors or for the adolescent to gain insight requires integration and translation to treatment goals and objectives.

Those therapists with a strong interest in the psychodynamic model of practice can find much psychodynamic and symbolic meaning in the child's stories and may seek to translate this meaning for the child through using the child's characters and setting to create stories with psychoanalytic interpretation. This may have therapeutic potential for the adult and perhaps for the adolescent; but the use of more surface-oriented stories providing the child with workable behavioral adaptations seems to be more effective with younger children. The telling of a story by a child can certainly provide catharsis for anger, frustration, and sadness and can also provide a sharing of "just feeling good"!

The therapist bridges a challenging situation when working in the pediatric cognitive–psychosocial domain. He or she must be able to experience the child's world and the child's interpretation of that world, while providing the benefit of the adult's experience in creating multiple options that are more adaptive and functional than the self-defeating ones the child may have chosen or that the child's disability may have imposed. This is certainly a therapy benefiting from the therapists' positive life experience. However, if the therapist loses sight of the task and pleasure of being a child, the therapy is not effective.

PERSONALIZED STORYMAKING

Making stories to fit a particular child's situation is not unlike what has been described previously except that it is not necessarily initiated by the child's story but is rather the therapist's construction based on the circumstance and perceived emotions of the child. Robertson and Barford (1976) see this kind of storymaking as appealing to the child's realm of fantasy and offering, vicariously, a means of acting out feelings that cannot be expressed in reality. Their work with children in hospital settings not only provides a release for the child's feelings but also encourages the child to get well. When a child is experiencing a long-term and painful illness the use of fantasy scenarios to help in alleviating pain and to maintain focus on wellness is useful. The therapist's use of fantasy scenarios can be broadened to include cartoons, comic books, television, and action figures.

Adults live their lives based on a personal story they have composed for themselves or, sometimes, based on stories others have composed for them. Adults' stories include a past, present, and future. Smith (1989) believes that adults' personal stories have three components: experiences, concepts, and themes. "Experiences are the people, places, and events that are a part of our history . . . . Concepts are beliefs or ideas we have about ourselves and others that we use to screen and interpret experiences and to guide our behavior…and themes are general, abstract principles that summarize and consolidate experiences and concepts . . . themes give unity to personal stories" (p. 7). These, then, would be the components that therapists would use to construct personal stories. The selection of themes would be based on mutually agreed upon therapeutic goals.

FANTASY, GUIDED AFFECTIVE IMAGERY, RELAXATION, AND THE USE OF METAPHORS

Fantasy and Imaging

What is meant by "imagery"? Images appear to be associated with the right hemisphere of the brain and its functions, which include the ability to construct visual and auditory "pictures," spatial representation, and fantasy. Generating images, imaging, and imagination, according to Sherrod and Singer (1984), are not necessarily the same things. Images may be thought of as internalized representations of sensory information with no actual stimulation. Thus people are able to recreate a picture or image of their living rooms or a significant other in their mind's eye. When people manipulate these images in their mind's eye, to imagine, for example, that maybe the sofa would be better in front of the window, this is imaging. Imagination requires the generation of images and manipulating them with a level of sophistication that may include generating thoughts about alternate scenarios, and the actual creation of a script or story for action. It is this capacity for imagination that we observe in the play of a child when he or she includes dolls and toys in acting out various daily activities (eating pretend lunches, diapering a doll, or driving a truck to the store). There is some support for the idea that children's imaginary companions are a result of their capacity for eidetic imagery. According to Piaget and Inhelder (1971), a characteristic of children with imaginary playmates may be that they enjoy imaginative play with more positive outcomes than negative ones.

Daydreams are a familiar representation of imaging and the processes of imagination known to most of us (Singer, 1988; Starker, 1982). In Mihaly Csikszentmihalyi's (1984) work with the daydreams and fantasies of children and adolescents he describes the process as a form of information processing having to do with the self, whatever one is currently concerned about, and general problem solving. When working with children and adolescents therapists must ask at what point in development the ability to image actually makes an appearance. Piaget (1962) believed that images made an appearance in the later part of the sensorimotor period of life, between the ages of 18 and 24 months, or at approximately the time that object permanency fully emerges. During the preoperational stage, about the age of 2 or 3 years, some pretend or make-believe play begins to develop. Between the ages of 4 and 6 years true symbolic play or the substitution of one object for another in play can be observed quite frequently (Piaget & Inhelder, 1971). It is at this point in development that children can express imaging not only through language but also through drawings, vocalizations, and movement (e.g., An elephant walks and sounds like this).

Later, during the stage of concrete operations, approximately ages 7 through 12 years, children begin to move away from imaginative, make-believe play, favoring more rule-bound games in groups. The ability to image is, of course, still there and many children at this stage begin to develop very sophisticated language and graphic representations of fantasy and imaging. The child begins to move into the stage of formal operations at around 12 years of age, and continuing into adolescence and adulthood the ability to image and daydream is at its peak (Singer, 1986; Singer & Singer, 1990). Adolescents may spend a great deal of time daydreaming about future plans and "trying out" different potential life roles.

With a cognitively delayed child it may be difficult to determine exactly how they receive, manipulate, and incorporate fantasy and imaging. One of the best measures may be to elicit verbal descriptions of events and to note if the descriptions contain images, or to ask for drawings that represent fantasy and imaging. Singer (1973, 1986) suggests the use of visual–spatial ability tests or, more simply, asking the child such direct questions as "What's your favorite game?" "What do you do when alone?" or "Do you have an imaginary playmate?" (1973). The therapist can also observe the free play and activity of the child and note whether imaginative play occurs. Noting the child's ability to manipulate imagery is important when selecting types of stories and storytelling techniques for therapeutic purposes.

Rosenfeld and colleagues (1982) developed a measure of fantasy to evaluate first and third grade children. In their research three fantasy styles were identified: active–intellectual, dysphoric–aggressive, and fanciful–intense. They determined that the children's styles of daydreaming were much like that of adults but with some differences in perception of content. It appeared that such things as ghosts and "evil" fairy tale figures were considered to be far less negative for the children than for adults. In the author's experience when children retell stories they've seen on television or in the movies they minimize the "evil" capacity of truly horrific characters (at least horrific in the adult's interpretation). Vampires may be expressed as "mean bloodsuckers" by a child, complete with gleeful demonstrations of neck biting, but they're seldom treated with fear or disdain. If there are rats in the same story, they're usually treated with more real interest!

McIlwraith and Schallow (1982-1983) found a positive correlation between extensive and unmonitored television viewing and dysphoric, hostile, ruminative fantasies. They did not, however, find that television viewing substituted for or replaced self-produced fantasies. In this author's work television and movie characters certainly influence the stories children choose to tell, including events recently witnessed on the news, although the children's stories never seem to reproduce exactly the events or stories they've observed. Instead, these characters and events only seem to provide impetus or color for the stories. Applebee (1978) provided analysis of children's stories and determined that children ages 2 to 5 years had difficulty separating fact and fantasy. The stories of boys at these ages tended to venture farther from home than did the stories of girls at similar ages.

Guided Affective Imagery and Relaxation Techniques

Guided affective imagery, historically, was a psychoanalytically oriented technique that was used with children as young as age 6. The topics presented to the child through imagery were not directly linked to the presenting problem but were indirect scenarios of similar content (Leuner et al., 1983). The technique continues to be used in this way, particularly in European psychiatry. Rosentiel and Scott (1977) indicate several major points that one must consider when utilizing imagery: (1) The scenes used in imagery must be geared to the cognitive abilities of the child; (2) the therapist should select the natural imagery of the child as a basis for the therapeutic exchange because the use of familiar characters allows the child more comfort with this technique; and (3) the therapist must be alert to the child's breathing patterns and changes in facial expressions to note any anxiety that may be created by the particular images selected.

The use of guided imagery is closely linked to relaxation techniques and may be considered an extension to basic muscle relaxation and the generation of relaxing, peaceful images. This characteristic of the technique may be the most useful, particularly when it is coupled with a therapeutic story. The child (or children in small groups) is encouraged to sit comfortably or to lie down. The room may be darkened. Relaxing images may include a place the child has described as particularly pleasant (i.e., grandma's kitchen, riding in the car). The scene may be set with an object such as a snow dome or music box (Fazio, 1992).

Sometimes it may be more effective to use a scene with which the child has no association. Steps in the process involve relaxation, setting the scene, and the telling of the story (by either the therapist, the child, or a combination of both). Frequently, if a state of relaxation occurs the child prefers that the therapist tell the story. The use of imagery can be effective as a way to retell a child's story with alternate solutions to problems being presented by the therapist. The therapist can assist the child in imaging how the solutions can be carried out and what the outcomes may be, or not be. Used in this way, guided affective imagery creates a very focused, calming way to present alternative solutions to problems presented by the child, or interpreted by the therapist. If the child has difficulty (depending on developmental age) keeping his or her eyes closed and "creating pictures" in his or her head, it can be useful to encourage this process by suggesting that the child create a film strip or video or see him- or herself on a stage or screen. Most children can relate to this and have little difficulty creating images of themselves doing or saying things that the therapist suggests. Singer (1993) refers to "mind play" in describing therapeutic imagery. This is a term that children can relate to.

In the use of basic relaxation the therapist asks the child to relax his or her muscles, usually through a sequential tightening and relaxing of muscle groups; eyes are closed. The child is then asked to image a quiet, pleasant, peaceful scene. Deep breathing is demonstrated and modeled by the therapist. The child may be seated comfortably or lying down. Lusk (1992) provides an excellent resource for relaxation and imagery scripts that may be adapted for adults, adolescents, or children. Relaxation training has been used fairly widely with children of all ages and in a variety of settings. Singer (1993) refers to the work of Setterlind in using relaxation training in a physical education program for normal children aged 10 through 18 years. These children were found to experience an increase in measures of positive self-insight, self-control, and self-influence.

Martin and Williams (1990), in describing therapeutic work using guided imagery with adolescents and adults, note that it may be effective to substitute a positive image when the client is experiencing an anxiety-producing negative situation, or an exaggerated image that carries far worse consequences than the client's fears. For children, the thera-

pist can provide images of potential coping mechanisms in the form of a person or persons who the child believes can handle anything. Often this is an actual person that the child knows, and sometimes it is a fantasy figure that the child admires. The child can then image him- or herself modeling the admirable behavior. Sometimes an image can be created to make a potentially threatening person or situation less threatening in the child's eyes (for example, the doctor trying to ride the child's tricycle or badly executing a skateboarder's maneuvers).

The work of Achterberg and Lawlis (1984) in helping cancer patients to create "cancer-destroying" images is similar to the approaches described above. Figure 15-2, *A* and *B*, represents drawings by children experiencing chronic illness. The "illness" was most often represented by small, menacing figures of bugs, scorpions, and spiders who were subdued by the child. In these drawings one child "used a long, really sharp knife to cut them down," and the other "formed a radiation screen that made them unconscious, and then dead."

Kazdin (1988), Spivack and Shure (1982), and Meichenbaum and Goodman (1971) describe combinations of ther-

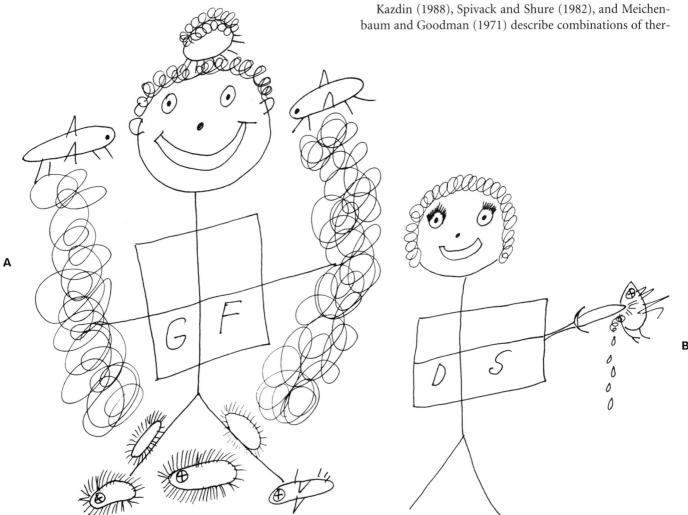

FIG. 15-2 Drawings by chronically ill children. **A,** The child explained the drawing by saying, "This is a germ fighter; radiation comes out of his fingers and kills germs; the germs look like centipedes, ugly flies, and even tarantulas!" **B,** The child's depiction of the drawing was, "This is a disease saver sword-girl; the sword sticks into bacteria until they die!"

apeutic techniques that are based in cognitive therapy. Children are instructed in how to make positive "I" statements that are repeated out loud. The therapist can then reinforce these statements through stories that are different from the child's situation but require similar strengths, followed by stories with the child as the central character, using his or her positive statements to achieve desired goals. Sometimes imagery may provide an experience for a child that he or she may be excluded from in real life because of physical or cognitive limitations or social isolation.

The following transcription provides an example of how a guided affective imagery session can be used for the rehearsal of alternate ways to cope with a potentially anxiety-producing situation. Kim is a 12-year-old girl who has been referred to therapy by her parents because of negative and failing school behaviors and difficulties in making friends. Kim is seated in a lounge chair with feet up; the therapist is seated nearby. The transcription begins after general muscle relaxation is accomplished:

Therapist: You're very relaxed now; feeling a little sleepy and heavy… I'm going to slowly count to 10 and as I do, I want you to see the numbers in your head like soft clouds. With each count you're one step closer to your special place…one…two…three… feeling more and more relaxed (counting continues slowly with reinforcement phrases)…you're in the place you like best… feeling very relaxed, and very safe; take a minute to look around you…feeling very good to be here…Now you're ready to think about the performance you'd like to do for the talent show…staying very relaxed; your hands are resting in your lap; your face is relaxed, no tightness anywhere. See yourself back-stage, waiting to go on. How do you look?

Kim: I look okay; I'm wearing a black, short dress. But I'm nervous; I feel sick.

Therapist: Freeze the picture and focus on relaxing; make your stomach very, very tight; so tight. Now let out your breath very slowly. Breathe deep and relax your stomach. Go back to your picture. You look good; can I start the tape?

Kim: Go ahead, I think I'm ready.

Therapist: Sing the song in your head; make it real; move around, lift your hands; it's just you and the song . . . in your safe, secure place. Take as much time as you need.

The imagery ended with counting in the reverse and reinforcement of feeling relaxed, safe, and secure. There were several sessions like this, followed by an actual dress rehearsal for the therapist. Kim performed at the talent show, the first school event in which she had participated.

Other sessions of this kind were conducted with other children and included the rehearsal of numerous actions and events to include test taking, kicking a soccer ball, talking to a girl, and reading out loud in class. Barell (1980) and Finke (1989) support the idea that "there is a subtle tendency for movements to be initiated automatically whenever such movements are imaged" (pp. 215-

216). Imaging may be particularly facilitative when the coordination of hands and feet are desirable in an action or series of actions. Rosenberg (1987) suggests similar links between imaging an activity or action and carrying it out. Performers and athletes frequently talk about "psyching" themselves out and imaging an activity before actually doing it.

Metaphorical Forms in Storytelling

Metaphors can assume many forms: proverbs, fairytales, poems, parables, and numerous combinations and variations of these. The use of metaphorical stories to transmit a lesson or selected "words of wisdom" is in every culture's repertoire of subtle teaching tools. Even very young children understand metaphors and, if not, seem particularly challenged to figure them out. They are, after all, puzzles to be unraveled.

Metaphors, when used in therapy, are indirect; they are most effective when they reflect the primary elements of the client's problem and one or more solutions to the problem, but the content of the metaphorical form is very different from the actual problem (Dolan, 1986; Frey, 1993; Gordon, 1978; Mills and Crowley, 1986). Religious teachings rely heavily on metaphor through proverbs and parables. Fairytales and metaphorical stories are an excellent way to engage a therapeutic group because they can relate to such a wide variety of problems and concerns. Films geared toward adolescent audiences such as *Pretty in Pink* (Deutch, 1986) and *Rumble Fish* (Coppola, 1983) can be extremely useful when functioning as an impetus for group therapy interactions. There are many cartoons, for all ages, that also meet this purpose. Mills and Crowley (1986) refer to the use of clay, paint, drawing, and puppetry to assist in the production of therapeutic metaphors.

Nursery rhymes and songs can be useful with young children:

> "The itsy bitsy spider climbs up the water spout…down came the rain and washed the spider out…out came the sun and dried up all the rain…and the itsy bitsy spider climbed up the spout again"…and again, and again, and again!

Accompanied by hand motions and facial expressions this little song speaks to anyone who has ever worked hard to achieve a goal, regardless of age or circumstances.

Cartoons such as *Calvin and Hobbes, Ziggy, Charlie Brown,* and *The Farside* present metaphorical messages that appear to be universal considering their continued popularity and appeal. Frey (1993) notes that "universal metaphors focus on issues that are common to human existence…such themes as anger, embarrassment, irrational thoughts, or procrastination" (p. 228). Frey goes on to suggest that the use of goals separates the use of metaphors in therapy from other settings. Therapeutic metaphors may "offer new choices, show different ways of perceiving a situation, and tap a variety of dormant beliefs, attitudes, and values of the child" (p. 223).

Oaklander (1978) suggested combining fantasy and drawing. When using the idea of a special place in facilitating relaxation, some children like to extend this to drawings or paintings using favored colors, shapes, and people. These drawings can be used to encourage the sharing of personal "special places" with other children in therapy or with siblings or other family members. A series of drawings can be produced and bound in a scrapbook or, if drawing is not the child's forte, magazine photos, actual photos, found objects, and construction paper can be used to produce a "special place/special things" collage.

Singer (1993) supported the use of motoric imagery; for example "repeating a word such as 'monkey' and demonstrating what a monkey can do" (p. 215). This serves to facilitate a child's cognitive functioning by coupling enactment with a story to assist in comprehension and memory tasks.

Stories Combined with Other Media

Younger children may find it difficult to involve themselves in storytelling activities without some accompanying opportunity for action. This may also be true for older children, particularly those who are attention-deficit disordered, developmentally disabled, or emotionally disabled. However, storytelling can also be a calming activity. After school, or after sports, therapy sessions can frequently be effective because the child is exhausted and ready for a snack and a story.

For some children it is easier to engage in storytelling themselves if they can tell the story through a doll or puppet. It may be particularly hard for them to tell stories about themselves or family members. Constructing a hand puppet that represents the child can be very useful, first as a way to help the child "see" the self and then as a tool to enhance "self" stories. These puppets are placed in a special place and are not used by other children. They can be taken down whenever the child wishes. An autistic child was observed using her hand puppet in self-talk. The therapist was able to use this observed opportunity to assist the child in a similarly fashioned communication with another child in therapy. The children continued to play together through their puppets and, in later sessions, often wore the puppets on their hands but frequently played together without the benefit of the puppets "doing the communication."

Sitting on the floor, telling a "serial" story through puppets, is an excellent way to engage several children in a group play activity. It may be easier to initiate such an activity with puppets designed around a commonly known fairytale. There are numerous such puppets available in toy stores or they can be constructed by the child and/or the therapist. The therapist can initiate the story with each child continuing it; the therapist can then construct the ending based on his or her interpretation of the most therapeutic outcome. Through either selective memory, personal interpretation, or creativity, the stories are seldom the ones the therapist may have expected! Bettelheim (1976) points out that "the child will ex-

tract different meaning from the same fairy tale, depending on his interests and needs of the moment" (p. 12).

Older children are usually able to engage in this kind of activity without benefit of puppets. They particularly enjoy the telling of "fractured fairytales" (an approach you may recall from the *Rocky and Bullwinkle* television cartoons). The intent seems to be who can be the most outrageous and the funniest. The perceptive therapist can learn a great deal about the child's real concerns, hopes, and fears from these stories and can return to these issues in further therapeutic exchanges. Richard Gardner's *Fairy Tales for Today's Children* (1974), *Modern Fairy Tales* (1977), and *Stories About the Real World* (1972) are good resources for stories that put a contemporary twist on a familiar tale. Adolescents find these stories entertaining and an opportunity to compare their observations of the world with those of other group members. No one ever quite agrees on the choices the hero or heroine may make and this initiates excellent content for group communication and interaction. The therapist is responsible for maintaining these sessions as a safe environment for children to try out their perceptions of the world and examine their positions in it. This is perhaps one of the most challenging tasks for the therapist: avoiding a "free for all" without setting overly demanding limits. Usually rules for the group sessions are agreed on between the children and the therapist. For the therapist to maintain a safe environment and to protect the therapeutic integrity of the group it must be maintained at no more than four or perhaps five children, depending on the diagnosis and dynamics of each child.

Games to enhance the telling of stories can also be a novel way to elicit personal narratives. The Ungame, Storytelling Card Game, and even picture Lotto cards can be used to initiate stories. The therapist may also consider constructing his or her own storytelling "grab bag." This would consist of phrases (typed or printed on small cards) that were selected to be personally meaningful to the child or children; these could then be blindly selected from the bag or box to help the child focus on issues that could be developed in a mutual story with the therapist. Children might also type their own cards on the computer to create boxes or bags of their own. A box of "happy" or "positive" phrases (selected by the child) can be comforting when the child comes to therapy after a school day full of what may seem to be insurmountable problems.

Singer (1993) describes the use of exercises or games to assist children in gaining control over the circumstances in their lives. Such games and exercises are also useful in facilitating the child's ability to use his or her imagination in a playful and pleasurable way. *Put Your Mother on the Ceiling* by deMille (1973) is an example. His exercises include imaginative ways to deal with images of school, pain, parents, and so forth; the game is not malicious but offers a safe way (the child's imagination) to deal with difficult events. The child can learn that controlled imagination and fantasy can be a fun way to help with real problems that may not be of the child's making.

Pantomime is another resource for developing alternate ways to tell stories. This can be particularly engaging for a child who is not as comfortable with verbal communication or for children who tend to rely on verbal communication. For these children an opportunity to "act out" a story may offer an emotional release of energy that would be therapeutically more facilitative. *The Magic If* by Kelly (1973) offers an example of stories suitable to pantomime.

Maurice Sendak is a masterful creator of children's stories that speak to the child's fears and concerns. The reading of Sendak's *Where the Wild Things Are* (1963) offers an opportunity for children to relate to the character's struggle to tame the menacing "monsters" (whatever they might be for each child). Coupling this story with guided imaging of the child's own particular "monsters" helps the story to be individually therapeutic. Many fairytales are initiated with a "journey" and this can become a significant metaphor for children and for adults. Starting out on a quest or adventure seems to indicate an opportunity to change the way things are, to make them better, and to start over. And, even though we may not really believe that the hero and heroine live happily ever after, it's comforting to hear this ending to a story. Children, particularly, are optimistic that their personal stories will have a happy ending. And who's to say that incorporating that idea into one's belief system will not positively affect the outcome? So, "once upon a time," "set out on a very long journey," and he or she "lived happily ever after" are phrases people have come to expect in stories, and ones that are comforting to them.

Bettelheim (1976) reminds us of the realities that are expressed in the conventional fairy tale. Life is often a struggle, but if a person maintains a steadfast path it is likely that a positive end will be accomplished. In his interpretation, more contemporary stories for children often avoid these more existential issues. In fact, the child may benefit from suggestions in symbolic form as to how he or she may deal with the "slings and arrows" of daily living. The reality is that problems cannot be avoided, but they can be dealt with in a positive manner that gains positive outcomes for the child.

Another approach to the utilization of stories in therapy is that of the production of art forms. Kramer (1971) proposes that the "production of art contributes to the development of psychic organization that is able to function under pressure without breakdown or the need to resort to stultifying defensive measures" (p. xiii). Kramer also describes what she terms "pictographic communication" or the use of "graphic symbols to relieve immediate anxiety and restore confidence" (p. 60). Occupational therapists, because of their occupation-based perspective, see play as incorporating the very widest dimensions for activity selection. The playroom typically includes such a broad assortment of potentially "playful" media that the enhancement of therapy and of stories can be accomplished in multiple ways through toys, arts and crafts, and computers, to name but a few.

The scripting of stories, personal or otherwise, can also be accomplished with computer word processing or with drawing programs for creating visual stories. Adolescents particularly enjoy this kind of storymaking. Scripting followed by videotaping can be an excellent group process activity and can take on the form of a club when this kind of rule-bound, adult rehearsal activity is deemed developmentally and therapeutically appropriate.

The reading of existing children's stories is an excellent therapeutic activity, whether used independently or as an entre into storymaking. The therapist can read to the child, or the child to the therapist; or stories can be created in response to illustrations. The therapist can also suggest stories that the parent may share with the child at home (Fig. 15-3). Subject matter can be selected from an array of children's stories that best meets the therapeutic needs of the child, whether to assist with issues of perceived or real rejection by other children; failure in school; serious illness or death of a parent, grandparent, sibling, friend, or pet; divorce of parents; or foster home placement. Oaklander (1978) noted that children may not respond as well to stories that specifically try to get at children's feelings but are rather more engaged

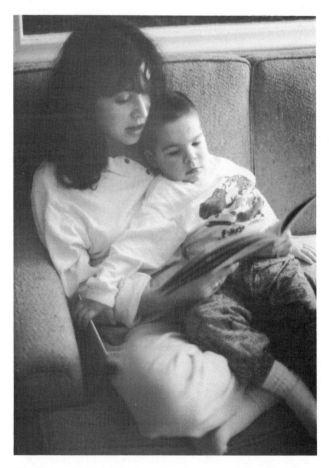

FIG. 15-3   The therapist can suggest specific stories that the parent might read to the child at home. (Courtesy Shay McAtee.)

by stories that are told to entertain the child. As mentioned previously, the symbolic or metaphorical interpretations prompted by the supposedly innocuous story may be the most meaningful to the child.

Smith (1989) refers to the multiplicity of messages that may be found in existing children's stories: "having a purpose, pursuing one's dreams, overcoming fears, learning to act decisively, coping with inevitable loss; sharing, generosity, and compassion; and understanding consequences and identifying alternatives" (p. 62). These are but a few of the themes that may be constructed from existing stories for children. Smith includes reviews of picture books that are appropriate for children from 2 to 8 years of age (pp. 269-285). Appendix 15-A is a list of children's books and stories, with brief descriptions, to assist therapists in developing their own libraries.

CONCLUSION

It has been the author's intention to stimulate the reader's interest in a form of play that has been with people from the beginning and one that is so obvious that therapists may have neglected it as they craft therapeutic play experiences. Stories, whether read or told, another's or one's own, independently constructed or shared, can be selected and adapted to the therapeutic goals of any child. Therapists should browse through the children's section of their local bookstores, enjoy old and new stories, and admire the beautiful illustrations. Many of the stories will seem appropriate to the therapist's experiences or those of someone they know. Many of them will seem to tell a metaphorical story of a child in one's therapeutic care. Practitioners can take them to their therapy settings and share them with a child.

REVIEW QUESTIONS

1. Describe what is meant by the term "imagery."
2. How is imagery expressed developmentally?
3. Provide examples of scripts that may be appropriate for use in guided affective imagery and relaxation.
4. Suggest some fairytales from your experience that provide potential therapeutic scenarios.
5. Describe how toys, games, and dolls may be used to enhance the therapeutic gains of storytelling and storymaking.

REFERENCES

Achterberg, J., & Lawlis, G. F. (1984). *Imagery and disease.* Champaign, IL: Institute for Personality and Ability Testing.

Applebee, A. N. (1978). *The child's concept of story.* Chicago: University of Chicago Press.

Austin, J. (1962). *How to do things with words.* Cambridge, MA: Harvard University Press.

Ayres, A. J. (1985). *Developmental dyspraxia and adult onset apraxia.* Los Angeles: Sensory Integration International.

Baldwin, B. (1995, August). The lost art of storytelling. *Better Homes and Gardens,* 32-36.

Bandler, R., & Grinder, J. (1975). *The structure of magic I.* Palo Alto, CA: Science and Behavior Books.

Barell, J. (1980). *Playgrounds of our minds.* New York: Teacher's College Press.

Bettelheim, B. (1976). *The uses of enchantment: The meaning and importance of fairy tales.* New York: Knopf.

Bruner, J. S. (1964). The course of cognitive growth. *American Psychologist, 19,* 1-15.

Bruner, J. S. (1990). *Acts of meaning.* Cambridge, MA: Harvard University Press.

Coppola, F. (Director) (1983). *Rumble Fish* (film). Universal City, CA: Hot Weather Films.

Csikszentmihalyi, M. (1984). *Being adolescent: Conflict and growth in the teenage years.* New York: Basic Books.

deMille, R. (1973). *Put your mother on the ceiling.* New York: Viking Press.

Deutch, H. (Director) (1986). *Pretty in Pink* (film). Hollywood, CA: Paramount Studios.

Dolan, Y. (1986). Metaphors for motivation and intervention. In: S. deShazer & R. Kral (Eds.). *Indirect approaches in therapy* (pp. 1-10). Rockville, MD: Aspen.

Fazio, L. (1992). Tell me a story: the therapeutic metaphor in the practice of pediatric occupational therapy. *American Journal of Occupational Therapy, 46*(2), 112-119.

Finke, R. A. (1989). *Principles of mental imagery.* Cambridge, MA: M. I. T. Press.

Florey, L. L. (1981). Studies of play: implications for growth, development and for clinical practice. *American Journal of Occupational Therapy, 35*(8), 519-524.

Frey, D. E. (1993). *Learning by metaphor. The therapeutic powers of play* (pp. 223-239). Northvale, NJ: Jason Aronson.

Gardner, R. A. (1971). *Therapeutic communication with children, the mutual storytelling technique.* New York: Science House.

Gardner, R. A. (1972). *Dr. Gardner's stories about the real world.* Englewood Cliffs, NJ: Prentice-Hall.

Gardner, R. A. (1974). *Dr. Gardner's fairy tales for today's children.* Englewood Cliffs, NJ: Prentice-Hall.

Gardner, R. A. (1976). Mutual storytelling technique. In: C. Schaefer, (Ed.). *The therapeutic use of child's play,* (pp. 314-321). New York: Jason Aronson.

Gardner, R. A. (1977). *Dr. Gardner's modern fairy tales.* Philadelphia: George F. Stickley.

Gordon, D. (1978). *Therapeutic metaphors.* Cupertino, CA: Meta.

Hassibi, M., & Breuer, H. Jr. (1980). *Disordered thinking and communication in children.* New York: Plenum Press.

Kazdin, A. E. (1988). *Child psychotherapy: developing and identifying effective treatments.* New York: Pergamon Press.

Kelly, E. (1973). *The magic if.* New York: Drama Book Specialists.

Knox, S. (1993). Play and leisure. In: H. Hopkins & H. Smith (Eds.). *Willard and Spackman's Occupational Therapy* (8th ed., pp. 260-268). Philadelphia: J. B. Lippincott.

Kral, R. (1986). Indirect therapy in the schools. In: S. deShazer & R. Kral (Eds.). *Indirect approaches in therapy* (pp. 56-63). Rockville, MD: Aspen.

Kramer, E. (1971). *Art as therapy with children.* New York: Schocken Books.

Leuner, H., Horn, G., & Klessman, E. (1983). Guided affective imagery with children and adolescents. New York: Plenum Press.

Lusk, J. (1992). *30 scripts for relaxation, imagery and inner healing.* Duluth, MN: Whole Person Associates.

Martin, M, & Williams, R. (1990). Imagery and emotion: clinical and experimental approaches. In: P. J. Hampson, D. F. Marks, & J. T. E. Richardson, (Eds.). *Imagery: current developments,* (pp. 268-306). London: Routledge.

McIlwraith, R. D., & Schallow, J. R. (1982-1983). Television viewing and styles of children's fantasy. *Imagination, Cognition and Personality, 2,* 323-331.

Meichenbaum, D. H., & Goodman, J. (1971). Training impulsive children to talk to themselves: a means of developing self-control. *Journal of Abnormal Psychology, 77,* 115-126.

Mills, J., & Crowley, R. (1986). *Therapeutic metaphors for children.* New York: Brunner/Mazel.

Oaklander, V. (1978). *Windows to our children.* Moab, UT: Real People Press.

Piaget, J. (1962). *Play, dreams and imitation in childhood.* New York: W. W. Norton.

Piaget, J., & Inhelder, B. (1971). *Mental imagery in the child.* New York: Basic Books.

Robertson, M., & Barford, F. (1976). Story making in psychotherapy with a chronically ill child. In: C. Schaefer (Ed.). *The therapeutic use of child's play* (pp. 323-328). New York: Jason Aronson.

Rosenberg, H. S. (1987). Creative drama and imagination. New York: Holt, Rinehart and Winston.

Rosenstiel, A. K., & Scott, D. S. (1977). Four considerations in using imagery techniques with children. *Journal of Behavior Therapy and Experimental Psychiatry, 8,* 287-290.

Russo, S., & Jaques, H. (1976). Semantic play therapy. In: C. Schaefer, (Ed.). *The therapeutic use of child's play* (pp. 391-398). New York: Jason Aronson.

Sendak, M. (1963). *Where the wild things are.* New York: Harper & Row.

Sherrod, L. R., & Singer, J. L. (1984). The development of make-believe play. In: J. H. Goldstein (Ed.). *Sports, games and play* (pp. 1-38). Hillsdale, NJ: Lawrence Erlbaum.

Singer, D. (1986). The development of imagination in early childhood: foundations of play therapy. In: R. van der Kooij & J. Hellendoorn (Eds.). *Play—play therapy—play research* (pp. 105-131). The Netherlands: Swets and Zeitlinger.

Singer, D. (1988). The conscious and unconscious stream of thought. In: D. Pines (Ed.). *Energy synthesis in science* (pp. 142-180). New York: John Wiley and Sons.

Singer, D. (1993). *Fantasy and visualization. The therapeutic powers of play* (pp. 189-216). Northvale, NJ: Jason Aronson.

Singer, D., & Singer, J. L. (1990). *The house of make believe: Play and the developing imagination.* Cambridge, MA: Harvard University Press.

Singer, J. L. (1973). *The child's world of make-believe.* New York: Academic Press.

Smith, C. A. (1989). *From wonder to wisdom.* New York: New American Library.

Spivack, G., & Shure, M. B. (1982). The cognition of social adjustment: interpersonal cognitive problem solving thinking. In: B. B. Lakey, & A. E. Kazdin (Eds.). *Advances in clinical child psychology, Vol. 5* (pp. 323-372). New York: Plenum Press.

Starker, S. (1982). *Fantastic thoughts: all about dreams, daydreams, hallucinations and hypnosis.* Englewood Cliffs, NJ: Prentice-Hall.

The following list of children's books, stories, and storytelling games is included to assist therapists to develop libraries of "storytelling" and "storymaking" resources (alphabetical by title).

APPENDIX 15-A

Books and Stories

- *The Brothers Lionheart,* by Astrid Lindgren. 1985. New York: Penguin Books.

  Originally published in Swedish, this is a story of a brother who courageously defends his younger brother against the treacherous Lord Tengil.

- *Country Angel Christmas,* by Tomie dePaola. 1995. New York: G. P. Putnam's Sons.

  The smallest child, and seemingly incapable one, is often excluded from plans and activities, but this story illustrates that there is something worthwhile for everyone to do.

- *Croco'Nile,* by Roy Gerraud. 1994. New York: Farrar, Straus and Giroux.

  Tale told of an Egyptian brother and sister; the value of compassion and friendship (beautifully illustrated).

- *Curious George,* by H. A. Rey. 1993. Boston: Sandpiper-Houghton Mifflin Books.

  A series of titles about the little monkey who always manages to get into trouble with only the best of intentions.

- *Daddy, Daddy Be There,* by Candy Dawson Boyd, illustrated by Floyd Cooper. 1995. New York: Philomel Books.

  Highlights important relationships between children and fathers . . . "Daddy, daddy be there, Tell me I am smart. Tell me I am special, Tell me I am able . . ."

- *The Emperor's New Clothes,* by Hans Christian Anderson, retold by Anthea Bell, illustrated by Dorothee Duntze. 1986. North-South Books.

  Classic story to demonstrate that common sense wins over vanity and envy.

- *Fairy Tales for Today's Children,* by R. Gardner. 1980. Cresskill, NJ: Creative Therapeutics.

  The Princess and the Three Tasks, Hans and Greta, The Ugly Duck, and Cinderelma.

- *The Girl, the Fish, and the Crown,* adapted and illustrated by Marilee Heyer. 1995. New York: Viking Press.

  Adaptation of a Spanish folktale of a selfish young girl who comes to know the value of compassion and generosity.

- *Goldilocks and the Three Bears,* retold and illustrated by Lorinda Bryan Conley. 1981. New York: G. P. Putnam's Sons.

  The story everyone is familiar with, beautifully illustrated.

- *Grandma's Shoes,* by Libby Hathorn, illustrated by Elvira. 1994. New York: Little, Brown and Company.

  A little girl copes with her grandmother's death by slipping into the woman's shoes and enjoying some special memories.

- *Hansel and Gretel,* retold by Rika Lesser, illustrated by Paul O. Zelinsky. 1984. New York: Dodd, Mead Publishers.

  A familiar story reflecting step-family dynamics and sibling unity.

- *It's a Spoon, Not a Shovel,* by Caralyn Buehner, illustrated by Mark Buehner. 1995. New York: Dial Books.

  This is an interactive, "What's the best answer" book for teaching manners.

- *It's Kwanzaa,* by Linda and Clay Goss. 1995. New York: G. P. Putnam's Sons.

  This little book celebrates African heritage through stories and illustrations. Good to stimulate cultural sharing in groups.

- *The Juniper Tree and Other Tales from Grimm,* translated by Lore Segal, illustrated by Maurice Sendak. 1973. New York: Farrar, Straus and Giroux.

  These are classic Grimm stories with the added beauty of Sendak's illustrations. Published in a two-volume collector's edition.

- *Leo the Late Bloomer,* by Robert Kraus, illustrated by Jose Aruego. 1973. New York: E. P. Dutton.

  It sometimes takes a while to catch up, developmentally; but you may shine when you do!

- *The Little Engine That Could,* by Watty Piper, illustrated by George and Doris Hauman. 1954. New York: Platt and Monk.

  Classic story of perseverance.

- *Mrs. Cole on an Onion Roll and other School Poems,* by Kalli Dakos, illustrated by JoAnn Adinolfi. 1995. New York: Simon and Schuster Books for Young Readers.

  All kinds of things that can happen at school, good and bad; prompts children to share school experiences.

- *Mufaro's Beautiful Daughters. An African Tale,* by John Steptoe. 1987. New York: Lothrop, Lee and Shepard Books.

  Pride frequently goes before a fall; kindness wins out at last . . . at least in this story. (Caldecott Honor.)

- *Multicultural Fables and Fairy Tales,* by Tara McCarthy. 1993. New York: Scholastic, Inc.

  Stories, and accompanying activities to help children formulate their own fables and morals.

- *My Favorite Things,* by R. Rodgers and O. Hammerstein II, illustrated by James Warhola. 1994. New York: Simon and Schuster Books for Young Readers.

  "When the dog bites, when the bee stings, when I'm feeling sad, I simply remember my favorite things and then I don't feel so bad!"

- *Night of the Gargoyles,* by Eve Bunting, illustrated by David Wiesner. 1994. New York: Clarion Books.

  This has the potential of being scary; but even scary things can be funny.

- *Nightmare in My Closet,* by Mercer Mayer. 1968. New York: Dial Press.

  Recognition of a child's fear of "What's hiding in the closet?"

- *One-Hundred-And-One Read-Aloud Classics,* edited by Pamela Horn. 1995. New York: Black Dog and Leventhal Publishers.

  Great collection of stories!

- *Pippi,* by Astrid Lindgren. 1992. Stockholm: Raben and Sjogren.

  The tales of Pippi Longstocking make for great reading. It happens that this edition is written in a cartoon format captioned in Swedish. Neither this author nor her clients have been able to read it, but they've told some wonderful stories based on the pictures. The stories are, of course, published in many languages, including English.

- *Reynard the Fox,* adapted from classic folk tale, and illustrated by Alain Vaes. 1994. Atlanta: Turner Publishing, Inc.

  Reynard the fox, trickster and deceiver, gets his in this story and discovers the secrets of being just and good.

- *Sad Underwear and Other Complications,* by Judith Viorst, illustrated by Richard Hull. 1995. New York: Atheneum Books, Simon and Schuster.

  One of a series of poetry collections that examine a wide variety of feelings and problems (potential, and real) from a childs' point of view. Such chapters as: Fairy Tales, Stuff You Should Know, Pals and Pests, and Knock Knocks.

- *Smoky Night,* by Eve Bunting, illustrated by David Diaz. 1994. San Diego, CA: Harcourt Brace and Company.

  The Los Angeles riots prompted this story for children about the value of cooperation no matter what ones' background or nationality. (The Caldecott Medal.)

- *Spinning Tales Weaving Hope,* edited by E. Brody, J. Goldspinner, K. Green, R. Leventhal, and J. Porcino, 1992. Philadelphia: New Society Publishers.

  Topics included are living with ourselves, others, and protecting our environment.

- *The Steadfast Tin Soldier,* a Hans Christian Anderson tale retold by Tor Seidler, illustrated by Fred Marcellino. 1992. New York: Harper Collins Publisher.

  A timeless story of love, vanity, patience, and virtue.

- *Stellaluna,* by Janell Cannon. 1993. San Diego, CA: Harcourt Brace and Company.

  This is a lovely little story about a somewhat frail and unattractive little bat who is trying to figure out what it means to be a bat and, in the process, learns about friendship. (American Booksellers Book of the Year in 1994.)

- *The Story of the Three Kingdoms,* by W. D. Myers, illustrated by Ashley Bryan. 1995. New York: Harper Collins Publishers.

"From that day on the People held their heads high, never forgetting to sit by the fire and tell their stories. Never forgetting that in the stories could be found wisdom and in wisdom, strength." (Preface.)

- *Stranger in the Mirror,* by Allen Say. 1995. Boston: Houghton Mifflin Company.

  This is a story about a young Asian boy, his and others' perception of aging, and the physical differences between people.

- *Talking Walls,* by M. Burns Knight, illustrated by Anne Sibling O'Brien. 1992. Gardiner, ME: Tilbury House Publishers.

  Introduction to many cultures through the concept of "walls"; illustrates the impact of walls on people who build them and are divided or unified by these partitions. Older children find this one stimulating.

- *Tanya and Emily in a Dance for Two,* by Patricia Lee Gauch, illustrated by Satomi Ichikawa. 1994. New York: Philomel Books.

  This book celebrates cooperation, individual strengths and skills, and the importance of spirit and discipline.

- *Tell Me A Story,* adapted by Amy Friedman, illustrated by Jillian Hulme Gilliland. 1993. Kansas City: Andrews and McMeel.

  Nineteen folk tales and legends from around the world.

- *Time for Bed,* by Mem Fox. 1993. San Diego, CA: Gulliver Books, Harcourt Brace and Company.

  A picture book of animals preparing their babies for sleep; good for when a child needs to be quietly cuddled.

- *A Tooth Fairy's Tale,* by David Christiana. 1994. New York: Farrar, Straus, Giroux Publishers.

  A beautifully illustrated tale of hope, dedication, and perseverance.

- *The Ugly Duckling,* by Hans Christian Anderson, retold by Marianna Mayer, illustrated by Thomas Locher. 1987. New York: Macmillan Publishers.

  Beauty is truly in the eye of the beholder.

- *The Velveteen Rabbit,* by Margery Williams, illustrated by William Nicholson. 1975. New York: Avon Books.

"What is REAL?" asked the Rabbit. The Skin Horse replied "Real isn't how you are made, it's a thing that happens to you. When a child loves you for a long, long time."

- *The Waiting Day,* by Harriett Diller, illustrated by Chi Chung. 1994. New York: Green Tiger Press, Simon and Schuster.

  A ferryman in ancient China works furiously to please his customers, but an apparently idle beggar teaches him a lesson in how to appreciate the beauty of "what is."

- *Where the Wild Things Are,* by Maurice Sendak. 1963. New York: Harper and Row.

  Monsters aren't necessarily much different from you!

Games for Generating Communication and Self-Stories

- *Stop, Relax and Think.* Childswork, Childsplay. The Center for Applied Psychology. 1-800-962-1141.

  A board game to help impulsive children learn to focus and think before they act. The feelings cards ask the child to respond to a situation with how he or she might feel in that situation. Recommended for ages 6 to 12.

- *The Storytelling Card Game.* Richard Gardner. 1988. Creative Therapeutics, 155 County Road, Cresskill, New Jersey, 07626-0317.

  Twenty-four picture cards; twenty are scenes free of humans or animals, and four are blank; fifteen human figurines for the board game with arrow spinner.

- *The Ungame.* Talicor, Incorporated. Post Office Box 6382, Anaheim, California, 92816.

  This is a noncompetitive game, appropriate for older children through adults, that explores a wide range of human experience through "draw" cards. Structured on two levels, one that is relatively superficial, and one with potentially more sensitive statements or questions. Examples: "If you could relive one year of your life, what year would it be? Why?"; "Complete the sentence: Something I really like about myself is _____."

GLOSSARY*

achievement **1.** Performance that is linked to public expectancies or standards of excellence. **2.** Something accomplished, especially by ability or special effort; connotes final accomplishment of something noteworthy; an attainment.

achievement behavior **1.** Performance that involves competition with self or others in pursuit of a public standard of excellence. **2.** Reilly's third hierarchical stage of play behavior, in which the player is driven by competition with self or others in pursuit of a public standard of excellence. In this stage, play involves extrinsic motivation; play is characterized by risk taking and strategizing; and play generates courage.

adaptation **1.** A change or response to stress of any kind; may be normal, self-protective, and developmental. **2.** A change in the fit between organism and environment that is beneficial to the organism. **3.** A change in routine, materials, or equipment that enables a person with a disability to function independently or to participate more fully in an activity.

adapted car An automobile that has been modified or enhanced with special equipment in order to enable a person with a disability to drive independently.

adaptive equipment Any structure, design, instrument, contrivance, or device that enables a person with a disability to function independently or to participate more fully in an activity.

adaptive response A successful or appropriate reaction to an environmental challenge.

adaptive sports equipment Any structure, instrument, contrivance, modification, or device that enables a person with a disability to participate in a sport.

alternative communication Modes of transferring messages or information from one person to another in place of oral communication; alternative media may be verbal or nonverbal, direct or remote.

arousal An organism's state of alertness or readiness to act; state of excitation of the central nervous system.

---

*Definitions adapted from Anderson, K. N., Anderson, L. E., & Glanze, W. D. (Eds.). (1994). *Mosby's medical, nursing, and allied health dictionary* (4th ed.). St. Louis, MO: Mosby; Case-Smith, J., Allen, A. S., & Pratt, P. N. (1996). *Occupational therapy for children* (3rd ed.). St. Louis, MO: Mosby; Singer, D. G., & Singer, J. L. (1990). *The house of make-believe*. Cambridge, MA: Harvard University Press; Rojek, C. (1995). *Decentring leisure*. London, UK: Sage; *Webster's unabridged dictionary of the English language* (1989). New York: Portland House; Yerxa et al., (1989). An introduction to occupational science, a foundation for occupational therapy in the 21st century. *Occupational Therapy in Health Care*, 6, 1-17; and chapters within this volume.

arousal modulation theory An explanation of play that defines it as intrinsically motivated behavior that directly affects the level of excitation (arousal) within the central nervous system (CNS); the function of play is to return the CNS to an optimal state of arousal through stimulus-seeking behaviors when the CNS is underaroused or through stimulus avoidance when the CNS is overaroused. Prominent arousal modulation theorists include Berlyne, Ellis, Hutt.

assistive technology Refers to those mechanisms, devices, or methods of "doing something" with added assistive adaptations to enhance performance and independence.

associative play Ludic activity that requires participation in relatively simple social interactions with peers, with no division of labor or product; from Parten's classification of social play in early childhood. See also **solitary play, parallel play, cooperative play.**

auditory Pertaining to the sense of hearing.

auditory defensiveness A type of sensory integrative disorder in which there is a tendency to react with distress to ordinary sounds; a tendency to overreact to sounds that are not disturbing or uncomfortable for most people.

augmentative communication Modes of transferring messages or information from one person to another to supplement, enhance, or support oral communication; alternative media may be verbal or nonverbal, direct or remote.

autism A severe pervasive developmental disorder with onset in infancy or early childhood, characterized by impaired social interaction, impaired communication, and a remarkably restricted repertoire of activities and interests; thought to result from brain dysfunction. Also called infantile autism.

autotelic Intrinsically motivated; done for its own sake.

Bundy's model of playfulness Graphic depiction of playfulness as determined by three elements, each in a continuum: intrinsic motivation, internal control, and freedom to suspend reality. A summation of each of the three elements determines the degree to which playfulness is present in a given transaction.

centering the family in care See **family-centered care.**

cerebral palsy A motor function disorder caused by a permanent, nonprogressive brain defect or lesion present at birth or shortly thereafter. The disorder is usually associated with premature or abnormal birth and intrapartum asphyxia, causing damage to the nervous system.

classical theories of play Theories of play that originated before World War I, specifically the late 19th and early 20th centuries.

Prominent classical theorists of play include Schiller, Spencer, Lazarus, Patrick, Groos, and Hall.

cognitive developmental theory   An explanation that focuses on the emergence of mental processes such as problem solving and creativity in infancy and childhood. Prominent cognitive developmental theorists who address play include Bruner, Sutton-Smith, Piaget, Gardner.

competence   The state of being adequate to meet the demands of a task or situation.

competency behavior   **1.** Play that involves practice or repetition of fragments of activity sequences in pursuit of mastery of skills. **2.** Reilly's second hierarchical stage of play behavior, in which the player is driven by effectance motivation and practices tasks repeatedly in pursuit of competence and mastery of skills. In this stage, play builds on trust in the environment and generates self-confidence.

connected knowing   A way of understanding a person as a person by entering the other person's perspective to discover the premises for his or her point of view.

constructive play   Ludic activity that involves building, or putting together objects to make a new whole object (as in stacking blocks to make a tower, or combining special materials to make a pretend house). This kind of play usually is heavily dependent upon manual dexterity, praxis, and visual perceptual skills. It is prominent in children's play from approximately 2 to 7 years, during which time it becomes increasingly more complex and symbolic. Constructive play may be involved in favorite occupations throughout life (e.g., building detailed model cars), and it may be an important precursor to particular types of work skills.

context   The situation in which an event occurs; includes physical, symbolic, social cultural, and historical dimensions.

cooperative play   Ludic activity that requires participation in highly organized and complex peer interactions for a purpose, such as making something or engaging in a game with rules; from Parten's classification of social play in early childhood.

creativity   The ability to be original in thought or expression.

development   The gradual process of change and differentiation from a simple to a more advanced level of complexity; in humans the physical, mental, and emotional capacities that allow complex adaptation to the environment and function within society and are acquired through growth, maturation, and learning.

developmental effects   Sequelae of some event, trauma, disease, or disorder such that progress in physical, motor, mental, social, or emotional capacities is slowed or changed in comparison to most children.

dramatic play   An imitative activity in which a child fantasizes and acts out various domestic and social roles and situations, such as rocking a doll, pretending to be a doctor or nurse, or teaching school. It is the predominant form of play among preschool children. See also **sociodramatic play.**

dyspraxia   A type of sensory integrative disorder in which a child has difficulty with praxis that cannot be attributed to a medical condition, developmental disability, or lack of environmental opportunity. See also **praxis.**

effectance motivation   An inherent drive to have an effect on the environment; to take pleasure in being a cause of some action or event.

environmental control system   Any structure, design, instrument, contrivance, or device that enables a person with a disability to effect changes in the surroundings in which daily routines take place and thereby gain more functional independence. Environmental control systems may consist of simple switches that operate appliances or turn on lights, or they may be complex microprocessor-controlled systems that enable the person to operate multiple appliances.

environmental negotiation   Those transactions required to succeed in moving through, over, or around obstacles in the physical surroundings; involves the organization of space, time, and social interactions.

exploration   Behavior that involves investigation of the environment. In arousal modulation theories, exploration is usually interpreted as the organism's attempt to reduce stimulation by becoming familiar with properties of the environment. In this view, exploration is characterized by serious affect and investigation of a novel environment. This is distinct from play, which involves stimulus-seeking behaviors, a relaxed attitude in a familiar environment, and experimentation with different actions on the object.

exploratory behavior   **1.** In arousal modulation theories, exploration as distinct from play behavior. See also **exploration.** **2.** In Reilly's conceptual framework, play that is completely intrinsically motivated and directed toward the environment, involving pleasurable sensory experiences; occurs only under conditions of low anxiety or pressure of need; also called sensorimotor play. **3.** Reilly's first hierarchical stage of play behavior, in which the player is driven by intrinsic interest in the environment and pure pleasure in doing something for its own sake. This predominates in infancy in early childhood, but also later in life when an event is very new or different. In this stage, play is a vehicle of rule learning and generates hope and trust in the environment. See also **rule learning, sensorimotor play.**

family   A group of two or more individuals who provide the primary nurturing environment within which the child physically develops, matures, and learns. The family is an interactional system that can be described through its members, organization, and behavior; it has routines and traditions that give cohesion and stability; it has its own rules and boundaries that let members know how to behave; and it moves through a life cycle over time.

family-centered care   A philosophy in which the child is viewed by the therapist as a member of a family unit; the family is instrumental in the retrieval of information for assessment and in the dissemination of intervention.

family play   Ludic, leisure, or recreational activity that is performed by the family as the primary unit, rather than by individual family members in isolation. Family play is strongly influenced by the values, culture, and setting of the family; it may arise spontaneously or be highly organized and preplanned.

family story   A narrative formulated by a child's family members that conveys their understandings, concerns, and values in relation to the child.

fantasy   **1.** The usually pleasant process of subjectively creating free and unrestrained thoughts or emotional inventions. **2.** A mental image. **3.** Subjectively solving complex problems by imagining them in concrete symbols and images.

fantasy play   Private, internal imaginative activity that may involve daydreaming or interior monologue. Fantasy play is thought to be the result of a developmental process in which the overt, action-oriented imaginative play of early childhood is transformed into private imagery and covert language during middle childhood.

framing 1. The giving and receiving of social cues that mark a given situation as playful; an essential aspect of playfulness, according to Bundy; see also **metacommunication. 2.** The therapeutic process of considering a circumstance or set of circumstances within the person's emotional and social life, usually to create realistic and positive outcomes; may utilize a narrative approach to redefine a person's life situation. **3.** Changing the conceptual and/or emotional viewpoint in relation to which a situation is experienced and placing it in an alternative frame that fits the "facts" of a concrete situation equally well, thereby changing its entire meaning (also called reframing).

freedom to suspend reality The ability to create new play situations and to interact with objects, materials, space, and people in ways that are fluid, flexible, and not bound to the constraints of "real life." See also **Bundy's model of playfulness.**

fun That which provides mirth and amusement; enjoyment; playfulness.

game 1. An amusement or pastime; an activity characterized by play. **2.** A competitive activity involving skill, chance, or endurance on the part of two or more persons who play according to a set of rules, usually for their own amusement or for that of spectators.

games with rules Play activities that require an individual to abide by explicit, socially sanctioned regulations governing conduct, action, or procedure; usually involves two or more players. The name of the highest level in Piaget's hierarchy of games.

goal fit The degree to which a therapeutic occupation contributes to treatment goals; term coined by Pierce.

gravitational insecurity A type of sensory integrative disorder in which the individual feels irrational fear, anxiety, or distress in relation to movement or a change of position; a tendency to react negatively and fearfully to movement experiences, particularly those involving a change in head position and movement backward or upward through space.

guided affective imagery The therapist's process of aiding and assisting the client's production of images to create alternative solutions to problems.

habits Skills that are performed so routinely that they have become automatic; allow for efficiency in daily occupations.

ideation The ability to conceptualize a new action to be performed in a given situation; a cognitive process that involves generating an idea of what to do; requires understanding the possibilities for actions in relation to objects and other people in the environment; generally precedes motor planning, which addresses the plan for how to do the action.

illicit play 1. Ludic activities that are illegal. **2.** Term used in the context of school to denote ludic activities enjoyed by children yet prohibited by adults, such as passing notes and making faces in the classroom.

imagery The formation of mental concepts, figures, ideas; a product of the imagination.

imaginary play See **imaginative play.**

imaginative play Ludic activity that involves symbolism; may consist of relatively simple symbolic games or complex sociodramatic play; may be solitary or highly social; may be a precursor to fantasy in later childhood and adolescence. See also **symbolic games, symbolic play, sociodramatic play.**

imitation 1. The act of following, copying, or mimicking another person or group of people in action or manner; often seen within the context of childhood play. Piaget distinguished imitation from play; imitation involved accommodation to reality whereas play was assimilation, a joyful exercising of existing schemata. **2.** A dimension of the Revised Knox Preschool Play Scale that addresses the ways children gain an understanding of the social world; includes factors of imitation, imagination, dramatization, music, and books.

instrumental play Term used in the context of school to denote activities that involve enjoyment on the part of the students but are controlled and organized by the teacher to achieve goals of the curriculum.

internal control The extent to which an individual is in charge of his or her actions and, to some extent, the outcome of an activity; an essential element of play in Bundy's model of playfulness.

intrinsic motivation A prompt to action that comes from within the individual and is not prompted by outside influences; drive to action that is rewarded by the doing of the activity itself rather than some external reward. Intrinsic motivation is widely accepted as an essential ingredient of play.

leisure 1. Freedom from the demands of work or duty. **2.** Free or unoccupied time; a block of time in which there is no external pressure to generate a product. **3.** Unhurried ease. **4.** Play, particularly play in adulthood; leisure in this sense is usually associated with a conviction that it is necessary for individual life satisfaction and maintenance of social order and that there are legitimate times, spaces, and practices associated with leisure. **5.** A nonobligatory activity that is intrinsically motivated and engaged in during discretionary time, that is, time not committed to obligatory occupations such as work, self-care, or sleep.

ludic Of or pertaining to play; playful; usually connotes an activity or experience that is highly autotelic, spontaneous, and flexible.

mastery The state of being competent; having adequate skills to exert some degree of control over one's environment and situation.

material management A dimension of the Revised Knox Preschool Play Scale that addresses the manner in which children handle materials and the purposes for which materials are used; process through which children learn control and use of material surroundings; contains factors of manipulation, construction, interest or attention to specific types of activities, purpose or goal, and attention span.

metacommunication A message about communication; term coined by Gregory Bateson in relation to the message "This is play," a signal that subsequent behavior is playful, not instrumental.

metaphor A figure of speech in which a term or phrase is applied to something that it does not literally denote to suggest a resemblance, as: "He isn't my cup of tea." Metaphor is used in some psychosocial therapies to carry indirect, potentially therapeutic meaning.

Meyer's philosophy of occupation The idea that health and adaptation to the complex demands of society require a rhythmic temporal pattern in occupations, and a dynamic balance of work, rest, play, and sleep; developed by psychiatrist and prominent founder of occupational therapy, Adolph Meyer, in the early part of the twentieth century.

middle childhood   The period of development that extends approximately from 6 through 11 years of age; 6 through 8 year olds are considered to be in the early period of middle childhood, whereas middle to late childhood encompasses the ages 8 through 11 years.

mobility device   **1.** Any structure, instrument, contrivance, equipment, or mode of transportation or action that enables individuals with disabilities to move independently from one location to another in the environment. **2.** Adaptive orthotic equipment that enables upper extremity function to accomplish certain activities of daily living.

modern theories of play   Systematic explanations of play that were developed after 1920. These include works by Bateson, Bruner, Ellis, Erikson, Huizinga, Hutt, Mead, Piaget, Schwartzman, and Sutton-Smith.

motivation   The state or condition of being prompted or moved to act in a certain way.

motivational properties   Those elements or characteristics of environments and/or objects that prompt interest and action.

motor planning   The process of mentally organizing a novel action; a cognitive process that precedes observable motor performance; involves the organization of timing and sequencing of actions.

multicultural play activities   Ludic activities that represent the diverse ways in which groups of people interact within a shared cultural context; these include patterns of behavior and technology communicated from generation to generation.

mutual storytelling   A form of therapeutic storytelling in which the child and the therapist each share in the development of a story. The therapist utilizes the child's responses in directing the story toward positive therapeutic outcomes. This technique was developed by a psychiatrist, Richard Gardner.

narrative   **1.** A story that conveys the personal meanings that an individual imbues on life events. **2.** Technique of presenting information in the form of a story.

narrative approach   A strategy in which a person is understood within the context of his or her story of personal life events. This approach may be used both in assessment to identify an individual's interpretations of experiences and in intervention through a process of renegotiation of meanings via transactions between the storyteller and the listener.

neonatal intensive care unit (NICU)   A section of a hospital containing sophisticated technological equipment and highly specialized medical intervention for the management and care of newborn infants who are premature, ill, and/or at risk for medical or developmental problems.

neuroregulatory ability   The capacity of an infant to maintain or regain a stable, well-modulated balance among autonomic, motor, state, and attentional systems; involves interaction with the environment, for example, signaling and responding to caregivers in a manner that reduces infant stress.

novelty   Newness.

object play   Ludic manipulation of tangible things.

occupation   A specific chunk of activity within the ongoing stream of human behavior that is named in the lexicon of the culture; engagement in occupations is thought to influence health, either positively or negatively.

occupational appeal   The attractiveness of a therapeutic activity to the patient; term coined by Pierce.

occupational behavior   **1.** A lifespan developmental continuum of play and work. **2.** A frame of reference for occupational therapy practice, founded by Mary Reilly, emphasizing mastery, achievement, and ultimately, health through engagement in play and work occupations.

occupational intactness   The degree to which an activity used in intervention is whole; the degree to which an intervention activity preserves the natural conditions under which it typically occurs in relation to the patient's experiences of choice, social situation, time, and space; term coined by Pierce.

occupational patterns   Those configurations of temporally organized occupations that make up an individual's daily round of activities and that give meaning to individual lives.

occupational role   The expected pattern of behavior associated with occupancy of a distinctive position in society and that contributes to society in an economic sense. Examples of occupational roles include player, preschooler, student, worker, homemaker, retiree.

occupational role of player   The expected pattern of behavior associated with occupancy of a distinctive position in society, specifically the position of being an infant or young child whose responsibility it is to acquire skills and habits in play that are essential for competence in later life roles.

occupational scaffolding   Guidance, task modification, or assistance provided by an adult that enables a child to participate as much as possible in a particular occupation; perceived by the child as play even in occupations that conventionally are classified as work, for example, a household chore.

occupational science   An academic discipline designed to provide a knowledge base regarding the nature of the human as an occupational being and intended to be useful for the clinical practice of occupational therapy.

parallel play   Ludic activity in which the young child is beside peer(s) and engages in a similar activity, but does not interact with peer(s); from Parten's classification of social play in early childhood.

parent–infant play   Self-initiated, intrinsically motivated, and often spontaneous interactions and exchanges between caregiver and infant that bring satisfaction and pleasure to both.

participation   **1.** To take or have a part in an activity or event. **2.** A dimension of the Revised Knox Preschool Play Scale that addresses the amount and manner of interaction with persons in the environment and the degree of independence and cooperation demonstrated in play activities; contains factors of type or level of social interaction, cooperation with others, and language.

peer relations   Interactions and exchanges between persons who are considered to be "age mates," or companions, or associates at roughly the same level of development; may relate to any domain of development or achievement, such as same-age preschoolers or college classmates of varying ages.

personalized storymaking   **1.** The process of creating stories about one's real-life events and actions. **2.** The process of inserting oneself as the main character in existing stories or fairy tales and projecting different outcomes.

play   **1.** An attitude or mode of experience that involves intrinsic motivation; emphasis on process rather than product and internal rather than external control; and an "as-if" or pretend element; takes place in a safe, unthreatening environment with social sanctions. **2.** Any spontaneous or organized activity that provides enjoyment, entertainment, amusement, or diversion.

play-based interventions The therapist's use of the child's natural propensity to engage in pleasurable, intrinsically motivated activities to achieve therapeutic outcomes.

play deficit **1.** A condition in which a child's play skills are immature for the child's chronological age. **2.** A mismatch between play skills and play preferences, such that the child chooses to do activities for which he or she lacks skills; this leads to frustration and poor self-esteem. **3.** Limited involvement in play because of very low playfulness.

play deprivation A condition or circumstance in which the child is prevented from engaging in developmentally appropriate play opportunities; may be environmental, or a result of illness or injury.

play history **1.** An interview schedule in which a caregiver and/or child is asked to furnish information about the child's past and current interests and patterns of participation in play. **2.** A specific assessment instrument developed by Takata that enables the therapist to develop a play diagnosis and prescription based on a caregiver's history of the child's play.

player role See **occupational role of player.**

playfulness **1.** The tendency to seek out opportunities for play; or to respond to overtures of play with interest and pleasure. **2.** A behavioral or personality trait characterized by flexibility, manifest joy, and spontaneity. See also **Bundy's model of playfulness.**

play skills The capacities needed to play qualitatively and quantitatively in an age-appropriate manner; these capacities are dependent upon underlying motor, cognitive, and social components.

practice games Ludic activities that involve the doing of actions purely for the pleasure of exercising them, without elements of make-believe or socially shared rules; term coined by Piaget to denote the most primitive type of game playing. This type of play is also called **sensorimotor play** and dominates the first two years of infancy.

praxis The ability to conceptualize, organize, and execute non-habitual motor tasks.

preexercise theory A classical theory of play attributed to Groos, who explained play as the primary vehicle through which instinctive behavior is expressed and gradually refined into mature behaviors. Play is viewed as a product of an evolutionary biological process, and is associated with the learning of behaviors critical to adaptation in adulthood.

prenatal drug exposure The subjecting of an embryo or fetus to chemical substances taken by the mother orally or via injection; usually in reference to maternal abuse of illicit drugs. Common drugs involved in prenatal drug exposure include heroin, methadone, cocaine, amphetamines, and phencyclidine (PCP).

pretend play Ludic activity that involves symbolic games and suspension of reality. See also **freedom to suspend reality, symbolic games, symbolic play.**

pretense-symbolic A dimension of the Revised Knox Preschool Play Scale that addresses the ways children learn about the world through imitation and make-believe; contains factors of imitation and dramatization. This dimension replaces the imitation dimension of earlier versions of this scale.

proprioception **1.** Sensation pertaining to stimuli originating from within the body regarding spatial position and muscular activity or to the sensory receptors that they activate. **2.** The perception of position of body position, including the position of limbs in relation to each other. Sensory receptors primarily are located in the muscle spindle but also in tendons and joint capsules; proprioception is processed in centers throughout the central nervous system and interacts closely with vestibular and visual systems.

proprioceptive Pertaining to the sensations of body movements and awareness of posture, enabling the body to orient itself in space without visual cues; see also **proprioception.**

psychodynamic theory Explanations of play that build on Freud's concepts of play as a vehicle for wish fulfillment and mastery of traumatic events. Erikson is a prominent psychodynamic theorist of play.

recapitulation theory A classical theory of play attributed to Hall, who explained the function of play as to rid the organism of primitive and unnecessary instincts; children's play was thought to replicate the evolutionary stages of the human race and allowed inherited instincts to be played out and weakened.

recreation **1.** Refreshment by means of some pastime, agreeable exercise, or the like, as after work. **2.** A pastime, diversion, exercise, or other resource affording relaxation and enjoyment; its function is thought to "recreate" or refresh the individual to prepare him or her to return to work. Sometimes used interchangeably with **leisure.**

recreation theory A classical theory of play attributed to both Lazarus and Patrick, who explained the purpose of play as replenishing spent energy; play was thought to occur after fatigue builds up in the child in response to the demands of new tasks; play serves to renew or relax the child.

recreational play **1.** Ludic activities that are highly group oriented, such as group singing, team sports, and service club activities; characteristic of adolescents. **2.** Term used in the context of school-based programs to denote ludic activities that occur outside the curriculum and classroom but within the boundaries of school; for example, recess or playground activities.

relaxation theory See **recreation theory.**

Revised Knox Preschool Play Scale An assessment instrument that utilizes observations of play in natural environments of children from birth through approximately 5 years of age. Observations are organized into four broad categories of child abilities: space management, material management, imitation or pretense symbolic play, and social participation. Earlier versions of this instrument are also known as the Play Scale and the Preschool Play Scale. See also **space management, material management, imitation, participation.**

role The expected pattern of behavior associated with occupancy of a distinctive position in society.

role theory An explanation of human behavior that emphasizes the social expectations associated with a distinctive position in society.

rules **1.** Symbols or mental representations that codify experience; concepts acquired in play; see also **rule learning. 2.** Socially sanctioned, explicit regulations governing conduct, action, procedure, or arrangement; see also **rules of games.**

rule learning The process by which the child acquires symbols or mental representations of experience; takes place during play, particularly in what Reilly called the exploratory behavior phase of play; involves ludic exploration of the properties and patterns of body actions, objects, materials, and social interactions. Rule learning entails the generation of actions or subroutines of behavior that correspond to stored mental representations; for example, dumping and pouring are behavioral subroutines associated with substances that have the properties of liquids.

rules of games Socially sanctioned, explicit regulations governing conduct, action, procedure, or arrangement during a competitive activity involving skill, chance, or endurance on the part of two or more persons.

rules of motion Symbols or mental representations that codify experiences related to one's own body movements.

rules of objects Symbols or mental representations that codify experiences related to tangible things in the environment.

rules of people Symbols or mental representations that codify experiences related to social interactions.

school-based practice Occupational therapy assessment and intervention that takes place in the context of the school environment.

sensorimotor play Purely autotelic experiences focusing on motion and sensations, without the elements of make-believe or socially shared rules; characteristic of the first 2 years of infancy. Also called **practice games** or practice play.

sensory integration 1. The organization of sensory input for use. 2. A frame of reference for occupational therapy practice, founded by A. Jean Ayres, that focuses on the neurological organization of sensory information for functional engagement in occupations. See also **sensory integrative therapy.**

sensory defensiveness A condition characterized by hyperresponsivity in multisensory systems; a tendency to react aversely to stimuli that most individuals tolerate easily.

sensory integrative disorder 1. Dysfunction in the brain's organization of sensory information for functional behavior. 2. One of several types of dysfunction in children that involve difficulties with sensory modulation or perception. See also **sensory defensiveness, dyspraxia, gravitational insecurity, vestibular–bilateral integration disorder.**

sensory integrative therapy A specialty area of occupational therapy practice that involves sensory stimulation and adaptive responses according to a child's neurologic needs. The goal is to improve the brain's ability to process and organize sensations. See also **sensory integration.**

skills Consolidations of rule-based subroutines of behavior that produce goal-directed behavior; for example, the subroutines of grasping the handle of a pitcher, pouring and holding a glass are combined in the skill of pouring a drink. Skills, when practiced repeatedly until automatic, become **habits.**

sociocultural theory An explanation that focuses on human collective behavior; sociocultural theories of play address how play gives rise to culture and how culture influences play. Prominent sociocultural theorists of play include Bateson, Huizinga, Mead, and Schwartzman.

sociodramatic play Ludic activity involving the enactment of dramatic scenarios with peers; involves sequences of imaginative or pretend play with peers, often portraying adult occupations or events from the players' everyday lives.

solitary play Ludic activity in which the infant or young child is at a distance from peers and does not interact with them; from Parten's system of classifying social play in early childhood.

space management A dimension of the Revised Knox Preschool Play Scale that addresses the ways children learn to manage their bodies and the space around them through experimentation and exploration; contains factors of gross motor activity, territory or area used in play, and exploration.

spatial organization The arrangement in space of materials and persons within a given area; the relative locations of various people, objects, materials, and equipment in a treatment room.

spontaneity The state or quality of tending to act without effort or premeditation, driven by internal forces independent of external causes. Spontaneity in childhood is thought to be related to increased variability of behavioral responses and creativity.

storytelling The development of a narrative, either true or fictitious, in prose or verse, designed to amuse or interest the hearer or reader. When used in therapy, storytelling may have the additional intent of providing the recipient with alternatives in thought or behavior.

strategies of inclusion The parent's structuring of play and work occupations in the home such that child play is embedded in adult household work, as when the parent simultaneously performs housework and play with the child, or when the parent allows the child to participate playfully in the adult work task; concept coined by Primeau. See also **occupational scaffolding; strategies of segregation.**

strategies of segregation The parent's structuring of play and work occupations in the home such that child play is separated spatially and/or temporally from adult household work; concept coined by Primeau. See also **strategies of inclusion.**

surplus energy theory A classical explanation of play that assumes that the organism possesses a finite quantity of energy that must be expended; play is non–goal directed behavior that serves to expend energy left over after obligatory activities have been accomplished for self-preservation. This theory is attributed to both Schiller and Spencer.

suspension of reality The degree to which an individual in play chooses to assume identities, act out events, or control materials in ways that diverge from the usual constraints of real life; an essential element of play in Bundy's model of playfulness.

symbolic games Ludic activities that have an imaginative element, involving make-believe or pretend; term coined by Piaget to denote the second level in his hierarchy of games. This type of play is dependent on mental representation, which emerges between 12 and 24 months of age.

symbolic play Ludic activities that have an imaginative element, involving make-believe or pretend. The hallmark of symbolic play is the ability to represent an absent object with another object that is dissimilar or with a mental image only. See also **symbolic games.**

symbolism The representation of an idea, action, or object by the use of another, as in systems of writing, poetic language, or dream.

systems approach A philosophy that views concepts as interrelated and interacting; useful in developing theories and analytic methods that link interdisciplinary concepts.

tactile Of or pertaining to the sense of touch; involves processing by sensory receptors in the skin, and by structures throughout the central nervous system, including specialized areas in the diencephalon and cerebral cortex.

tactile defensiveness A type of sensory integrative disorder in which there is a tendency to have strong negative emotional responses to ordinary touch sensations.

temporal organization The arrangement of activities or occupations in time, including duration and sequencing of activities; chronological pattern of activities.

Test of Playfulness (ToP) An assessment instrument developed by Bundy to operationalize play and playfulness in young children via observational ratings. See also **Bundy's model of playfulness,** on which this instrument is based.

therapeutic Beneficial to the patient; pertaining to treatment.

therapeutic use of objects, materials, and activities The therapist's strategic presentation of tangible things in the environment to facilitate treatment goals via the child's active engagement in organized play; includes reducing the number of objects in the environment and carefully selecting when and how to present materials that are motivating to the child.

therapeutic use of self The therapist's conscious or unconscious utilization of personal traits and interactions as a tool to facilitate treatment goals; may include strategies such as initiating an activity, providing emotional support and assistance, giving positive feedback and encouragement, exhibiting a playful attitude, and giving assurance of safety.

therapist design skill The ability of the occupational therapist to create activities that are tailored to meet the unique needs and goals of each child; term coined by Pierce.

therapist's story A narrative formulated by a therapist that conveys his or her interpretations and concerns in relation to the child, based upon professional knowledge and clinical experience.

transition The passage from one place or state to another; in school-based practice, transition signifies the passage from one phase of education to another (elementary to middle school, or junior high to high school), or from school to adult work.

transition program School-based practice that focuses upon helping the student adapt to changes involved in passage from one phase of education to another, or from school to work.

vestibular sensation Information regarding one's head position and motion in relation to gravity. The vestibular sensory system classically is viewed as a type of proprioception. The word "vestibular" in this sense refers to the vestibule of the inner ear, where the receptors of this system are located; vestibular processing in the central nervous system primarily involves the brainstem and indirectly influences many other parts of the brain. Vestibular sensation interacts closely with vision and with proprioception arising from muscles to regulate posture, balance, and visual field stability.

vestibular–bilateral and sequencing disorder A type of sensory integrative disorder characterized by poor postural mechanisms, inadequate coordination of the two sides of the body, and difficulties with motor sequencing; thought to be related to dysfunction in central processing of vestibular sensations.

visual Pertaining to the sense of sight; involves processing by receptors in the retina of the eye, as well as large subcortical and cortical fields in the central nervous system.

INDEX